Symposium on problems and complications in aesthetic plastic surgery of the face

Volume twenty-three

Symposium on problems and complications in aesthetic plastic surgery of the face

Editors

BERNARD L. KAYE, M.D., F.A.C.S.

Clinical Professor of Surgery (Plastic),
University of Florida School of Medicine;
Chief, Plastic Surgery Service, Baptist Medical Center,
Jacksonville, Florida

GILBERT P. GRADINGER, M.D., F.A.C.S.

Associate Professor of Surgery (Plastic),
Stanford University, Stanford, California;
Assistant Clinical Professor of Surgery (Plastic),
University of California, San Francisco, Medical Center,
San Francisco, California; Chairman, Division of Plastic and
Reconstructive Surgery, Peninsula Hospital and Medical Center,
Burlingame, California

Proceedings of the Symposium of the Educational Foundation of the
American Society of Plastic and Reconstructive Surgeons, Inc.,
and the American Society for Aesthetic Plastic Surgery, Inc.,
held in Monterey, California, January 27-30, 1980

with 660 illustrations

The C. V. Mosby Company

ST. LOUIS   TORONTO   1984

Editor: Karen Berger
Assistant editor: Terry Van Schaik
Manuscript editor: Judith Bange
Design: Staff
Production: Carol O'Leary, Barbara Merritt, Ginny Douglas

Volume twenty-three

Printed in the United States of America

The C.V. Mosby Company
11830 Westline Industrial Drive, St. Louis, Missouri 63146

Library of Congress Cataloging in Publication Data

Symposium on Problems and Complications in Aesthetic
  Plastic Surgery of the Face (1980: Monterey, Calif.)
    Symposium on Problems and Complications in Aesthetic Plastic Surgery of
    the Face.

    (Proceedings of the Symposium of the Educational Foundation of the
American Society of Plastic and Reconstructive Surgeons, Inc. and the
American Society for Aesthetic Plastic Surgery, Inc.; v. 23)
    Bibliography: p.
    Includes index.
    1. Face—Surgery—Complications and sequelae—
Congresses. 2. Surgery, Plastic—Complications and sequelae—
Congresses. I. Kaye, Bernard L. II. Gradinger, Gilbert P.
III. American Society of Plastic and Reconstructive Surgeons. Educational
Foundation. IV. American Society for Aesthetic Plastic
Surgery. V. Title. VI. Series: American Society of Plastic and
Reconstructive Surgeons. Educational Foundation. Symposium.
Proceedings of the Symposium of the Educational Foundation of the
American Society of Plastic and Reconstructive Surgeons, Inc. . . . ; v. 23.
[DNLM: 1. Face—Surgery—Congresses. 2. Surgery, Plastic—
Congresses. 3. Postoperative—Complications—Congresses. WE 705
S99203s 1980]
RD119.5.F33S95 1980   617'.520592   83-11454
ISBN 1-8016-2624-2

C/MV/MV 9 8 7 6 5 4 3 2 1   02/C/260

Contributors

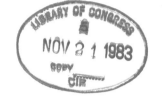

SHERRELL J. ASTON, M.D., F.A.C.S., P.C.

Associate Professor of Plastic Surgery, Department of Plastic Surgery, New York University School of Medicine; Attending Surgeon, Department of Plastic Surgery, Manhattan Eye, Ear and Throat Hospital, New York, New York

DANIEL C. BAKER, M.D.

Associate Professor of Surgery (Plastic), New York University School of Medicine; Assistant Attending Surgeon, Institute of Reconstructive Plastic Surgeons, New York University Medical Center; Associate Attending Surgeon, Manhattan Eye, Ear and Throat Hospital, New York, New York

THOMAS M. BIGGS, M.D., F.A.C.S.

Clinical Associate Professor, Division of Plastic Surgery, Baylor College of Medicine; Academic Chief, Department of Plastic Surgery, St. Joseph Hospital, Houston, Texas

SALVADOR CASTAÑARES, M.D.

Formerly Division of Plastic Surgery, Department of Surgery, University of Southern California; formerly Chief of Plastic Surgery Division, Hospital of the Good Samaritan, Los Angeles, California; formerly Chief of Plastic Surgery Division, Hollywood Presbyterian Hospital, Hollywood, California

EUGENE COURTISS, M.D.

Associate Clinical Professor of Surgery (Plastic), Boston University School of Medicine; Clinical Instructor, Department of Surgery, Division of Plastic Surgery, Harvard Medical School, Boston, Massachusetts; Chief, Plastic and Reconstructive Surgery, Newton-Wellesley Hospital, Newton Lower Falls, Massachusetts

ALBERT F. FLEURY, Jr., M.D.

Clinical Instructor, Georgetown University Hospital, Washington, D.C.

SIMON FREDRICKS, M.D., F.A.C.S.

Clinical Professor, Department of Plastic Surgery, Baylor College of Medicine; Chief of Service, Department of Plastic Surgery, St. Luke's Episcopal Hospital, Houston, Texas

MATTHEW C. GLEASON, M.D., F.A.C.S.

Clinical Professor, Department of Surgery, Division of Plastic Surgery, University of California, San Diego; Chief of Division of Plastic Surgery, Mercy Hospital, San Diego, California

JOHN M. GOIN, M.D.

Clinical Professor of Surgery, Division of Plastic Surgery, University of Southern California School of Medicine; Chief of Plastic Surgery, Department of Surgery, The Hospital of the Good Samaritan, Los Angeles, California

MARCIA KRAFT GOIN, M.D., Ph.D.

Clinical Professor of Psychiatry and the Behavioral Sciences, Department of Psychiatry, University of Southern California School of Medicine; Coordinator of Residency Training, Psychiatric Outpatient Department, Los Angeles County General Hospital, Los Angeles, California

MARIO GONZALEZ-ULLOA, M.D.

Medical Faculty, Plastic Surgery, La Salle University; Director General, Department of Plastic, Reconstructive, and Aesthetic Plastic Surgery, Dalinde Medical Center, Mexico D.F., Mexico

v

MARK GORNEY, M.D.

Clinical Associate Professor, Department of Surgery (Plastic), Stanford University, Stanford, California; Chief of Plastic Surgery and Director of Residency Program, Department of Plastic Surgery, St. Francis Memorial Hospital, San Francisco, California

GILBERT P. GRADINGER, M.D., F.A.C.S.

Associate Professor of Surgery (Plastic), Stanford University, Stanford, California; Assistant Clinical Professor of Surgery (Plastic), University of California, San Francisco, Medical Center, San Francisco, California; Chairman, Division of Plastic and Reconstructive Surgery, Peninsula Hospital and Medical Center, Burlingame, California

JOSÉ GUERREROSANTOS, M.D., F.A.C.S.

Professor and Chairman, Division of Plastic and Reconstructive Surgery, University of Guadalajara, Medical College, Guadalajara, Jalisco, Mexico

MICHAEL M. GURDIN, M.D., F.A.C.S.

Associate Clinical Professor Emeritus, Department of Surgery (Plastic), University of California, Los Angeles, Medical Center; Senior Attending, Department of Plastic Surgery, Cedars-Sinai Medical Center, Los Angeles, California

CHARLES E. HORTON, M.D.

Professor of Plastic Surgery, Eastern Virginia Medical School, Norfolk, Virginia

NORMAN E. HUGO, M.D.

Professor, Department of Surgery, College of Physicians and Surgeons, Columbia University; Chairman, Department of Plastic Surgery, Columbia Presbyterian Medical Center, New York, New York

BERNARD L. KAYE, M.D., F.A.C.S.

Clinical Professor of Surgery (Plastic), University of Florida School of Medicine; Chief, Plastic Surgery Service, Baptist Medical Center, Jacksonville, Florida

JOHN R. LEWIS, Jr., M.D.

Clinical Professor, Department of Surgery (Plastic), University of Kentucky, Lexington, Kentucky; Associate Clinical Professor, Department of Surgery (Plastic), Emory University School of Medicine, Atlanta, Georgia; Chief of Plastic Surgery, Department of Surgery, Doctors Memorial Hospital, Atlanta, Georgia

VERNER V. LINDGREN, M.D.

Clinical Professor of Surgery, Department of Plastic and Reconstructive Surgery, Oregon Health Sciences University; Staff Member, Department of Plastic and Reconstructive Surgery, Good Samaritan Hospital, Emanuel Hospital, and Physicians and Surgeons Hospital, Portland, Oregon

J. BRIEN MURPHY, M.D.

Clinical Assistant Professor, Division of Plastic Surgery, Hospital of the University of Pennsylvania; Staff Member, Lankenau Hospital and Bryn Mawr Hospital, Pittsburgh, Pennsylvania

ROSS H. MUSGRAVE, M.D.

Clinical Professor of Surgery (Plastic), University of Pittsburgh School of Medicine; Senior Staff Member, Department of Plastic Surgery, Montefiore Hospital and Presbyterian-University Hospital; Consulting Staff, St. Francis Hospital, Veterans Administration Hospital, Pittsburgh, Pennsylvania

ALVARO OLMEDO, M.D.

Department of Plastic and Reconstructive Surgery, Clinica Londres, Mexico D.F., Mexico

FERNANDO ORTIZ MONASTERIO, M.D.

Professor of Plastic Surgery, Graduate Division, Medical School, Universidad Nacional Autonoma de Mexico, Mexico City, Mexico; Head of Division of Plastic Surgery, Plastic and Reconstructive Surgery, Hospital General Del Sur, Mexico, D.F., Mexico

JOHN Q. OWSLEY, Jr., M.D., F.A.C.S.

Clinical Professor of Surgery, Division of Plastic Surgery, University of California, San Francisco, Medical Center; Chairman, Department of Plastic Surgery, R.K. Davies Medical Center, San Francisco, California

GEORGE C. PECK, M.D., F.A.C.S.

Associate Clinical Professor, Department of Surgery (Plastic); College of Physicians and Surgeons, Columbia University, Columbia Presbyterian Hospital, New York, New York; Beth Israel Hospital, Passaic, New Jersey

IVO PITANGUY, M.D., F.A.C.S., F.I.C.S.

Chief and Full Professor, Department of Plastic and Reconstructive Surgery, Catholic University of Rio de Janeiro; Chief, Department of Plastic and Reconstructive Surgery, Santa Casa de Misericórdia General Hospital (Thirty-eighth Infirmary), Rio de Janeiro, Brazil

JULIEN REICH, M.D.Sc., F.R.A.C.S., F.R.A.C.D.S.

Director, Kooyong Clinic for Plastic Surgery, Melbourne, Victoria, Australia

LARS M. VISTNES, M.D., F.R.C.S.(C)

Professor of Surgery and Head, Plastic Surgery, Department of Plastic Surgery, Stanford University School of Medicine, Stanford, California

DONALD R. WEIS, M.D.

Clinical Instructor, Department of Ophthalmology, Harvard Medical School; Associate Surgeon, Department of Ophthalmology, Massachusetts Eye and Ear Infirmary, Boston, Massachusetts

Preface

The highly successful Symposium on Problems and Complications in Aesthetic Plastic Surgery of the Face was held in Monterey, California, January 27-30, 1980, under the sponsorship of the Educational Foundation of the American Society of Plastic and Reconstructive Surgeons, Inc., and the American Society for Aesthetic Plastic Surgery, Inc. In response to many requests from those who attended this symposium, as well as from many who could not attend, we, as co-chairmen, along with the faculty members, decided to publish its transactions. Some additional material has been used for updating, and additional authors have contributed chapters for completeness.

Challenges in aesthetic plastic surgery of the face that currently confront the plastic surgeon can be divided into problems and complications. For the purposes of this book, *problems* are defined, for the most part, as those conditions that the patient brings to the surgeon prior to surgery. They may be straightforward and readily solved by conventional surgical methods, such as sagging jowls or excess eyelid skin. Conversely, they may be difficult to solve, such as the "witch's chin." Some may be insolvable at present and require the development of new knowledge and new techniques for their solution. We believe that such a problem approach is realistic, because the problem approach is the method that the practicing surgeon consciously or unconsciously uses each time he confronts a new patient. Usual postoperative problems are also discussed.

Complications present another major challenge in aesthetic facial surgery. In this book we define *complications* as those unfavorable conditions that may result after surgery. A significant portion of the material in this book is devoted to complications of aesthetic facial surgery, their avoidance, and management. By devoting our symposium and this book solely to aesthetic facial surgery, we hope to expand on this material even further.

Medicine is not an exact science, and aesthetic plastic surgery is as much art as science. The aesthetic plastic surgeon is dependent not only on his own skill and knowledge, as well as the cooperation of his patients, but also on variables and vicissitudes of nature, many of which are beyond his recognition or control. Although the incidence and seriousness of complications following facial aesthetic surgery are less than those encountered in other types of surgery, in the foreseeable future there will continue to be some incidence of complications because of nature's role in the healing process. Many such complications can occur even though the care rendered is optimal, and they can and have occurred in the best of hands. Indeed, among well-trained, well-qualified plastic surgeons, complications may occur without any negligence whatsoever on the part of the surgeon; in the vast majority of such cases, the occurrence of a complication is not indicative of negligence or malfeasance. It is hoped that by continuing to study such complications, we may reduce the incidence of postoperative complications and improve our management of them when they occur.

An additional goal of this book is to provide an update and exposition of newer techniques in aesthetic facial surgery. While not intending to make this an atlas or surgical text, we have welcomed the presentation of some of the latest concepts and techniques in aesthetic facial surgery insofar as they are presented within the framework of problems and complications.

We wish to thank our distinguished faculty members and contributors who generously shared their expertise and their experience. We are grateful to Linda Campbell, Victoria Doretti, and the staff of the Educational Foundation of the American Society of Plastic and Reconstructive Surgeons, Inc., for their invaluable assistance and cooperation in making this symposium and book possible.

This book would never have been completed without the patient, always pleasant guidance of Karen Berger, Senior Editor, Medical and Dental Division, and the amicable and meticulous attention of Judi Bange, Senior Manuscript Editor, of The C.V. Mosby Company.

Bernard L. Kaye
Gilbert P. Gradinger

Contents

Part VI

Surface surgery

Symposium on problems and complications in aesthetic plastic surgery of the face

Patient selection and patient dissatisfaction

Chapter 1

Learning to say no

Ross H. Musgrave

A good friend of mine who, a number of years ago, was a visiting plastic surgeon in Africa told me that in the French Cameroun he observed surgery performed by some brilliant young native (nonphysician) surgeons, sometimes working four to an operating room (shades of MASH), with a supervising senior surgeon in charge. These "surgeons," after 4 years of nurses' training, had picked up their surgical techniques in a matter of months and were handling not only trauma cases, but hysterectomies and herniorrhaphies as well. These young men had mastered the technical skills required for surgery but had had no experience in learning the equally challenging skill of knowing *when* to operate.

Similar observations might be made for many of the residency programs in plastic surgery in the United States today; in these training programs most of the time is spent in teaching young trainees how to handle tissues carefully, how to apply dressings, how to suture, how to graft, and how to delay a flap and transfer it; proportionately little time is spent on the matter of when to operate and when not to operate. This topic, however, deserves attention. Patient selection can greatly affect the ultimate success of the surgery. In the field of elective aesthetic surgery, the decision as to whether to proceed with surgery or to say no takes on an even greater importance. Because we, as plastic surgeons, are dealing with deformities that are inextricably linked with emotional factors, we must adhere to a practice of thorough preoperative screening and patient selection.

PATIENT SELECTION

For even the most inexperienced physician or resident in the field of plastic surgery, obviously disturbed patients are easy to spot and reject; it is the shady, gray-zone, emotionally labile, demanding, perhaps overdramatic patient who is difficult to judge. Sometimes the patient is an affluent or prominent citizen or a local politician's (or physician's) wife; then the decision for or against elective surgery gets a little more complicated. The mere fact that a patient has a correctable deformity and that the surgeon knows how to perform a correctable procedure does not necessarily mean that the surgeon is obligated to be the catalyst who brings the two elements (sometimes cataclysmically) together. Choosing the right patient is as important as selecting the correct procedure. Goldwyn[1] has adeptly noted those patients who should cause the surgeon to be on the alert for possible trouble:

- The patient who writes an excessively long letter to arrange for the initial consultation
- The rude or pushy patient
- The unkempt patient
- The patient who makes the surgeon's office his or her home
- The patient who praises the surgeon excessively and denigrates colleagues
- The patient who hides the fact that he or she is under some form of treatment, either mental or somatic
- The indecisive or vague patient
- The patient with minimal deformity
- The patient who refuses to undress for proper examination
- The patient who does not wish to be photographed
- The perfectionist
- The shopper
- The plastic-surgiholic—the seeker or bearer of multiple operations
- The acquiescing patient

- The paranoid or depressed patient
- The patient with a recent loss
- The patient in psychotherapy
- The male patient
- The patient whom the surgeon does not like
- The important patient (VIP), in which case surgical judgment may defer to the patient's status

Each of us would and should have our own particular list. In addition to the aforementioned list of patients, certain other general guidelines apply for patient selection. The surgeon needs to be cautious about doing surgery to satisfy someone other than the patient. For instance, if the patient, an attractive elderly woman, is seeking a face-lift not because she personally desires it but because her husband is distressed by her wrinkles and wants her to look like the woman he married 39 years ago, then the surgeon should beware. Also, the surgeon should be wary of the patient who repeatedly interrupts him before he has finished answering the last question or finished explaining some particular facet of the proposed surgery. This inability to listen to the full explanation indicates that the patient has selective hearing and will later swear on a stack of Bibles that he or she was never informed of the possibility of numbness, hair loss, nerve damage, or thickened scars. The surgeon should also be wary of the patient who seeks elective cosmetic surgery in order to hold onto a wayward lover or spouse. The most skillfully wielded scalpel cannot overcome a once-sharp Cupid's arrow long since dulled by infidelity or boredom.

Care should also be taken in selecting the older, plain-Jane patient who wants to be "tightened up" and requests a face-lift to make her "beautiful." A face-lift has never yet made anyone beautiful who was not beautiful to begin with (unlike a rhinoplasty or a chin implant). Beauty is only skin deep, but ugly is to the bone. We can all recall certain unattractive, yet charming, talented and prominent women of the world, such as Eleanor Roosevelt, Golda Meir, Indira Gandhi, and Margaret Meade, who became truly more attractive as they grew older. We all have the Margaret Meades and the Eleanor Roosevelts in our practice who want a face-lift in order to look "gorgeous." It does not require much pulling of the skin upward and backward, thus eliminating the soft draping effect of the natural aging process, to bring out the stark reality that a patient's bone structure was and is abysmal, and a face-lift will

make this more obvious; the patient will appear as she was at 30, only now with myopia, dentures, sparse dyed hair, arthritis, and a slumped posture. If, after much discussion, the surgeon is finally persuaded to operate on one of these women with "bad bones," he must point out and carefully emphasize in advance that what he is doing is not going to make her beautiful, but only more wrinkle free and hopefully more rested in appearance. The patient must understand the goals of the surgery before agreeing to it.

For elective surgery, the preliminary interview session should impart information about the surgery and the patient's desires. This session should also include the taking of appropriate patient photographs to allow the surgeon time to carefully evaluate the patient and the patient's motives. The patient should be asked to return for a second session after the photographs have been developed and evaluated. Even though there are cameras available that provide instant prints, the time period between consultations can be of great value for both surgeon and patient, allowing both time to consider suggestions and questions brought up at the first interview.

TELLING THE PATIENT NO

There are many ways of turning a patient down gracefully without flatly saying no. One method is to establish rigid goals for patient cooperation as a sine qua non before one performs elective surgery (e.g., weight loss, cessation of smoking, or reduction of alcohol intake). Frequently, an enthusiastic but borderline or questionable candidate can be deterred by the way the surgeon describes the possible complications of a proposed procedure. For instance, for a patient requesting a face-lift, the surgeon could dwell on the possibilities of scar tissue, skin slough, hematomas, nerve damage, hair loss, and unsightly scars. The possibility of ectropion should be noted for all potential blepharoplasty patients. These complications can be emphasized or deemphasized, depending on the patient.

When all of the surgeon's strategies for discouraging the patient have been apparently exhausted and the patient is still interested in surgery that the surgeon feels would be ill advised, the surgeon may have to resort to the "bludgeon" technique of telling the patient that enough of an improvement cannot be made to make surgery worthwhile in terms of time, money, and suffering, to say nothing of the consequences of any unforeseen complication. The surgeon can explain that he has given this decision a great deal of thought and that from his experience he does not feel that the patient has the emotional stamina to stand up under any serious complication. Consequently, he does not want to operate. This is a difficult thing to say to a patient, and sincerity is crucial. It frequently takes longer (and it is tougher) to say no than to say yes.

GENERAL COMMENTS

One certainly cannot adequately select patients with a 10- or even 15-minute preoperative consul-

tation, at the end of which time the patient is scheduled for surgery for the following morning. It takes time and soul searching (on the part of both surgeon and patient), and it takes more than one visit. I tell my residents that we earn our living by the patients we operate on, and we earn our reputations by the patients we refuse to operate on.

REFERENCE

1. Goldwyn, R.M.: Patient selection: the importance of being cautious. In Courtiss, E.H., editor: Aesthetic surgery: trouble—how to avoid it and how to treat it, St. Louis, 1978, The C.V. Mosby Co.

Chapter 2

Medical-legal criteria

Mark Gorney

The term *malpractice* is defined in our legal lexicon as "treatment of a patient in a manner contrary to accepted medical standards with injurious results to the patient." Whereas, most of these actions are based on laws governing negligence, the law recognizes that medicine is an inexact art and that there can be no absolute liability, The cause of action is usually the "failure of the defendant/ physician to exercise that reasonable degree of skill, learning, and care and treatment ordinarily possessed by others of his profession in the community." Whereas, in the past there was a tendency to accept the term *community* in the geographical sense, this is no longer true. On the supposition that all physicians keep up with the latest developments in their field, the term *community* is now regularly interpreted as the specialty community; the standards are the best standards of the specialty without regard to geographical location. This is what is usually referred to as *standard of care*.

Standard of care has some special implications in plastic surgery, since there are a great many variations to achieve the same end; to a certain extent, then, the plastic surgeon has more latitude than other surgeons.

Warranty

By merely contracting to render surgical treatment, the plastic surgeon warrants, or so the law holds, that he has the learning and skill of the average member of the specialty, and that he will apply that learning and skill with ordinary and reasonable care. This warranty of due care is legally implied and need not be mentioned by the physician or the patient. However, this warranty is one for service and not for cure. It is still the burden of legal opinion that the physician does not imply the success of this operation or, for that matter, favorable results or that no medical errors will occur, provided that they are not due to a lack of skill or care. In other words, there is no warranty against mistakes, and most judges will instruct a jury on this important point.

If the surgeon, however, binds himself even by provable implication to a certain result, then the whole picture changes, and the patient may recover damages for breach of warranty. Many surgeons, out of a sincere desire to demonstrate what can be done, or at the patient's insistence, still show photographs of their work or from the literature. This has been interpreted by the court not as implied, but as *expressed* warranty.

Some surgeons like to use drawings. In today's medical-legal climate, the inclusion of these drawings in the patient's record should be discouraged, since they can become part of the permanent record and can be used against the surgeon in court. A chalk board in the examining or consultation room, however, may be the best $3 to $5 investment ever made. It is, in the fullest sense, a sincere attempt to educate the patient.

Patients who request to see pictures of previous work will usually accept the fact that these are part of the confidential record. Ultimately, a statement to the effect that whoever shows pictures is obviously only going to show the best results (which is unfair) will be understood and accepted. There is nothing inherently wrong in showing pictures, provided one shows a cross-section of results, good to indifferent.

INFORMED CONSENT

For centuries, English common law has respected the individual's rights to the integrity of his or her person. An unauthorized "harmful or offensive touching" constitutes technical battery. A physician who treats a person without that person's consent is usually guilty of battery. Note that battery, unlike other forms of medical liability, does not require an expert witness to testify to the standard of care. It is therefore becoming increasingly more common as a basis for legal action against physicians. It is the physician's word against the patient's.

How does *informed consent* differ from consent that is routinely obtained? The patient must have sufficient understanding of the nature, purpose, and risk of the procedure about to be performed, so that he or she can make an intelligent decision about accepting or rejecting it. Obviously, in discussing the element of risk, a certain amount of discretion must be employed. Is this consistent with a full disclosure of facts necessary for informed consent? Unfortunately, the answer to this question has never been fully delineated, and there are many areas subject to interpretation. The emphasis seems to be on the word *informed*. In the key case, on which most legal theory of informed consent is based, the court, attempting to define the yardsticks of disclosure, divided medical and surgical procedures into basically two categories:

1. The common procedure or one that carries minor or very remote serious bodily harm (e.g. the administration of antibiotics)
2. Procedures involving serious risks for which the physician has an affirmative duty to disclose the potential of death or serious bodily harm and explain in lengthy terms the complications that might possibly occur

The term *affirmative duty* means that one does not wait until the patient asks. The physician is under obligation to disclose all voluntarily. The court goes on to say that there emerges from this decision a necessity and requirement for divulging to the patient all information relevant to a meaningful decisional process. It is, in other words, the prerogative of the patient, not the physician, to determine the direction in which the patient believes his or her interests lie. For the patient to be able to chart his or her course knowledgeably, familiarity with therapeutic alternatives and their hazards is essential, and it is therefore an integral part of the physician's overall obligation to the patient to disclose the available choices with respect to the proposed therapy and the dangers inherent in each.

This, then, requires the prudent plastic surgeon to adopt the following guidelines:

1. Do disclose the identity of the proposed procedure.
2. Do disclose the identity of the chief surgeon when this person is someone other than the attending physician.
3. Do disclose the risk of death or serious harm when applicable.
4. Do disclose peculiar risks associated with the specific procedure.
5. Do disclose the risks to a greater extent when the proposed procedure is experimental, new or novel, ultrahazardous, capable of altering the patient's sexual capacity or fertility, or purely cosmetic in purpose.
6. Do disclose the intent to perform procedures incidental to the principal procedure.
7. Do not inform the patient that the proposed procedure is simple.
8. Do not inform the patient that no complication will occur.
9. Do not expect to obtain an informed consent by merely answering the patient's questions.
10. Volunteer information. Do not expect a nurse or paramedical person to make disclosures required in an informed consent.

There is probably an eleventh guideline that may be more important than the rest: *write it down!*

Obviously, as important as what is said is how it is said. Contrast these two answers to a common question: "Doctor, is there any danger in this operation?"

Answer 1: "Don't worry about a thing! We do lots of these every year! There's nothing to it. You'll do just fine."

Answer 2: "Any operation, no matter how minor, carries with it a certain amount of risk. This is an operation that we do quite commonly. The vast majority of our patients obtain satisfactory results, and I see no reason why you should be any different."

By no means is this a warning that you are not to comfort your patient. You would be a poor physician if you did not. Measure your patient's intelligence, however, and tailor your words accordingly. When in doubt, always give the family the true picture, and your motivation can never be questioned.

In elective aesthetic surgery of the face, one should avoid arcane medical terminology and the use of painful words. Instead of *incise, chisel,* or *fracture,* one can use the terms *open, take down,* or *remodel.* Easily understandable metaphors should be used. One should discuss the use of a local anesthetic and the reason for it, the degree of anticipated pain, the postoperative course, the duration of disability, and the immediate postoperative appearance. There should be a discussion of the change in balance of facial features, with heavy emphasis on the matter of natural asymmetry of the human face and the tendency of the mirror to exaggerate this. This is particularly important in blepharoplasty or rhinoplasty cases. Obviously, the most common complications should be volunteered frankly and openly (e.g., the possibility of motor nerve injury or significant hematoma in face-lift surgery).

GENERAL COMMENTS

Although it may seem to be the ultimate platitude, the best way to stay out of trouble is to be honest, warm, and compassionate. If you use your common sense and behave toward the patient as you would want another physician to behave toward your spouse, it is highly unlikely that you will have need of this information.

Chapter 3

Patient selection criteria: an ounce of prevention

Mark Gorney

The desire to appear normal or aesthetically pleasing is older than plastic surgery. The puritan ethic that had until recently dominated our culture and disapproved of narcissism is rapidly breaking down. The growing popularity of aesthetic plastic surgery has, unfortunately, created in our country a carnival-like atmosphere in which advertising by unqualified practitioners is only one aspect. In this climate it becomes imperative to establish clear criteria for patient selection; without these, there will be an inevitable parallel increase in patient dissatisfaction and litigation.

Who, then, is the "ideal" candidate for aesthetic surgery? There is no such thing, but the surgeon should certainly seek out those personality factors that will enhance the physical improvements sought. There are in most cases clear indications of who will do well and enjoy the results. A person who is obviously intelligent, preferably educated, and who listens (instead of merely hearing) and clearly understands the pros and cons of what is sought is a good candidate. Individuals who have a clearly discernible physical problem about which they have an understandable but not neurotic concern are good candidates. Those whose jobs require them to look alert and well or who must compete with younger people are probably good candidates. Someone with a sense of humor is always a better candidate than a dour, anxious individual. All these attributes are generally true with the notable exception of rhinoplasty patients. They are in a category by themselves and should be evaluated with the utmost care. Generally speaking, men make more difficult patients

than women. They do not tolerate pain as well and are generally more fussy.

There are basically two major categories for rejection of a patient seeking aesthetic surgery. One is anatomical unsuitability, and the other is emotional inadequacy. Both of these are dealt with elsewhere, but since emotional inadequacy is by far the most important, it is reviewed here purely on a pragmatic basis. The inexperienced surgeon must learn early to differentiate between healthy and unhealthy reasons for seeking aesthetic improvement. In the male patient it becomes absolutely critical to develop a sixth sense regarding motivation, since, by far, the vast majority of poor results in this group are on the basis of emotional dissatisfaction rather than technical failure.

In our civilization, there is still a certain stigma attached to seeking aesthetic improvement. This may add a significant element of guilt to a preexisting distorted body image. Jacobson et al.[1] neatly liken the body image to a gyroscope. When it is functioning well, we do not notice it. It does not decide the course or steer the ship. In a storm, however, the ship becomes difficult to steer if the gyroscope is not functioning. The concept of body image is a familiar one to most plastic surgeons, but not to lay people. It can be easily explained to the patient by using the following analogy: when one thinks of oneself in the third person, in dreams or fantasies, one tends to think of the best period in one's life — be it age 20 or 30, for example. With advancing age, the image in the mind stands in sharp contrast to the image in the mirror. The greater the disparity between these two images, the more likely the disruption of one's function within one's peer group. Obviously, every patient seeking rhinoplasty cannot be referred for a psychiatric evaluation, nor is it necessary. Patients seeking plastic surgery believe that they are trying to do something positive about their problems. If they are asked to see a psychiatrist, they may consider themselves failures. It is very seldom that patients have sufficient self-awareness to realize that their problems lie more in their minds than in the physical parts that they wish corrected.

There are no objective criteria in this gray zone. The criteria are not only subjective, but totally different to patient and physician. The patient has an idea of what he or she wants; the surgeon knows, more or less, what can be done. The problem is for the two to communicate as accurately as possible beforehand. It is much easier to arrive at a prior mutual understanding than look back sadly in retrospect.

Obviously, there is a significant difference in the psychodynamics of the male versus the female cosmetic surgery patient. Jacobson et al.[1] have pointed out that both sexes have positive psychological expectations and a conscious wish for attractiveness. Women, however, more obviously wish to change themselves to feel more attractive, whereas men seem more interested in changing others' attitudes toward them.[1,3] The male patient, again according to Jacobson et al.[1], often shows:

1. A family or cultural background conflicting with his present life
2. Difficulties in heterosexual adjustment
3. A self-deprecating attitude and feelings of inadequacy
4. Familial conflict and either conscious or unconscious shame related to ethnic background.

Often there are identifiable common traits in certain types of aesthetic surgery candidates. Patients with outstanding or "lop" ears often show a hostile, aggressive, "chip on the shoulder" attitude. Most often, they have inherited this deformity from a parent who also suffered ridicule in childhood. Patients seeking rhinoplasty, on the other hand, frequently show a guilt-tinged second-generation rejection of their ethnic background masked by some excuse such as not photographing well. Often it is not so much a desire to abandon the ethnic group as it is to be viewed as individuals and to rid themselves of class attributes.[2,4,5]

Motivation, rather than specific psychodynamics, should be the plastic surgeon's overriding concern. Is there a pragmatic desire to improve appearance, or is there a pathological projection of subconscious problems onto a physical fault? Contrast these two commonly heard statements:

- I don't like my nose. It's too big for my face and I don't photograph well.
- I've always been terribly self-conscious about my nose. My father's family all have noses like this. I hate it!

Many patients can say anything convincingly, but the second statement should trip a red flag and invite further inquiries into the patient's real motivation.

Strength of motivation is important and has a startlingly close relationship with patient satisfaction. A strongly motivated patient will have less pain, a better postoperative course, and a significantly higher index of satisfaction, regardless of the result.

PATIENT SELECTION AND LIABILITY POTENTIAL

Despite all this, it is possible to establish some nearly objective criteria of patient selection and liability potential in order of descending importance.

Objective deformity versus patient concern

Fig. 3-1 shows graphically a plot of the patient's objective deformity as judged by the surgeon versus the patient's degree of concern with that deformity. Two opposite extremes of patient selection are as follows:

1. The patient with major deformity but minimal concern (*lower right-hand corner*)·
2. The patient with minor deformity causing extreme concern (*upper left-hand corner*)

The latter represents the poorest candidate. One seldom sees the patient in the lower right-hand corner, but the broad group of patients seeking aesthetic surgery falls somewhere on a diagonal band between the contralateral corners. The decision to accept or reject a patient for surgery must be the surgeon's ultimate responsibility. I have found it very useful to note sometime during the initial visit on a "tic-tac-toe" type of diagram (Fig. 3-1), my coded impression of where the patient falls. Then when a patient whom I dimly recall expresses interest in proceeding with the surgery, a glance at the chart with the X in the appropriate square serves as a reminder as to this patient's candidacy.

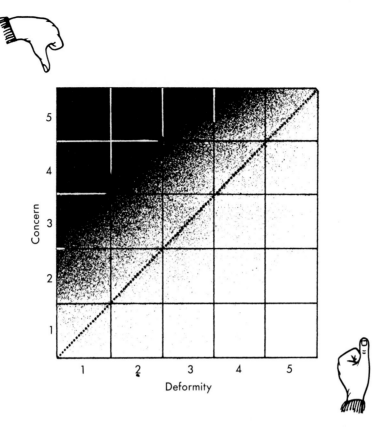

Fig. 3-1. Plot of patient's objective deformity as judged by surgeon versus patient's degree of concern with that deformity.

Great expectations

Increasing experience invariably teaches the plastic surgeon to avoid patients who expect surgery to change their whole lives. If the surgeon operates on someone with a large, crooked nose and large hang-ups, the result is likely to be someone with a smaller, straighter nose and larger hang-ups, or worse. Certainly, a reasonable degree of positive change is expected and usually occurs. However, aesthetic surgery, regardless of excellence, is dubious therapy for severe personality disturbances.

The demanding patient

The individual who brings pictures, drawings, and exact specifications should be refused as a general rule. Such a person has little insight into the realities of reconstructive surgery and, by definition, forces the surgeon into very narrow parameters that often cannot be fulfilled. More than likely, this type of patient is very explicit, very fussy, and very demanding about tiny imperfections and will not understand the fact that the surgeon is working with human tissue, not clay.

The indecisive patient

We have already spoken about the relationship between motivation and result. To the question, "Doctor, do you think I ought to have this done?" the correct answer is, "This is a decision that I cannot make for you. I cannot encourage or discourage this operation. I can only tell you what I think we can accomplish. If you have thought about it carefully and feel strongly that you would like to have it done, you will probably be satisfied with the results. If you have any doubts at all, I strongly recommend that you think about it further or not have it done at all." It is very difficult to dissuade a jury or an arbitration panel when one of the patient's principal claims is that he or she was "talked into" the surgery.

The immature patient

For reasons other than growth and development, one should carefully evaluate the degree of maturity in the young applicant. There is, of course, no linear relationship between maturity and age. Some of the most immature 3-year-olds are actually 50 years of age or older. Immature individuals often have excessively romantic and unrealistic expectations of the effects of the change. When confronted with a mirror postoperatively, they sometimes exhibit disconcerting shock reactions and alarming behavior. If they have been talked into the surgery by a relative or friend, this only compounds the problem.

The "important" patient

Beware of patients who make a conscious effort to impress others with their stature, profession, standing in the community, peer groups, and the like. Such individuals often suggest that a successful result on them will immediately bring on a flood of referrals and undying fame. They will also turn out to be very difficult patients with weak egos needing constant shoring up. They are difficult to satisfy and are prone to forget their financial obligations.

The secretive patient

Some applicants make a fetish of absolute secrecy about their surgery. Besides the fact that such arrangements are difficult to guarantee, exaggerated concern over this aspect of the operation indicates a suspicious degree of guilt concerning what they are about to do.

Familial disapproval

I much prefer the immediate family to be in agreement with the proposed operation and often refuse to do it if they are not. Too often, failure of communication or an unsatisfactory result produces an automatic "See, I told you so!" reaction. This only deepens the patient's guilt and dissatisfaction, and the associated headaches.

Failure to establish rapport

An experienced aesthetic surgeon can usually determine within minutes of entering the examining room if the individual sitting in the chair will become a patient. Within a very few moments of the opening conversation, there are often discernible "bad vibes." One of the fatal mistakes in plastic surgery is to take on as a patient someone whom one truly dislikes. A clash of personalities cancels out all other factors, regardless of the "challenge" of the case.

The truly ugly patient

The patient whose deformity borders on the monstrous usually has grave mental or deep psychiatric problems. With the exception of those who may be helped by the brilliant craniofacial surgery techniques of Tessier, such individuals are rarely candidates for aesthetic surgery in the traditional sense. Once again, the challenge may prove to be too much of a temptation, and in the end, one winds up converting the merely grotesque into the simply ridiculous.*

The surgiholic

Beware of the patient who has had multiple or repeated aesthetic procedures. Such a patient obviously has a severe and probably incorrigibly distorted body image. Aside from the technical difficulties involved, you will suffer from comparison with the other surgeons. If you are more successful, you may wind up like Sir Harold Gillies' favorite image of the patient running alongside your coffin, pleading for "one more, please."

AN OUNCE OF PREVENTION

There should be a frank discussion of fees and costs— if not by the surgeon, then by someone in the surgeon's office. Experience has shown that payment in full and in advance for cosmetic surgery tends to diminish subsequent unhappiness with the final results.

It is an ironclad rule in my office never to accept patients at the first visit. I ask them to go home, think about what I have told them, and return (at no fee). I ask them to write down any questions and, at the second visit, I go over the highlights of our original conversation and cover, once again, the most significant complications that may occur. When I am convinced that the patients are well and truly motivated and understand clearly what I have told them, then, and only then, do I allow them to book the surgery.

At surgery, it is axiomatic that all patients under local anesthesia should be adequately sedated. No permit should be signed after sedation is administered, since it may be held to be invalid. All members of the surgical team should understand clearly that the patient, under the influence of narcotics, can misinterpret the most innocent words or jokes and that these can come back to haunt them. Under no circumstances should there be any arguments of any kind, even in jest. There should be no swearing for any reason. Assistants and/or observers should be warned to save questionable doubts for later. There is no such word as *oops* in the operating room, whether the

---

*EDITOR'S NOTE: "Beauty is only skin deep, but ugly is to the bone." (See Chapter 1.) (B.L.K.)

surgeon drops a hemostat or comminutes the nasal bones. It helps to talk to the patient and be highly visible at the beginning and end of the procedure. It is extremely therapeutic to have music in the operating room if the surgery is being performed with the patient under local anesthesia: it not only diffuses the unfamiliar and terrifying atmosphere, but also tends to cover up the sounds of the operating room, which in themselves are extremely anxiety producing.

At the end of the operation, the surgeon should always report to the family immediately. If they are not present, a telephone call may be the least expensive investment the surgeon ever makes. A visit on the evening of the operation is immensely reassuring to the patient. The surgeon should be the last thing the patient sees before going under the anesthetic and the first face that the patient focuses on in the recovery room. Discharge instructions should be clear and specific, and in writing. Availability during the first few days is essential. If the surgeon signs out, it should be to someone equally competent, and the patient should be notified of this ahead of time.

When dressings come off, there will be innumerable questions, all of which require simple, reassuring answers. These questions will be fewer in number and the patient will be less anxious if they have been answered preoperatively.

GENERAL COMMENTS

Litigation and misunderstanding between patient and physician in plastic surgery have as a common denominator, not poor results but poor communication. Underlying all dissatisfaction is a breakdown in rapport between patient and surgeon. This vital relationship is often shattered by the surgeon's arrogance, hostility, or coldness (real or immagined), but mostly by the patient's feeling that "the surgeon didn't care." There are only two ways to avoid this debacle. One is to make sure that the patient has no reason to feel that way. The other is to learn to avoid the patient who is going to feel that way no matter what is done.

REFERENCES

1. Jacobson, W.E., et al.: Psychiatric evaluation of male patients seeking cosmetic surgery, Plast. Reconstr. Surg. **26**:356, 1960.
2. MacGregor, F.C., and Shaffner, B.: Screening patients for nasal plastic operations, Psychosom. Med. **12**:277, 1950.
3. Meyer, E., et al.: Motivational patterns in patients seeking elective plastic surgery (women who seek rhinoplasty), Psychosom. Med. **22**:193, 1960.
4. Palmer, A., and Blanton, S.: Mental factors in relation to reconstructive surgery of nose and ears, Arch. Otolaryngol. **56**:148, 1952.
5. Stern, K., Fournier, G., and LaRiviere, A.: Psychiatric aspects of cosmetic surgery of the nose, Can. Med. J. **76**:469, 1957.

Chapter 4

Patient counseling

Eugene Courtiss

Patient counseling has different meanings for different surgeons. Although the dictionary provides several definitions of *counsel* (i.e., [1] mutual exchange of advice or opinions, [2] opinion or guidance on what to do, and [3] recommendations), the first, "mutual exchange of advice or opinions," most clearly defines the ideal because it includes the word *mutual,* which is the key to proper patient-doctor relationships.

This chapter appropriately follows one on patient evaluation. After the evaluation (a one-way process), the patient is counseled (a two-way, mutual process). However, both are ongoing processes that complement each other. In addition to exchanging advice with the patient, the surgeon should provide guidance. This means that the surgeon must inform the patient as to what to expect, what can and what cannot be achieved, and what may go wrong with the surgery: the expectations, limitations, and complications. After having been *informed* of these essential parameters, the patient *consents. Informed consent* is a process that carries great legal meaning. In addition to the potential for legal action, if surgery is done on an uninformed patient, nonlegal problems may ensue in the form of patient disappointment and dissatisfaction.

EXPECTATIONS

There are two types of expectations: procedural, which relate to the mechanics of having surgery, and surgical, which refer to the technical aspects of the operation. Some surgeons provide patients with booklets that cover these points; however, most prefer to counsel verbally.

Procedural expectations

Procedural expectations include such mundane but important questions as whether the patient should fast after midnight; whether the patient should report to the office, the outpatient department, or the admitting office; what laboratory studies will be done; who will be present in the operating room (residents, nurses, observers); how much time the operation is expected to require; whether the patient will go to a recovery room, then how long before the patient leaves the facility—to go home, to a hospital, a nursing home, or a hotel; how long the patient will be out of work and at home; and the costs, including insurance coverage. Neglecting to cover financial matters prior to surgery can lead to many serious problems. Some surgeons find these discussions difficult; they should recognize this fact and delegate it to their staffs.

Without exception, cosmetic surgery fees should be paid in advance. When the procedure has been paid for previously, a major area for conflict is eliminated and the patient is more satisfied with the results. (The paid-for denture fits better than the unpaid-for one.)

Surgical expectations

Surgical expectations include the type of anesthesia used and whether there will be pain, ecchymosis, edema, or scars. Discussing scars is vitally important: every plastic surgery procedure (except, it is hoped, dermabrasion and chemical peel) produces scars. The myth that scars disappear, or that a plastic surgeon can remove them, must be dispelled with emphasis and clarity. Furthermore, surgeons cannot predict, with any certainty, the appearance of a given patient's scar.

Another important expectation involves symmetry. The Lord does not make individuals symmetrical; neither can plastic surgeons. Inability to achieve symmetry is not only important in relation to paired organs, such as the eyelids, ears, and breasts, but also in relation to the face and nose, which, although not paired, have two sides in juxtaposition to each other. My operative permit includes: "I understand that the two sides of the human body are not the same and can never be made the same."

Another myth, that plastic surgery—particularly aesthetic surgery—is magic, must also be dispelled. These are specific operations, which alter specific human features. And, of course, the operations do not provide instant results. The patient should be made aware that weeks, months, and even years may be required before healing is complete and swelling and erythema have resolved.

Patients should expect to still look like themselves; the only difference is that a given feature will be changed (e.g., the excess skin in the eyelid will be gone, or the neck will have a more desirable contour).

Patients expect to have the surgeon's genuine interest and concern. They expect that the surgeon will endeavor to obtain the best possible result. The surgeon can guarantee that. However, that is the only guarantee that should be given. Guarantees are legal contracts that should be avoided, because aesthetic plastic surgery is inexact and unpredictable.

Showing photographs of other patients preoperatively is controversial. Some justify the practice as being educational for the patient and feel that it helps to better inform the patient. However, others worry that this practice suggests commercialism (like picking something out of a catalog) and could imply salesmanship (rather than information and education); it may be misleading if the surgeon shows only the best results, and these photographs may be construed as a contract for the patient. The photographs the patient wants to see (what he or she will look like after the surgery) cannot be shown.

LIMITATIONS

All operations have limitations. These should be discussed in great detail. If scarring has not been covered previously, it should be explained at this time. Also, the fact that the surgeon cannot make one person look like another (or "have" anyone else's nose or eyes, for example) deserves emphasis. The fact that a patient undergoing a face-lift may not look "younger" should be noted.

Patients should understand that the scars of all surgery are permanent.

COMPLICATIONS

The complications of the contemplated surgery constitute the major component of patient counseling and therefore of informed consent. Literally books have been written on the topic, which is as broad as it is controversial. Certain questions are relevant: "What complications should be discussed?" "Should they all be discussed?" "What if the surgeon omits the one that the patient gets?" The answers follow two basic philosophies: one either tells everything possible or says very little. Few advocate that patients should know everything about all potential complications. Besides requiring an inordinate amount of time to accomplish, this type of explanation would cause most patients to forgo surgery. On the other hand, those surgeons who advocate not discussing complications do not answer the patient's needs, nor do they properly inform the patient, who must consent. A middle ground is more appropriate; the surgeon should discuss those complications that are important either because of their high frequency (e.g., numbness in the ear after rhytidectomy) or because of their severity (e.g., blindness after a blepharoplasty). Discussion of these complications should include their frequency, treatment, and permanence.

GENERAL COMMENTS

Patient counseling should not be hurried. For most patients a single interview will suffice; however, either the patient or the surgeon may feel that a second interview would be beneficial. In that case, it should be arranged and encouraged. The surgeon should beware of the patient who requires a third interview. Such patients are often looking for impossible guarantees and frequently have such emotional uncertainties that they can never comprehend the true nature of the procedure, its expectations, limitations, and complications. Patients such as these are at high risk for postoperative disappointment and dissatisfaction. Just as in baseball, "three strikes and you're out" is a safe policy.

In minimizing medical liability, good medical records are second only to good medical care; thus the surgeon should note in the patient's chart what expectations, limitations, and complications have been discussed.

Chapter 5

Problems in management of the aesthetic surgery patient

Julien Reich

Whilst the purely technical achievements in aesthetic surgery during the relatively short time of its evolution have been quite remarkable, it must not be forgotten that certain nontechnical aspects represent the very foundation on which this specialty rests. If we remind ourselves that there is a human being under the drapes on the operating table, it becomes incumbent on us to be aware, not only of the individual psychological makeup of patients, but also of the interpersonal and sociopsychological factors to which the patients are subject as members of the community in which they live. Basically, then, we are concerned with individuals who have decided that aesthetic surgery has something to offer them. The surgeon who agrees that this is so and who accepts an individual as a patient will invariably be faced by problems of management quite apart from the purely technical challenge of the operative procedure.

Surgeons vary, of course, in the extent to which they are aware of these problems of management. This is related to the amount of contact that they have with the day-to-day management of the patient, the feedback from their staffs, as well as the degree of empathy that they are capable of generating. Nevertheless, it is the way in which these problems of management are handled that largely determines the overall result of aesthetic surgery. It behooves us, therefore, to consider the main participants as well as the various stages of the patient-surgeon encounter in some detail.

THE AESTHETIC SURGERY PATIENT

The patient consults the surgeon because of dissatisfaction with some aspect of his or her ap-pearance. The patient desires a change in appear-ance that, it is hoped, will lead to other desirable changes in the life-style or quality of the patient's life.

Dissatisfaction with one's appearance is pri-marily related to adverse interpersonal relation-ships, especially unfavorable comments or atti-tudes, either during childhood or more recently. This feeling of dissatisfaction is reinforced, first, by self-comparison with others; second, by the mirror image; third, by failure in achievements, especially in a competitive situation, and, fourth, by a change in the life situation (e.g., a loss of em-ployment or a failure to gain it, divorce, or be-reavement) that represents a major crisis in the life of the individual and that the individual tries to deal with in a positive manner.

The individual as a member of society is also subject to the changes that affect it. In our society there is an emphasis on youthfulness, outdoor ac-tivities, physical fitness, and ready-made fashions for standard figures, and we are all exposed to the forces of advertising that constantly assail our minds. There can be little doubt that the predom-inant motivation for aesthetic surgery, in our so-ciety, is sociological—namely, to improve the pa-tient's acceptability to others. This is particularly the case where other "social approval" factors such as power, wealth, social position, and per-sonal achievement are less evident. Migration, whether forced or voluntary, and its associated ethnic problems are also assuming increasing im-portance. What, then, does the patient wish to achieve by seeking a surgical improvement in ap-pearance? Five goals present themselves: first, to escape being regarded as different; second, to be an inconspicuous member of a group; third, to re-establish a previously satisfactory appearance; fourth, to avoid being discounted as a useful member of society; and fifth, to satisfy a need to be admired, which is possibly the best definition of vanity in this context.

Preoccupation with one's appearance needs to be resolved in some way, whether this takes the form of a visit to a beauty parlor, dieting (whether supervised or one of the more erratic crash diets), a physical exercise program, or a request for a surgical improvement in appearance. Patients who fail to obtain relief from their preoccupation will sooner or later display manifestations of conflict related to their appearance. By far, the most frequent manifestation is the appearance of *anxiety* or, to a lesser extent, *depression*. These may be regarded as manifestations of a psychological conflict—namely, how they see themselves in the mirror as opposed to how they would like to look or how they think they ought to look. Another manifestation is *focusing*, wherein an aspect of appearance assumes gigantic proportions to the point where the patient looking in a mirror sees nothing else but that particular feature.* Other patients practice *concealment* in an attempt to hide an unacceptable feature. This may include the wearing of high collars or scarves, the fringing of the hairline, the wearing of wigs, and the excessive use of makeup. Again, there may be *denial* of the existence of some unfavorable aspect of appearance, occasionally combined with focusing on some other aspect that they now regard as unfavorable, even though it may not be as obvious to an observer.

Whilst the above-mentioned motivational factors and manifestations related to a dissatisfaction with one's appearance apply to all aesthetic surgery patients, variations may be noted in relation to the personality type of the individual. The patient's personality type assumes crucial importance in his or her management as an aesthetic surgery patient. The surgeon should be aware of the characteristics of the different personality types and the steps to be taken to ensure a smooth course during the treatment period. Let us briefly consider these.

Possibly the most important personality type, from our point of view, is the *obsessive* type. These individuals are usually well organized, orderly, and rigid or ritualistic. They manage their feelings intellectually and become anxious when uncertain. These patients need to be supplied with precise details about the operation and the postoperative period and need to be given regular progress reports during the time that they are under care. If anxiety develops in these patients, explanation should be used rather than sedation.

The *dependent* personality type constantly needs the support of others and expects their assistance. Such individuals are usually cooperative and grateful if they feel that support is available. They may, however, bcome manipulating or demanding on surgeon or staff. They are prone to display helplessness, anxiety, depression, or anger if support is not available when they want it. On the other hand, they may display pseudoindependence, in which case they may not carry out specific orders given to them even if this impairs the result. If problems arise, it is best to meet their demands to a reasonable extent or coax them into cooperation, as one would with a child.

The third personality type to be considered is the *hysterical* type. These individuals are warm and responsive and are able to express their feelings easily. They relate freely with others, even if somewhat superficially. Their thinking may be vague and quite unpredictable. They are of interest to us because they are often preoccupied with attractiveness. Although quite definite in their desire for surgery, they nevertheless regard it as a threat that may generate anxiety. Having undergone surgery, they become apprehensive about dressings, areas of bruising, crusts, swellings, the removal of sutures, and, indeed, the outcome of the operation. These patients do best with frequent reassurance and the repetition of information, even if this has already been supplied to them on printed sheets.

Of greater significance from a management point of view, is the *paranoid* personality type. These often sensitive and shy individuals may be suspicious, resentful, and even hostile. They take offence easily, are distrustful, and tend to blame others for any problems. This applies especially to surgeons who have previously operated on them. These patients require care and patience if they are accepted for surgery. A neutral attitude must be maintained in the face of complaints and accusations. It is most important not to give these patients any guarantee or to confront them or cause them to feel trapped. There have been several instances where a plastic surgeon has been physically attacked, and even killed, by this type of patient.

---

*EDITOR'S NOTE: This manifestation can also appear with intense ferocity in the postoperative patient who is unhappy with a particular result. (B.L.K.)

Recognition of the paranoid individual is not usually difficult if the surgeon is prepared to observe and listen, instead of talking down to the patient. One must remember that a psychotic illness is not synonymous with mental deficiency. Psychotic individuals can be highly intelligent and successful people who are quite impressive in interpersonal contact. Objectivity on the part of the surgeon is essential.

In dealing with a paranoid patient, the surgeon has a choice between bluntly refusing to operate because the person is psychologically unsuitable or agreeing that there is an operable deformity; however, there are usually associated psychological problems in this type of case. It would be harmful and dangerous to simply reject such a patient. My policy is to hold out some hope if circumstances change and to arrange for psychiatric help on the basis that concern with one's appearance, although often quite normal, may be a manifestation of a deeper problem and that evaluation by a person skilled in this field would be invaluable in helping to achieve the patient's objective.

Finally we must consider the *schizoid* personality type. These are generally shy individuals who give one the feeling of remoteness or perhaps eccentricity. It is not unusual for them to appear at successive consultations demanding entirely different procedures and appearing totally oblivious of previous requests and discussions. They display a passive attitude in relation to the requested operation and will usually be found to be unappreciative no matter how good the result. Their remoteness makes it quite difficult to establish any close patient-surgeon relationship with them, and the nursing staff can expect little appreciation for their efforts.

It is important to point out that variations and combinations of the above personality types are not unusual. It is most important to stress that a psychiatric label is not as significant to the aesthetic plastic surgeon as an understanding of how a patient feels, why the patient feels that way, and what can be done about it.

THE SURGEON

Since the aesthetic surgery experience involves both a patient and a surgeon and the establishment of a satisfactory relationship between them, one must consider both sides of the equation. Whilst numerous papers have been written on the psychological makeup of aesthetic surgery patients, few mention that of the surgeon.

When one considers that the surgeon's attitude may range from exalted omnipotence and aggressive extroversion to the professional insecurity of a recently qualified surgeon, it is obvious that surgeons represent, by virtue of their personalities, a significant variable in interpersonal relationships.

Whilst it may have been considered undesirable in the past to look at the surgeon in an analytical way, times have changed. As members of the medical profession, surgeons are open to scrutiny by the media and to abuse by politicians. These influences have not been lost on the public, and the physicians of today face attitudes and opinions about their motivations that would have been unthinkable even 10 years ago. It is thus proper that we, as surgeons, should look at ourselves from time to time, and keep in mind certain factors that enter into our relationships with patients.

Basically, of course, the surgeon wishes to help the patient, although, on reflection, we all have noticed considerable variations from surgeon to surgeon in the intensity of this desire to help. It is unlikely that any shortcomings in this direction are capable of modification, since we are dealing with a developed personality that has rationalized its attitudes and behavior pattern.

Among the other predominant motivational factors of surgeons, we must consider monetary reward and professional success. Surgeons, like other active members of a community, work to make a living. They wish to provide for their families and their own needs, to enjoy a life-style in keeping with the social position that they occupy in the community in which they live, and to achieve a degree of security that will enable them to live out their lives with dignity and without want. In addition, of course, they have to cover their overhead expenses and pay taxes. One does not need to be an economic expert to appreciate the increasing difficulties in achieving the above-mentioned aims and meeting one's obligations in these times in which we live. Monetary reward is thus an important consideration.

In considering the need for professional success, surgeons are concerned more specifically with peer approval, acceptance by their colleagues at home and abroad as at least being competent in their work, admiration by their patients, and a constant demand for their services.

All these may come naturally and effortlessly with time. However some surgeons may feel the need to achieve these objectives in a more active fashion. They join societies, seek office, participate in scientific programs, organize symposiums, write papers, and generally try to draw attention to themselves, under the pretext of "contributing." They establish contacts and exchange hospitality with those who seem to matter—all this largely to appease their egos and amount to "somebody." Less admirable is the propensity of some to advertise their services more directly in order to to achieve a greater share of the market.

How does all this affect the patient-surgeon relationship and, more important, the patient's well-being? It is generally agreed that contact with one's professional colleagues should prove of benefit to one's patients and is laudable as such. However, the matter is not as simple as that. Participation in intraprofessional activities exposes the surgeons of today to pressures not experienced by their professional fathers.

Thus the constantly expressed admonition to present something new, does not always lead to significant advances; it certainly interferes with long-term evaluation and, one fears, leads to a degree of dishonesty not worthy of professional endeavor. How many times does it happen that a more or less spectacular presentation of a technique, material, or method at a scientific meeting is followed by its indiscriminate application in the treatment of patients by large numbers of surgeons on return to their practices? A spate of unsatisfactory results or disappointments is followed by the inevitable denouncements of the breakthrough at some future meeting or in a journal—sometimes not until several other papers have been published reporting variations, modifications, or other applications of the original material, which would appear not to have been comprehended adequately in the first place. Clearly, then, these attitudes forced on surgeons may affect the well-being of their patients.

Certain less clearly definable subsidiary factors related to the surgeon's personality makeup may enter the patient-surgeon relationship. Thus we may note *moral judgment* of the patient or of the patient's motivation, *hostile reactions* to the patient's personality, *erotic feelings* toward the patient, and the existence of *latent sadism* that may affect the degree of gentleness during the whole period of patient-surgeon contact.

Finally, we must include the *prevailing mood* of the surgeon at the time of patient-surgeon contact. Both intrinsic and extrinsic factors influence this. Suffice it to say that intrafamilial problems with one's spouse or children, financial crises, ill health, and sundry irritations due to the ever-increasing growth of bureaucracy all influence how the surgeon feels on any one day and thus his attitude to any additional problems presented by his patients. We may indeed consider the proportionate relationship between these various factors as powerful influences on four desirable qualities of the surgeon working in this field: professional judgment, aesthetic judgment, ethical behavior, and the degree of care the surgeon is prepared to give to any particular patient.

THE PATIENT'S CONTACTS

It is appropriate here to consider the attitudes of contacts to an individual's desire to undergo aesthetic surgery. There may be resistance on the part of the family. This may be due to fear for the patient's safety, inability to see the need for an operation, insensitivity to the patient's feeling of deformity, moral or religious reasons, resentment that a familial feature is objectionable, the fear of losing the affection of the patient, and, finally, economic factors. On the other hand, the attitude of the family is sometimes favorable because of an awareness of the effects of the deformity, other family members perhaps having suffered the same feelings. They may have experienced the benefits of a surgical improvement in appearance. Sometimes they manifest guilt feelings because they feel a sense of responsibility for the deformity. Finally, they may agree to the operation in an attempt to increase the social and economic chances of the offspring who is recognized as being physically unattractive. In the case of adolescents, the opinions of close friends often equal or exceed those of the family. Close friends may consider the operation to be necessary if they have a feeling of empathy (i.e., they are able to imagine how the patient feels), or if they have a strongly developed sense of aesthetics, in which case the patient's appearance may in fact be offensive to them. Again, they may consider the operation to be unnecessary if they are able to look beyond the deformity, or if they have a possessive attitude with the underlying fear that an improvement in the patient's looks may increase the patient's popularity and lead to a loss of closeness in their friendship.

In the case of casual contacts, we are faced with emotional judgments of appearance. Such contacts may simply like or dislike a person's looks. These likes or dislikes are often the basis of impulsive character judgments and may have marked psychological or psychosocial effects on the individual. Casual contacts often feel the need to express an opinion as to the indication or otherwise of aesthetic plastic surgery. It does not occur to them that such a decision is a personal one. They probe for reasons and volunteer viewpoints, usually centered on their inability to see the need for an operation. The reason for this view is likely to be psychological. They may be dissatisfied with some aspect of their own appearance but have suppressed it successfully and now resent someone else who actively tackles a similar problem.

Most patients can cope with the attitude of casual contacts. However, there are two instances where such views can cause problems, and that is in the case of family physicians or the nursing staff with whom the patients come in contact during their hospital stay. Family physicians may express doubt about the proposed operation and may be frankly derogatory toward aesthetic plastic surgery. In general, they find it difficult to see the need for such elective surgery. This is not surprising in view of the fact that their main preoccupation is with the quantity of life rather than with the quality of it. Unfavorable comments by nursing or other staff who come in contact with aesthetic surgery patients while they are in the hospital reinforce guilt feelings built up by the patients because of family resistance, or because of the presence of sick people in the hospital where they undergo what may be regarded as unnecessary surgery, and they do not consider themselves worthy of taking up the time of the staff or using the facilities of the hospital.

THE CONSULTATION

The consultation is significant in that it is a meeting between a patient who has a problem and a surgeon who, apart from a desire and ability to help, will need to understand the patient's background in order to understand the problem. It is therefore quite clear that the consulting room is not to be regarded primarily as a booking agency for the operating theater. The two main aims of a consultation are, first, to establish mutual trust and, second, to ensure adequate communication.

In practice, one finds that although patients may be driven by a strong urge to attain an alteration in appearance, they are often reluctant to state their main concern. While this may be interpreted as embarrassment or self-consciousness, it is more likely to be due to the fact that when people first meet, they perceive each other by a process that involves categorization for type of personality, social background, and financial status, and observation for such factors as attitude, degree of involvement, and emotional state.

This act of mutual perception may be fairly rapid if the circumstances are favorable. However, in some cases it may not be possible to achieve an early assessment. The patient may appear nervous and insecure, contraindicating any in-depth discussions or probing. In such cases, it is best to confine oneself to an examination of what the patient mentioned initially as the reason for requesting the consultation. This will often be some insignificant skin lesion that is unlikely to have worried the patient, in view of the fact that this person has many other similar lesions that apparently cause no concern whatsoever. This type of management often helps to relieve tension and allows the patient to make an assessment of the surgeon. Eventually the patient will reveal the real problem or reason for requesting the consultation. Sometimes this only emerges as the patient is about to leave the consulting room; the patient may then turn, smile, and say, for instance, "Oh, by the way, Doctor, would you say that I am too young to have a face-lift?" Faced with this, it is best to smile, shrug one's shoulder, and say: "You are the only one that can make such a decision. If you eventually feel that a face-lift would be of benefit to you, you may care to call again, and I would be pleased to discuss this procedure with you in detail."

In the case of the patient who is able to arrive at an early and satisfactory assessment of the surgeon, a further step takes place in the patient-surgeon relationship. The patient will now talk freely and tell the surgeon of his or her real concern. The surgeon responds by listening and by offering certain verbal as well as nonverbal responses, such as appropriate facial expressions, as well as gestures. The patient perceives this as understanding on the part of the surgeon and experiences a satisfactory emotional reaction. Once this stage has been reached, adequate communication is possible.

It should be pointed out at this stage that instinctive liking or disliking can occur between patient and surgeon. Since these feelings are usually mutual, a decision should be made early as to whether it is wise to continue or discontinue the association.

Assuming that adequate communication is possible between patient and surgeon, it is important, first, to establish what the patient desires, the realism of the expectations, and the patient's ability to accept an imperfect result; secondly, the patient must be informed of the result that may be expected, the possible complications, the postoperative course, and the financial commitment.

A single consultation is often not a sufficient patient-surgeon contact on which to base the decision of whether or not to carry out elective aesthetic surgery with its far-reaching psychological implications. A second consultation (and, where any doubt remains, a third one) is generally indicated to evaluate the medical and family history, social situation, economic status, and the patient's understanding of the intended procedure and possible outcome. This also allows the patient to make the necessary social and financial arrangements for surgery.

If at all possible, the aid of a third party should be enlisted; this person should be made acquainted with the postoperative course and should be someone to whom the patient can turn when in doubt during that time. This is particularly important in outpatient surgery, where many days often elapse before the patient is seen again following the operation. A member of the family or a good friend may act in this capacity and is infinitely preferable to a member of the surgeon's office staff at the other end of a telephone.

When a meeting with one of the patient's daily contacts is possible (and with the agreement of the patient), the contact should be told about the various changes in appearance that may occur during the healing phase and how the contact can affect the patient's attitude toward the result of the operation. Most important, the contact's aid and cooperation should be enlisted even if this does not come easily to this individual. I usually point out that such an attitude of encouragement on the contact's part not only helps the patient, but will make the patient much easier to live with during the period of revalidation of the body image. This supportive attitude is also of great value when a complication occurs and delays the normal period of resolution. The value of this policy lies further in the prevention of guilt feelings in a patient who undergoes an operation against the initial wishes of an uninformed family member or friend. This prevents the major cause of postoperative anxiety or depressive reactions.

When there are unfavorable intrafamilial attitudes, or when the patient exhibits an emotional or otherwise unstable personality, it is best to decline to schedule the operation until the procedure has been discussed thoroughly with the patient and with one or more members of the patient's family. The resolution of unfavorable interpersonal attitudes, whilst appearing to take up valuable time, will pay worthwhile dividends by resulting in a smooth postoperative course and a satisfied patient.

Decision to operate

On the basis of what has been said so far, one should avoid operating (1) if the patient is subject to an unfavorable interpersonal or intrafamilial relationship, (2) if the patient has an unstable personality, (3) during a period of emotional stress, and (4) unless the financial aspect has been freely discussed and understood by the patient.

In relation to psychological aspects, it should be pointed out that neuroses or psychoses as such are not necessarily contraindications to surgery. Realistic expectations and the ability to accept an unfavorable result are infinitely more important in a decision of whether or not to operate on a patient than is any psychiatric label. Having considered all aspects, if one feels that a patient is not acceptable for surgery, one should not simply reject this person but should hold out some hope of a later operation if relevant circumstances change, or arrangements should be made for a professional assessment by a social scientist, psychologist, or psychiatrist, as the case demands. It can be explained to the patient that concern with appearance, whilst often quite normal, may be a manifestation of an emotional problem that everyone has at some stage and that a skilled evaluation is useful and important.

Informed consent

The question of patient information and informed consent should be approached in a positive manner. In my practice, a consent form is used for each of the aesthetic plastic surgery procedures, as well as a general form for any unusual or combined operation. Surgery is refused unless the patient has signed the relevant form, witnessed by an independent person who is not a member of the surgical staff. A copy of the form is given to the patient. In addition, information sheets concerning the hospital stay, the postoperative care, the precautions, and instructions to be observed during the postoperative phase are given to the patient. From a purely legal point of view, patients must sign the copies of the consent form stating that they have read and understood the contents and that the contents have been explained to them.

Before I used these forms, a large percentage of patients in my practice seemed to remember very little of what was said to them during the consultation. The drive to undergo a surgical improvement in appearance is so great that many patients do not wish to hear anything that might put them off. I hoped that the use of these forms would cause these patients to take notice and would eliminate those who were not prepared to accept the restrictions and possible complications of the procedure. From the questions asked later by patients, however, and from the questioning of patients during the postoperative period, it soon became obvious that most of them had signed the consent form either without reading it or without absorbing its contents. I have since adopted a policy of checking patient comprehension of the contents of these forms at a second consultation or in the hospital prior to the operation. This has greatly reduced the tiresome repetition of questions and answers, and it has increased patient acceptance of the various stages of the healing phase.

Closely related to the foregoing points is the question of financial obligation. It became evident during an analysis of the unfavorable reactions of the results of aesthetic surgery in my practice that the first evidence of dissatisfaction was often voiced when the bill was sent. In several other instances dissatisfaction was expressed in anticipation of the bill, accompanied by suggestions for a reduction or a waiving of the fee. A review of these patients and their behavior during the postoperative period revealed several instances of undue anxiety while they were in the hospital that could not be explained on the basis of any complication or unfavorable interpersonal relationship with the nursing staff. Following the actual disappearance of several patients who, during or shortly after hospitalization, left without having paid their accounts, I changed my policy. All my patients for aesthetic surgery are now informed that the fees are payable in advance before they enter the hospital. Since I have adopted this policy, there have been no instances of patient dissatisfaction that could be traced to the economic commitment, nor has there been any evidence of unexplained anxiety by patients while in the hospital.

THE PREOPERATIVE PERIOD

Once the surgeon has indicated his willingness to operate, one of two types of psychological reactions may be observed in the patient. There may be a sudden relief in the feelings of anxiety that have existed in this patient. This reveals itself as a change in the patient's facial expression to one of joy, a change in outlook to that of optimism, and a change in attitude to that of impatience. Any date proposed for the operation will seem too far away. This, of course, is the time for caution, lest the patient be allowed to rush into the operation with unrealistic expectations. Deceleration of the patient's sense of urgency in these cases will lessen the chances of patient dissatisfaction with the result of the operation.

Conversely, the surgeon may notice an actual development of or an increase in the patient's state of anxiety. In my experience, this has been due to one or more of four factors: first, the natural fear of the surgical experience; second, apprehension about the change in appearance that the patient is not able to approve of beforehand; third, guilt feelings because of lack of approval or actual disapproval by close contacts; and fourth, inability to afford the financial commitment.

It must be remembered that the urge to undergo a surgical improvement in appearance is so great that the individual is capable of rationalizing this action and of ignoring the above anxiety factors. There is no doubt that operating on a patient with unresolved anxieties due to this mechanism is a most important source of difficulties in the postoperative relationship, and a source of potential litigation.

THE OPERATION

To the surgeon, the aesthetic operation represents a creative and technical challenge. To the patient, on the other hand, undergoing the operation represents a dual crisis. First, there is the physiological trauma, which has its own psychological concomitants. Second and more important, there occurs an invalidation of the existing body image, which can lead to a temporary loss of the patient's points of reference in terms of concept. The patient's reaction may range from marked anxiety to a sense of depersonalization that constitutes a psychiatric emergency. There is no doubt that with the widespread use of local anesthesia in aesthetic surgery, one needs to be cautious about conversations in the operating room. Premedication may allow a patient to hear what he or she is unable to interpret. Amnesia, though usual, may not be complete. The unintentional induction of emotional conflicts at this stage is a very real possibility.

Outpatient surgical facility and patient care

My experience with patient care both in a hospital environment and in an outpatient surgical facility over a period of several years has left no doubt in my mind that an important part of the surgeon-patient relationship is lost in outpatient surgical facilities.

Apart from a short consultation, the patient

has no significant psychological interaction with the surgeon. Fees and procedures before, during, and after the operation are usually discussed with the patient by one of the staff members, and part of the patient information is communicated via a videoscreen.

On the day of the operation, patients arrive and are usually seen by another staff member, often at a small window in the waiting room, with other patients present. They sign certain papers and pay a preoperative fee. Led into a strange room, patients undress, they may or may not be given a premedication, and when they are eventually taken to the operating room, they are usually sedated to an extent that prevents them from expressing themselves coherently or logically. They undergo surgery, during which amnesia may or may not be complete. Several hours later they are wheeled to their car, still under the influence of sedatives, and left in the care of a friend or relative, usually a lay person.

Few surgeons see their patients for several days. Whilst phone contact is usually made the following day, it is often done by a member of the office staff, and routine inquiries are made. Patients may have doubts or problems that they really do not have the opportunity to discuss with the surgeon in order to reassure themselves. This impersonal atmosphere is not a satisfactory surgeon-patient relationship, and it would appear that a significant part of the immediate benefit of aesthetic surgery is lost.

There is no doubt that economic factors make this type of practice attractive. It is also convenient for the surgeon. From the point of view of patient care in aesthetic plastic surgery, however, it leaves a good deal to be desired.

THE EARLY POSTOPERATIVE PERIOD

The early postoperative period may be characterized in one of three ways. First it may be uneventful and pleasant. This is usually the case with patients who have a normal personality, realistic expectations, and satisfactory interpersonal relationships. Second, psychological disturbances may occur. Anxiety and, occasionally, depression are common in patients with a personality disorder or emotional instability, in patients who experience uncertainty about the outcome, and where unfavorable attitudes of contacts are a problem. These patients depend on others for reassurance about the wisdom of their decision and the outcome of the operation. Finally, there may be a provocation of the staff by a demanding and critical attitude

on the part of the patient. The real problem at this time is that the altered feature is usually covered by bandages or dressings, and the patient is unable to feel reassured that the outcome of the operation will be satisfactory. While in this stage of doubt and misgivings, the patient searches for reassurance. The attitudes of the surgeon and nurses are thus of utmost importancce. In suitable cases, removal of the dressings to allow the patient to see the early result of the operation, together with a reiteration of the changes to be expected during the stage of resolution of the operative trauma, does much to relieve the state of anxiety. It should be pointed out, however, that this early viewing may be distressing to some and should be used only in properly selected patients, in which case it will invariably prove reassuring.

A firm, confident, and encouraging attitude expressed frequently by the surgeon and nursing staff is essential. This, of course, requires frequent contact with the patient, at least on a daily basis. Unfortunately, a large number of surgeons consider this unnecessary and often do not see a patient for a week or more. Difficulties arise if there has been a lack of understanding of the patient's problems or actual opposition by the family or the patient's personal physician to the patient's desired change in appearance. If, as is usually the case, the patient decides to undergo surgery in the face of such opposition or advice, the development of a marked emotional upset is almost certain. These problems may be compounded by thoughtless though well-intentioned remarks by members of the nursing staff, or by their probing of the patient's motivations to satisfy their own curiosity.

It is important to ensure that all those who come into contact with aesthetic surgery patients should be familiar with the aims of such surgery and with the usual conscious motivations. They should also understand the psychological mechanisms whereby the anxiety may be made to grow into an excessively demanding or critical attitude. Unless these factors are understood, interpersonal irritations and counterirritations may turn the postoperative period into a virtual nightmare for all concerned.

The problem is no less important in the case of patients treated in an outpatient surgical facility. In fact, the likelihood of unfavorable postoperative reactions developing under such circumstances is perhaps even greater, since the patient is sent home fairly early after the operation and sometimes is not seen for several days, although telephone contact is often made the following day to inquire as to the patient's well-being. It is in these cases that the aid of a third party who is in constant contact with the patient will be found to be invaluable. A little time spent in interviewing these contacts is a very worthwhile investment in terms of both the patient's and the surgeon's peace of mind.

COMPLICATIONS

If the surgeon was honest with the patient during the consultation, the patient will know about the various common complications that may occur and what steps, if any, will need to be taken if they do occur. The patient who undergoes surgery with such knowledge almost expects something to happen and will be grateful if it does not. The patient who is not prepared for complications, however, does not expect them and will interpret their occurrence as lack of care on the part of the surgeon. This leads to resentment. My three cardinal rules in relation to the occurrence of complications are the following: first, prepare the patient for their possible occurrence; second, be honest and do not try to deny them when they occur; and third, if you are in doubt about their management, obtain another opinion.

In this context, it may be well to remember that if the patient of a colleague is referred to the surgeon for a second opinion about a complication, or if the patient consults the surgeon directly without the colleague's knowledge, it is the surgeon's duty to deal with the situation as professionally as possible. It is not the surgeon's job to sit in judgment on the colleague who carried out the primary treatment, since the circumstances that led to the complication can only be assumed. Guesswork based on assumption is unfair and a potential cause of wrongful litigation.

THE LATE POSTOPERATIVE PERIOD

The late postoperative period is the stage after surgery when the patient is able to assess the outcome in the mirror and observe the reactions of others to the final result of the operation. A new or amended body image is formed, and this may be accepted as satisfactory if there is rapid revalidation, coincidence of mirror and body image, a favorable response from contacts, and disappearance of preoccupation with appearance, and if the patient gets on with the task of living. It may be unsatisfactory if there is slow revalidation, a vacillating attitude to the result of the surgery, an unfavorable response from contacts, or a failure of aesthetic improvement, psychological improvement, or psychosocial improvement.

What about the dissatisfied patient? Transient dissatisfaction may lead to tension in the patient-surgeon relationship. Tact and firmness on the part of the surgeon and support from the patient's daily contacts may resolve the problem. Permanent dissatisfaction, however, may occur and represents a very important problem in the practice of aesthetic surgery.

Dissatisfaction with a technically good aesthetic result in plastic surgery is occasionally clearly related to the psychological makeup of the individual. In approximately 2% of patients, this dissatisfaction may be of a maliciousness that can be explained only by the psychotic nature of the individual's mental processes. In a large majority of patients, however, the degree of satisfaction with the results of technically good aesthetic plastic surgery is not clearly related to the patient's individual psychological status. The basis of such dissatisfaction, whether temporary or permanent, is predominantly the result of unfavorable interpersonal relationships during the preoperative, operative, and postoperative phases. In other words, the surgeon's preoccupation with the individual psychology of patients should be broadened to include certain aspects of social psychology, namely, the social changes that have occurred in our society and the ways in which people behave toward each other.

In my experience, the most common reaction of the immediate family to the result of an aesthetic operation has been one of reserve. This has applied not only to those families who expressed their disapproval before the operation, but also to those who encouraged the patient to undergo surgery. The reservation in expressing approval of the result of the operation appears to be due to two main factor: first, an aesthetic one related to the temporary postoperative distortion of the region and, second, one related to the actual change of the former appearance to which they had become accustomed. Gradually, however, I have found that approval by the family is forthcoming in almost all cases as they become used to the change in appearance and become aware of the beneficial effect on the patient.

The approval of close friends is important in determining the patient's attitude toward the result of the operation. This need for approval is a significant one, because it acts as a confirmation of the success of the operation through the medium of a trusted opinion. This is most helpful at a time when the unavoidable distortion due to tissue reaction and the confusion due to invalidation of the previous body image make it difficult for the patient to view his or her mirror image objectively. Such approval is also an important aid in the successful and speedy integration of the new body image, a process essential for achieving the desirable psychological result of such surgery.

Some of the patient's contacts may use this transitional period for their own purposes to satisfy their aggressive tendencies, jealousies, resentments, or guilt feelings and to consciously or subconsciously induce conflicts in the patient by their unfavorable comments. These responses may further undermine the patient's sense of security and produce an overwhelming state of anxiety in the patient during this difficult period of adjustment.* The behavior of these contacts may not only negate any potentially beneficial result of the operation, but may produce tensions and conflicts with which the patient may not be able to cope.

---

*EDITOR'S NOTE: These responses may be a principal cause of postoperative patient dissatisfaction with an otherwise good result. (B.L.K.)

A patient's dissatisfaction with the results of aesthetic surgery will be resolved in one of several directions; the patient will not allow it to persist. Thus it may lead to the appearance of attention-seeking devices, to accident proneness in relation to the site of the operation, to a search for further aesthetic surgery elsewhere, or to litigation in the spirit of retaliation in the patient's search for compensation for an imagined wrong. Psychotic individuals may even entertain or attempt destructive actions, directed at the surgeon as well as themselves.

SUMMARY

The aim of aesthetic plastic surgery is to enable patients to accept how they see themselves and, through this, to improve the quality of their lives.

The aesthetic surgery experience involves an interpersonal triangle consisting of the patient, the surgeon, and the patient's daily contacts. This chapter has concerned itself with patients' attitudes toward appearance and during the various stages leading to a surgical improvement in appearance.

Chapter 6

Dissatisfaction

Marcia Kraft Goin
John M. Goin

The labeling function of language is a necessary one. We cannot think clearly without categorizing. We have to be able to distinguish cows from asteroids and apples from amebae. But the very process of labeling leads to stereotyping—to the confusion of the word with the reality it symbolizes, the map with the actual physical terrain. The term *dissatisfied patient* implies a taxonomic and etiological uniformity that does not exist. Some dissatisfied patients are reasonable people whose operations have not come out well and whose results are not up to either their own unexceptional expectations or those of the surgeon. In such cases the fault usually lies in the selection of a poor anatomical candidate for surgery, inadequate patient counseling, substandard surgical technique and judgment, or a complication. In most cases, however, the effective counseling of patients will do much to alleviate dissatisfaction.

We know of one very large and highly respected group of specialized surgeons who employ a number of "nurse-counselors" to take on the time-consuming burden of the consultation. The assumption here seems to be that the function of a consultation is to give information to the patient and nothing more. "Here's where the incisions go; these are the risks; you'll be in the hospital this many days, off work that many." If this were true, which it is not, then nurse-counselors, glossy brochures, and videotapes or slide-sound productions narrated by those same sincere voices that convince television viewers of the virtues of cat foods and deodorants would be a sensible and efficient alternative to the traditional consultation. In our view, those who favor this type of purely information-giving consultation have lost sight of the dual functions of the true counselor: to gather data about the patient, which will be of use in decision making, as well as to transmit facts to the patient. It is difficult enough to predict whether a given patient will be satisfied with a given operation when you know all that you can possibly know about that patient's psychological state, mood, expectations, motivations, and goals. When you lack this information, you might as well select patients by tossing a coin. The initial consultation, which is discussed in greater detail elsewhere,[1] must be more than a routine dispensing of facts, more than the assessment of a condition amenable to surgery—it must be a searching investigation of an individual and his or her psyche, using every bit of spoken, inferential, and visual evidence available. During this session, four questions should never leave the surgeon-counselor's mind:

1. What will be the physical outcome of the operation?
2. What does the patient expect of the operation in terms of physical changes and life changes?
3. What psychological changes, if any, is the operation likely to produce?
4. How much of what I am saying is this patient actually hearing? The impossibility of obtaining a truly informed consent has been demonstrated again and again. Anxiety, denial, and lack of surgical sophistication are among the obstacles to patients being really informed. There are always gaps in these physician-patient communications—it is important for the surgeon to know as accurately as possible how big the gaps are.

Once these estimations are made—and they can be made only by listening as well as talking—there is a sound basis for counseling the patient about the advisability of an elective operation.

But we digress. Our subject is dissatisfaction—let us return to it. What about the dissatisfied patients whose operative results seem quite satisfactory to the surgeon? One useful way to think about these patients is in terms of the time of onset of their dissatisfaction. When this criterion is applied, three fairly distinct groups of dissatisfied patients emerge. Dissatisfaction may be manifested (1) immediately (within a few days of the operation), (2) 2 or 3 weeks postoperatively, or (3) sometime after 2 months.

IMMEDIATE DISSATISFACTION

One can be reasonably certain that patients who are in the immediately dissatisfied group have psychological problems of some sort, since in most instances patients are usually unable at this time—because of bruising, swelling, and dressings—to get much of an idea as to how their operations are going to turn out. Consequently, their dissatisfaction very frequently masks other concerns and feelings. Among these are (1) anxiety over the ultimate surgical result, (2) postoperative depression, and (3) regressive reactions—childlike dependency, often expressed through whining and petulance—common to postoperative patients of all kinds. These patients may be completely unaware of their real feelings, or they may realize that their distress is emotional; but, believing that the surgeon does not want to hear about emotional suffering, they convert their complaints into physical ones.

When immediate dissatisfaction is cloaking deep anxiety about the eventual result, there is a simple and effective remedy. Once we did a prospective psychological study of female face-lift patients. During the course of this study the office schedule dictated that some patients making early postoperative visits were seen by the psychiatrist before the surgeon. The psychiatrist routinely asked each patient what she thought of the results of her operation. Those patients who had not yet seen the surgeon almost always replied, "I don't know. I haven't seen the doctor yet." Those who were asked the same question after they had seen the surgeon usually said, "My result is very good; he told me so, and he seemed very pleased with how it's coming out." Patients at this stage are really not in a position to make an independent judgment—they may be a little depressed or enervated; they have no idea how much swelling and bruising is "normal," and it is hard for them to conceptualize the final result. Later on, of course, they can make a realistic appraisal of their appearance, but at this early stage almost everything must be taken on faith. This faith requires frequent reinforcement by reassurance—verbal and nonverbal—from the surgeon and the surgical staff. Such reassurances can have a truly remarkable effect on patients' perceptions of the success of their operations.

"Your operation really went very well." "You are not nearly as bruised as the average patient." "I was surprised by how much skin I was able to remove—you are going to have a very nice result." Such statements made with enthusiasm and a sincere smile may do as much as a little extra tightening of the superficial musculoaponeurotic system (SMAS) to produce a truly satisfied patient.

Of those who express immediate dissatisfaction because of postoperative regressive changes, the most difficult to deal with are those who become angry, hostile, and obnoxious. Here, the psychological assessment made during the initial consultation (and subsequent preoperative visits) is invaluable. The understanding of the patient's basic character structure gained through previous interviews will permit the selection of the right type of psychological management. Obnoxious, hostile patients usually fall into one of three groups: (1) paranoid, (2) pseudoindependent, or (3) sociopathic.

Paranoid patients, who are fundamentally frightened people, respond to their inner fears, anxieties, and distrust with self-protective attacking mechanisms. By projecting their own deep-seated feelings onto others, they achieve some degree of psychological comfort. In effect, they are saying, "It is not I who am baselessly and irrationally fearful and suspicious of you, it is you who are hostile and bear me ill will." The expressed concerns of these patients (e.g., about swelling, pain, and bruising) are real enough, but beneath these concerns, usually unexpressed, are anxieties about the surgeon's motivations, skill, character, and devotion. They need straightforward, frank answers to their expressed concerns—"The swelling is perfectly normal"; "Your melanoma was very close to the surface, less than half a millimeter thick, and the cure rate for such tumors is very close to 100%"—but these statements must be reinforced by others that clearly indicate that the surgeon knows exactly what he is doing and that he cares about this particular patient. "You are healing beautifully, but just to be on the safe side, I want to see you frequently for a while. Why don't you come in day after tomorrow, and I'll give you a fresh bandage." Or, "Despite the fluorescein test we did during your operation, there's a narrow rim of your flap that doesn't look too healthy. I've seen this before—it's not a disaster; at worst, your healing will be delayed a few weeks, and during that time I'll want to see you quite frequently to stay on top of things."

Pseudoindependent people (many VIPs fall into this group) are deeply shaken when their facade of independence crumbles away under the stress of an operation. Suddenly, they feel scared and vulnerable, feelings that they consider shameful. They react to these feelings of shame with irritable hostility. One of the women in our study of breast reconstruction patients exemplifies this group. On her first postoperative visit she happened to see the psychiatrist first. She was seriously annoyed with the surgeon. He had used some tape that he should have known would irritate her skin. A suction drain had been placed so that it made a transient indentation in her "normal" breast. She said she was "really going to give it" to the surgeon for his thoughtlessness and lack of care. She and the psychiatrist talked about how difficult it was for a dynamic person like herself to limit her activities, to have to depend on the ministrations of others, and how generally irritating this was. When she saw the surgeon, she not only failed to "give it to him," but she seemed completely pleased with everything. Obviously, this was because she had already had the opportunity to ventilate her feelings to the psychiatrist. When there is no convenient psychiatrist loitering around the office, the surgeon should do what the psychiatrist did in this case. Acknowledge the reality and validity of the patient's physical complaints, indicate that they will pass, and let the patient know that you, the physician, realize how irritating it must be for anyone as vital and vigorous as your patient to be temporarily incapacitated.

The obnoxious sociopath should be handled in quite a different way. These totally self-centered, conscienceless people respond best to an authoritative approach by which the surgeon acknowledges the patient's complaints but very firmly informs the patient that the postoperative course is normal and that the result is a good one. True sociopaths are rare. Patients who become belligerent and dissatisfied in the immediate postoperative period are usually members of the first two groups (paranoids or pseudoindependents).

DISSATISFACTION EMERGING DURING THE SECOND OR THIRD WEEK

During the second and third weeks postoperatively, two forces are at work that may lead to dissatisfaction. Patients with stronger than average dependency needs will be affected by the withdrawal of emotional support from those close to them that was provided during the immediate postoperative period. This support is of great importance to these patients. As they recuperate and bruising, swelling, bandages, and stitches disappear, so does the emotional support, leaving a disappointing void. Also, as early postoperative changes subside, patients are better able to evaluate their operative results. If a patient's dissatisfaction is justified, then a reasonable explanation of why the present result is the best that can be expected for that particular patient, or the presentation of a timetable for eventual revision, is in order.

If the dissatisfaction is not warranted, it is a good idea to take early postoperative photographs as soon as the first premonitions of disappointment are detected. Patients often find it difficult to compare preoperative photographs, particularly 2 × 2 inch transparencies, with their actual image in a mirror. Comparison of photographs, particularly good-sized prints, can often be a great help in demonstrating the amount of improvement that an operation has produced. Many patients and their families quite honestly forget their preoperative appearance within a few days of an operation. If their photographic demonstration of reality fails to improve the patient's dissatisfaction, one can move on to suggest that the real source of dissatisfaction may lie not in the operation but elsewhere in the patient's life.

DISSATISFACTION OCCURRING AFTER 2 MONTHS

Patients with objectively satisfactory results who express inappropriate dissatisfaction after 2 months—a relatively late time—may not be experiencing disappointment with the physical results of the operation per se. Rather, they are frequently disappointed because some secretly hoped-for change that they wished might occur as a result of the operation has failed to materialize, such as marriage or some other new relationship, improvement in a deteriorating marriage, career advancements, or actually *being* rather than looking younger.* One patient in our prospective study of face-lift patients had the operation with the irrational hope that it would cure her husband's impotence. When it failed to do so, she was disappointed, but, like most patients in this late dissatisfaction group, she was able to come to terms with what she really knew was an impossible hope and eventually was able to enjoy her improved appearance despite the operation's failure to achieve her real goal. This patient revealed her true motivation only to the psychiatrist, after trust and rapport had been painstakingly established during several hours of interviews. Had the study not been underway, the surgeon would never have understood fully the reasons for her dissatisfaction but could have suggested to the patient that she might look for other causes for disappointment in her life.

Surgeons are human too. They have their own psychological reactions to surgery and to patients. Very few things prick the surgical ego as deeply as disparagement of one's own surgical skills. A patient who is dissatisfied with an excellent operation can be more than just annoying. Only the surgeon knows how skillfully the procedure has been done. The natural response is anger, to attack, to lecture, even to reject the patient. The one, never-to-be-broken rule is, "don't get mad." You, the surgeon, are the expert, and you know you have done well. Therefore something is wrong with the patient's perceptions or expectations. For you as a physician, this is simply another complication to be dealt with.

An orthopedic colleague, a fine surgeon and a seemingly totally relaxed and easy-going man, once told us, "I never look at my schedule for the next day. "If I do, I always see a couple of names on there, and I think, oh God, and the rest of the day is ruined." This attitude is a giant step on the road to the unhappy land of dissatisfied surgeons. Complications—physical and psychological—and their management are part of the surgeon's job. Sometimes fixing a psychological complication can be as satisfying as a perfect cleft lip repair. These complications are not a pleasant part of life, but they need not dominate it. Satisfied surgeons have learned the trick of switching off the day's

triumphs and disappointments when they leave the office or hospital and not switching them on again until the next day's work begins.

SUMMARY

1. Patients who express dissatisfaction in the immediate postoperative period are often struggling with anxiety about the eventual outcome, or they may be undergoing regressive changes precipitated by the stress of the operation. Simple reassurance and recognition of the particular type of psychological regression are most helpful.

2. Dissatisfaction occurring around the second or third week postoperatively may be due to dawning recognition of the limitations of the operation and/or the gradual withdrawal of needed emotional support by others. Reality testing with preoperative and postoperative photographs and an invitation to discuss other, unrelated life disappointments will help to define and perhaps ameliorate the problem.

3. When dissatisfaction occurs at 2 or 3 months postoperatively the real culprit may be some life event and its failure to be changed by the operation rather than the operation itself. This is particularly true of patients in midlife. Being aware of the many fears, alterations, and problems of people in this age group—career changes, divorce, bereavement, children leaving home, anxiety about physical health, and fears of dependency—can help the surgeon to assist dissatisfied midlife patients in searching for nonsurgical causes for dissatisfaction.

It is no news that people are different, but often we overlook this obvious fact and, in particular, how great the magnitude of the differences in viewpoint, expectation, and perception can be. Flexibility in outlook and in the ability to regard the wildly differing perceptions of others with equanimity is the sine qua non of the successful management of dissatisfied plastic surgery patients.

There is a doubtless apocryphal story about Pablo Picasso that illustrates these qualities well. The story goes that a wealthy industrialist, madly in love with his beautiful young wife, decided to have her portrait painted, to hang in their exquisite Paris apartment. Knowing nothing about art, he made inquiries and found that Picasso was the most famous living artist. The portrait was commissioned, and after many months the long-awaited unveiling was scheduled to take place in the artist's studio. When the cloth was drawn from

---

*EDITOR'S NOTE: Also consider the possibility of unjustified but constant gnawing criticism of the result by an envious or disapproving spouse, relative, or friend. Few patients can stand up to this type of attack for any length of time. (B.L.K.)

the huge painting, the industrialist was staggered to see a greenish face floating at some distance from a lumpy body. The eyes were both on the same side of the nose, and an ear was disposed sideways across the forehead. The incredulous businessman pulled a photograph of his wife from his billfold.

"This painting, it is a joke, a terrible joke. Here, this photograph is what my wife looks like, not that monstrosity on your canvas."

The artist calmly took the photograph and studied it with great care. His eyes moved back and forth between the painting and the photograph. Finally, he handed back the photograph.

"You are right," said Picasso, "your wife is much smaller."

REFERENCES

1. Goin, J.M., and Goin, M.: Changing the body: psychological understanding and management of the plastic surgery patient, Baltimore, 1981, The Williams & Wilkins Co.
2. Goldwyn, R.M.: The patient and plastic surgeon, Boston, 1981, Little, Brown & Co.

Editorial comments
Part I

Generally, we find that with increasing time in the practice of aesthetic plastic surgery, we experience less patient dissatisfaction. Although we would like to attribute this to the improved surgical skill that comes with time and experience, probably most of it is due to improvement in the nonsurgical skills of plastic surgery: patient selection, preoperative counseling, postoperative support (which also requires that one's staff be made up of experienced, sincere, and empathic assistants—a sine qua non in the practice of aesthetic surgery), and skill in dealing with the various types of patient dissatisfaction that may occur postoperatively. With time and experience, we learn what patients want to know, what they need to know surgically and legally, and how many times we must tell them to make them know. (Also, we need to learn when to say no, as Dr. Musgrave has shown us.)

Anticipated results, unusual results, trade-offs, the postoperative course, and potential problems and their management, if discussed, emphasized, and reiterated preoperatively, may be accepted by the patient as part of the normal chain of events.

If brought up postoperatively for the first time, they may be misconstrued as excuses for imagined failures or shortcomings on the part of the surgeon. Reinforcement of the educational process may be desirable, and, as stated by Drs. Musgrave, Gorney, Courtiss, and Reich, more than one preoperative visit may be needed to accomplish this.

On the other hand, patient dissatisfaction may be due to factors other than those resulting from the surgery itself or complications. Drs. Goin, Goin, and Reich help us to manage specific problems in these areas through their perceptive observations and sage advice.

The preceding part may be one of the most important in this book for preventing and dealing with many problems in facial aesthetic surgery. The younger surgeon will benefit from reading and rereading it as he gains more experience in handling aesthetic surgery patients. The experienced aesthetic surgeon will benefit from this section by comparing his techniques with those of the authors, broadening or modifying them as he sees fit.

B.L.K.

Part II
Aesthetic plastic surgery of the face

Chapter 7

Aesthetic evaluation of the face: profileplasty

Mario Gonzalez-Ulloa

The profileplasty method was first described in 1960.[6] It was born out of an angry rebellion against the results I was obtaining, as well as those I saw published in plastic surgery journals, in which patients—usually women—almost always ugly in the preoperative stage, also looked ugly in the postoperative stage. Sometimes there had been some improvement in the shape of the nose but the total effect was still an ugly face. What was it that was missing to make those faces beautiful? It was the lack of a coherent, harmonious whole, of that integral sense of relation between the different segments of the face.

In works of art throughout the centuries, many faces have been portrayed that exhibit that striking quality which has enabled them to survive the harsh judgment of generations and still elicit in the viewer a reaction of appeal because of their beauty. These faces belong to different periods and to distinct cultures. Some are European, others African, Asiatic, or American.

In literature and philosophy, too, there have been numerous attempts to define *beauty*. But most of these definitions lack universality, being based on a specific canon, a subjective vision, acceptable to some but not necessarily to all (Fig. 7-1).

In my personal search for what constitutes true beauty, I have arrived at these conclusions:

- That the appreciation of beauty is an eminently individual equation, involving the creator's or observer's own ideals, aspirations, and symbols
- That outward appearance is but a mere clue in deciphering a personality

- That surgery is successful only if it results in patients' having an appearance in accordance with their expectations, agreeable to others and showing no trace of the operation
- That most individuals aspire to be "the best" within their type, to the point of wishing to be the prototype of beauty within their particular classification
- That to achieve this goal of being the best, they must possess other characteristics, unrelated to their appearance, that make them a "whole" person
- That sometimes, due to external pressures or a desire to improve their degree of acceptance, individuals desire a partial or total metamorphosis of their type[18]
- That the surgeon must have the capability to perform the varied corrective operations required and accept the risk for the adjustments to be made

For quite some time, but especially during the last 20 years, an extraordinary ethnical phenomenon, quite unique in history, has occurred: a massive blending of human groups, resulting in new values, customs, and life-styles, not to mention new physical types, no longer conforming to the classic ideal of beauty. These new prototypes, recognized in international beauty contests and fashion magazines, offer an expanded gamut for the appreciation of beauty. They require one to sharpen one's critical sense in order to detect the combinations of features that make up a pleasant whole, even though a particular feature might seem defective because it does not adhere to established patterns.

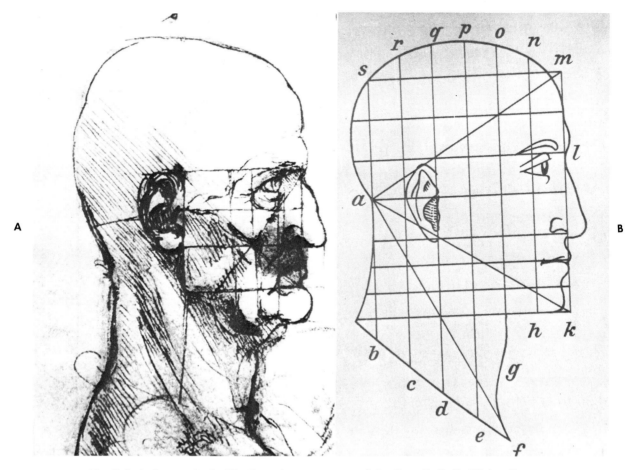

Fig. 7-1. A, Leonardo da Vinci's various segments of the face. **B,** Della Divina Proporzione. (**A** courtesy Maurice H. Goldblatt, University of Notre Dame. **B** from Albrecht Dürer's Della Symmetria Humana.)

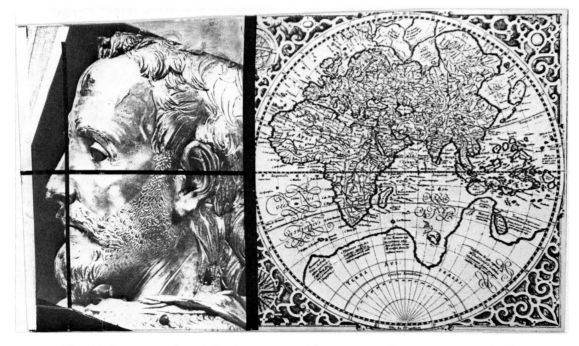

Fig. 7-2. Equator and meridian in a map and its corresponding measurement in the human face.

Now more than ever, aesthetic plastic surgeons must study these emerging prototypes so as to broaden their own definition of beauty and be able to find and bring it forth in those individuals discontented with their physical appearance. I believe that such continuous study of faces of all types, including measurement and evaluation of proportions, will increase the ability of surgeons to help solve their patients' problems.

The pursuit of beauty constitutes the ideal, the dream, the search, the fundamental endeavor of the artist-surgeon. But there are many paths to beauty, each of which is valid for the one following it, hence the dilemma of finding norms one can use to identify the characteristics that produce that aura, that spellbound sensation when a person encounters beauty.

To evaluate faces, I have developed two lines of reference that facilitate the study and comparison of various segments of the face. Interestingly, in applying these reference lines to hundreds of faces of the types traditionally considered beautiful, I have found certain principles worthy of note. The lines are designated as the *equator*—the horizontal line running from the upper ridge of the external auditory canal to the lower border of the orbit—and the *meridian 0*—the line perpendicular to the aforementioned, passing through the center point of the forehead, nasal root, nasal base, lips, and chin. Like the equator and meridian in geography, these lines enable us to measure, calculate, and obtain reference points. With them, we can estimate, create, or recreate beauty in a face within the parameters of its specifc prototype (Fig. 7-2).

TECHNIQUE

The study from which this concept emerged has been reported on previously,[2,6-9] but the technique of documentation is elaborated here in further detail. Basically, the surgeon must assume that a beautiful face corresponds to a beautiful facial skeleton and an ugly face to an ugly skeleton. So, to improve a face, it is in its "architecture" that the work must be done (Fig. 7-3).

With the use of the equator and meridian 0 lines, we can diagnose a frontal protraction, when the forehead protrudes beyond the meridian 0, or a frontal retraction, when the forehead is submerged behind the meridian 0. Similarly, we can define nasal, labial, and mental protraction or retraction for the nose, lips, and chin, respectively (Fig. 7-4). In addition to their diagnostic function,

these lines serve as guides in the surgical correction process (Fig. 7-5).

The first step in the profileplasty method is to obtain accurate documentation on the "geography" of the patient's preoperative face through the use of life-sized photographs and radiographs. The photographs are taken in frontal, lateral, and three-quarter positions against a dark background, with a camera in the horizontal position; the camera lens, 135 mm to avoid spherical aberration, is pointed toward the nasion. The lower border of the orbit and the upper margin of the external auditory canal of the patient's face are marked (Fig. 7-6). The patient's eyes must be open, focused on a mirror in front of the face to avoid tilting of the head.

Lights are placed as follows: one behind the patient, to differentiate the hair from the background; another at a 45-degree angle at a 3 m distance; and another at the same distance, angle, and level but with a dimmer intensity, focusing on the opposite side of the patient's face. Stroboscopic lights with a synchronized echo system are used.

The distance between the nasion and the lower part of the chin is measured with a pelvimeter. In the darkroom this measurement is used for enlarging the photograph to precisely life size.

With regard to the radiograph, I have termed the technique bustography.[14] It shows in a single take the bony structure and the soft tissues — and both with a high degree of accuracy (Fig. 7-7, *C*).

After all metallic objects around the head and neck have been removed, the patient is placed in a vertical position, lateral projection, in front of a radiological chassis, 35 × 63 cm. Cross-references are projected on the equator and meridian 0 of the face. Specifications are focal distance: 1.4 m, screen without intensifier; shutter time: 0.32 seconds; exposure factors: 8 kV, 100 mA, without filter, without Bucky diaphragm (Fig. 7-7, *A* and *B*).

Placed over an illuminated viewing box, the photographs and radiographs are then marked by the surgeon to indicate the equator and meridian 0 lines. The equator, as mentioned above, is traced with two reference points: the upper ridge of the external auditory canal and the lower ridge of the orbit. The meridian 0 is perpendicular to the equator, using the nasion as the reference point.

The lower pole of the face and the nasiolabial angle are then traced. These define the lower third of the face. The middle third is made up of

Text continued on p. 42.

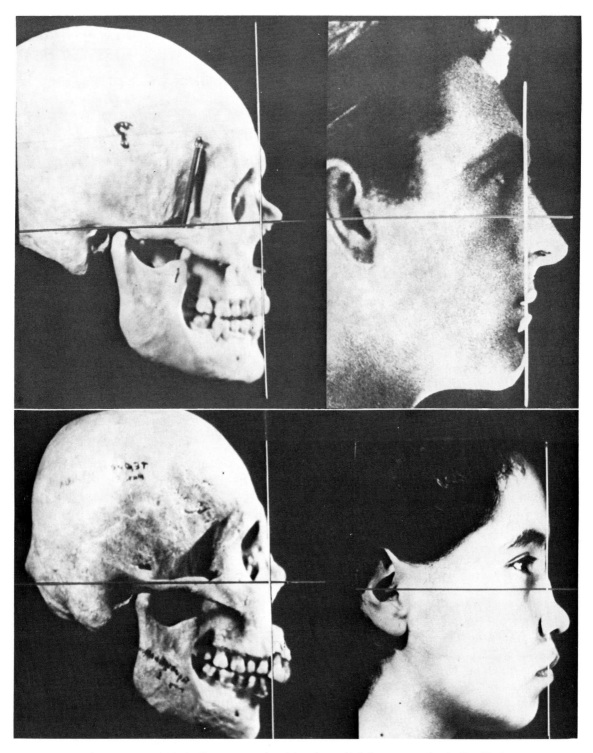

Fig. 7-3. A beautiful skull corresponds with a beautiful face; an ugly skull will always correspond with an ugly face.

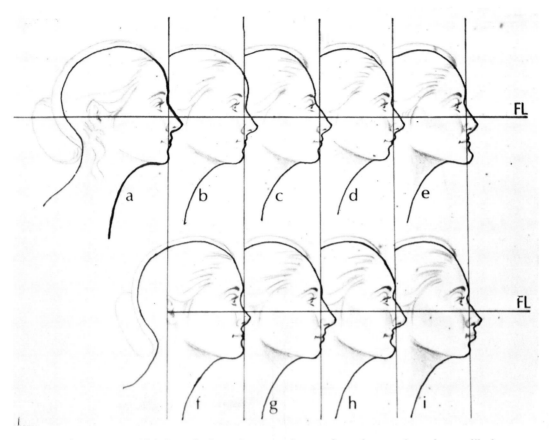

Fig. 7-4. *a,* Beautiful face; *b,* frontal protraction; *c,* frontal retraction; *d,* mandibular protraction; *e,* mandibular retraction; *f,* nasal retraction; *g,* nasal protraction; *h,* upper maxillary retraction; *i,* upper maxillary protraction. *FL,* Frankfort line.

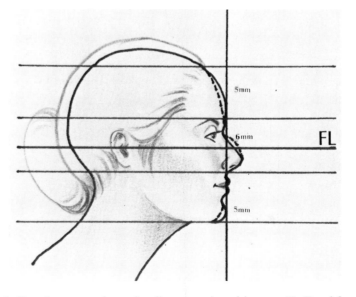

Fig. 7-5. Planning correction using lines mentioned in text. *FL,* Frankfort line.

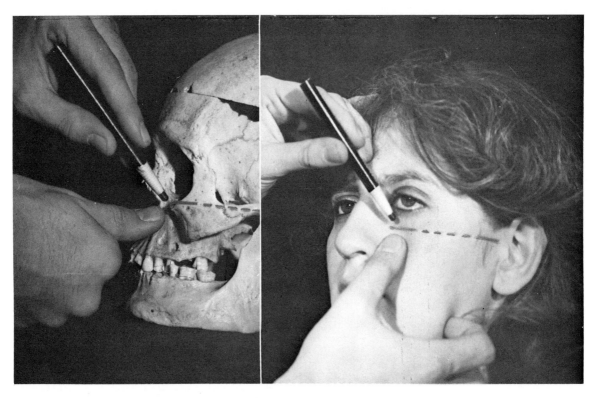

Fig. 7-6. Manner of palpation to obtain Frankfort line.

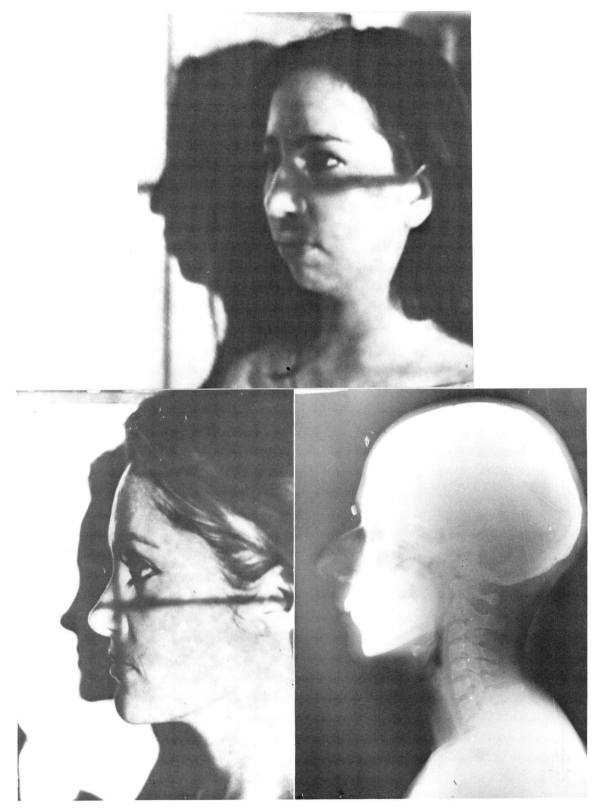

Fig. 7-7. Patient placed in front of radiographic shasis in which hair implant and eyebrow are marked, as well as external auditory canal.

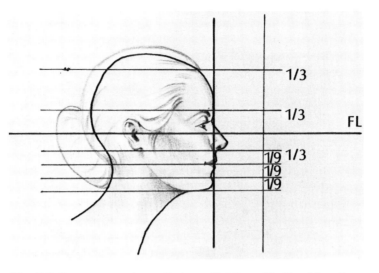

Fig. 7-8. Exact proportions of a beautiful face. *FL,* Frankfort line.

the area between the nasiolabial line and the upper border of the orbit. The upper third runs from this line to the root of the hair. The thirds should be of the same proportions to produce the effect of a harmonious face (Fig. 7-8).

The lower portion of the face, with the labial and labiomental line, is further subdivided in equal thirds: the two upper areas for the lips and the lower one for the chin, which should touch the meridian 0 line (Fig. 7-8). In women, this can be somewhat less, according to the evaluation of the patient's morphology and character, as well as the surgeon's taste.

These same lines are then traced on the radiograph. At this point the surgeon is equipped to evaluate the problem, plan for the correction, and determine the most adequate technique to cope with the particular problem.

CLASSIFICATION OF FACIAL PROBLEMS AND OTHER CONSIDERATIONS

Facial problems are many* and can generally be classified as follows:
A. Disproportions of the upper third of the face[10]
  1. Retraction or protraction of the forehead

---
*References 7-9, 11, 12, 16, 21, 24, 25.

  2. Hair significance in relation to the facial profile
B. Disproportions of the middle third of the face: retraction, protraction, or descent of the nose[4,20,23]
C. Disproportions of the lower third of the face[1-3,5,15,22]
  1. Retraction or protraction of the lips
  2. Retraction or protraction of the maxilla
  3. Retraction or protraction of the mandible
  4. Retraction of the chin
    a. First degree: mild retraction
    b. Second degree: moderate retraction
    c. Third degree: severe retraction
  5. Protraction of the chin—with or without descent

There are other considerations that affect the relative beauty of a face: its dynamic aspect, asymmetries, the central "T" of the face,[13] and the shape and position of the ears and teeth (these last two affecting the frontal profile of the face).[17-19]

SUMMARY

Beauty will continue to be a subjective matter. Nevertheless, the plastic surgeon who is charged with improving a patient's appearance must of necessity define certain characteristics, proportions, and facial relationships that produce a harmoni-

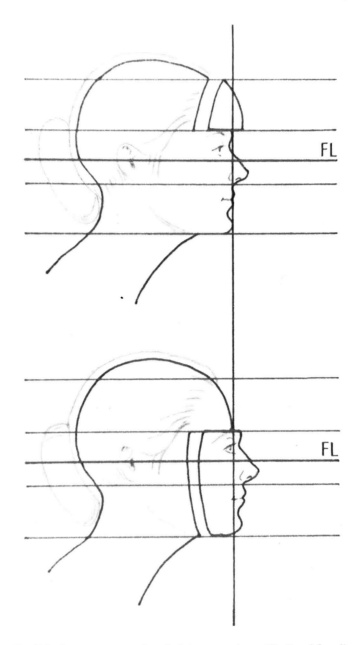

Fig. 7-9. Surgeon correcting facial proportions. *FL,* Frankfort line.

ous effect. In this task the profileplasty technique herein described can be of significant help. In redistributing millimeters (Fig. 7-9), the artist-surgeon has the touchy but ever-challenging job of perceiving and bringing forth that perennially sought quality of beauty.

REFERENCES

1. Gonzalez-Ulloa, M.: Temporomandibular arthroplasty in the treatment of prognathism, Plast. Reconstr. Surg. **8:**136, 1951.
2. Gonzalez-Ulloa, M.: Some important details in the treatment of prognathism by double condylectomy, Plast. Reconstr. Surg. **9:**391, 1952.
3. Gonzalez-Ulloa, M.: Late results in the treatment of prognathism by double condylectomy, Plast. Reconstr. Surg. **18:**50, 1956.
4. Gonzalez-Ulloa, M.: An articulated acrylic prosthetic structure for the repair of the flat nose, J. Int. Coll. Surg. **27:**359, 1957.
5. Gonzalez-Ulloa, M.: Mentoplasty with acrilic implants, Rev. Lat. Am. Cir. Plast. **3:**13, 1957.
6. Gonzalez-Ulloa M.: Basic studies in the preparation for profileplasty, Transactions of the International Society of Plastic Surgeons, Second Congress, London, 1960, Churchill Livingstone.

7. Gonzalez-Ulloa, M.: Planning the integral correction of the human profile, J. Int. Coll. Surg. **36:**364, 1961.
8. Gonzalez-Ulloa, M.: Quantitative principles in aesthetic surgery of the face (profileplasty), Plast. Reconstr. Surg. **29:**186, 1962.
9. Gonzalez-Ulloa, M.: A quantum method for the appreciation of the morphology of the face, Plast. Reconstr. Surg. **3:**241, 1964.
10. Gonzalez-Ulloa, M.: Grundlagen der profiloplastik, Handbuch der plastischen chirurgie, Berlin, 1965.
11. Gonzalez-Ulloa, M.: Profileplasty. In Goldwyn, R.M., editor: The unfavorable results in plastic surgery, Boston, 1970, Little, Brown & Co.
12. Gonzalez-Ulloa, M.: Experiencia de diez años en la ejecución de la perfiloplastia: reporte sumario, Rev. Esp. Cir. Plast. **4**(2), 1971.
13. Gonzalez-Ulloa, M.: The central "T" of the ageing face, Third Symposium of the American Academy of Facial Surgery, New York, May 1971.
14. Gonzalez-Ulloa, M.: Bustography, Twenty-fifth Symposium of the Dalinde Medical Center, Mexico, 1972.
15. Gonzalez-Ulloa, M.: Ptosis of the chin: the witch's chin, Plast. Reconstr. Surg. **50:**54, 1972.
16. Gonzalez-Ulloa, M.: Rhinoplasty: complications and how to avoid them—cadaver counterpoint, Instructional course, International Society of Aesthetic Plastic Surgery, Jerusalem, 1973.
17. Gonzalez-Ulloa, M.: Building out the malar prominencies (as an addition to rhytidectomy), Plast. Reconstr. Surg. **53:**293, 1974.
18. Gonzalez-Ulloa, M.: La tétrada basica para la belleza de la cara moderna, Rev. Plast. Latinoam. **1**(1), 1975.
19. Gonzalez-Ulloa, M.: Levantamiento de los huesos malares para producir un diferencial étnico y un perfil juvenil de la cara, Rev. Med. Mod. Mex. **15**(1), 1976.
20. Gonzalez-Ulloa, M.: Punch-rhinoplasty (as a complement to rhytidectomy), Aesth. Plast. Surg. **2:**291, 1978.
21. Gonzalez-Ulloa, M., and Stevens, E.: Implants in the face, Plast. Reconstr. Surg. **33:**532, 1964.
22. Gonzalez-Ulloa, M., and Stevens, E.: The role of chin correction in profileplasty, Plast. Reconstr. Surg. **41:**477, 1968.
23. Gonzalez-Ulloa, M., and Stevens, E.: Syndrome of retraction of the middle third of the face: its importance in profileplasty, Int. Surg. **51:**345, 1969.
24. Gonzalez-Ulloa, M., et al.: Reporte preliminar de la perfusión subcutánea del dimetilpolisiloxano para aumentar el volúmen y alterar el contorno regional, Cir. Cir. **33:**401, 1965.
25. Gonzalez-Ulloa, M., et al.: Preliminary report on the subcutaneous perfusion of dimethylpolisiloxane to increase volume and alter regional contour, Br. J. Plast. Surg. **20:**424, 1967.

Chapter 8

Upper facial nerve anatomy and forehead lift

Ivo Pitanguy

In this chapter the anatomy of the upper branches of the facial nerve and of the frontalis musculature is described, as well as a personal surgical technique for forehead lifting: criss-crossing of the aponeurotic expansion of the frontalis muscle. This technique has produced very satisfying results with extremely low complication rates.

ANATOMICAL CONSIDERATIONS

In the upper third of the face, the facial nerve divides into temporal and zygomatic branches at the anterior border of the parotid gland (Fig. 8-1). The topographical anatomy of these nerves varies frequently. In our analysis of 20 head halves, Silveira Ramos and I encountered four variations. The temporofrontal branch, innervating the upper third of the face, showed the most frequent variations, making it more vulnerable to injury. In these dissections we noted that in spite of great variations in the number and disposition of the temporofrontal branches, their direction was constant.[5,6] The course projected on the skin was a line starting from a point 0.5 cm below the tragus of the ear, extending toward the eyebrow, and passing 1.5 cm above the lateral aspect of the eyebrow (Fig. 8-2).[6] This line represents the course of the temporofrontal branch. Another anatomical guide to the temporofrontal branch of the facial nerve is the frontal branch of the superficial temporal artery, which, at the level of the lateral border of the frontalis muscle, sends a descending branch to the muscle that generally coincides with the penetration of the frontal nerve into the muscle. Anatomically, the identification of this vessel is helpful in directing the level of

dissection. The lack of subcutaneous mass at the level of the lateral border of the frontalis muscle makes the frontal branch of the facial nerve more superficial and more vulnerable to injury.

Subaponeurotic dissection superior to the frontal arterial branch provides better protection for the pilar bulbs, easier dissection, and less bleeding (Fig. 8-3).[6] The more superficial undermining inferior to the vessel diminishes the risk of frontal nerve injury. Between these two different planes exists a "no man's land" that, more

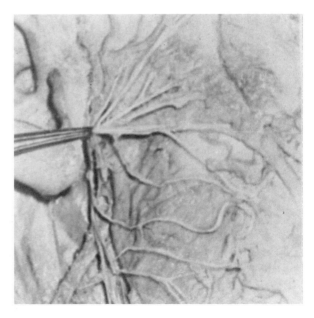

Fig. 8-1. In upper third of face, facial nerve divides into temporal and zygomatic branches at anterior border of parotid gland.

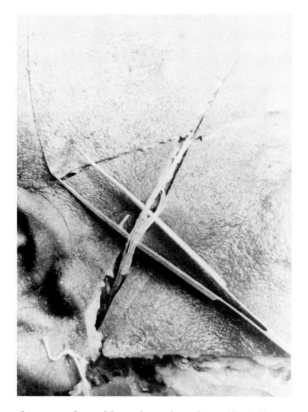

Fig. 8-2. Course of temporofrontal branch projected on skin is line starting from point 0.5 cm below tragus of ear, extending toward eyebrow, and passing 1.5 cm above lateral aspect of eyebrow. (From Pitanguy, I., and Silveira Ramos, A.: The frontal branch of the facial nerve: the importance of its variations in face lifting, Plast. Reconstr. Surg. **38:**352, 1966.)

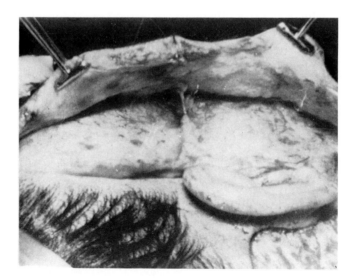

Fig. 8-3. Subaponeurotic dissection superior to frontal arterial branch provides better protection for pilar bulbs, easier dissection, and less bleeding. (From Pitanguy, I., and Silveira Ramos, A.: The frontal branch of the facial nerve: the importance of its variations in face lifting, Plast. Reconstr. Surg. **38:**352, 1966.)

than a simple pedicle, is an important anatomical area containing the frontal nerve(s). The importance of the temporofrontal nerve derives from the fact that it innervates the frontalis muscle, which is the main muscular entity of the forehead, being responsible for its parallel wrinkling.[1] The other muscles involved in the biomechanics of the frontoglabellar area are the corrugator, which is responsible for the oblique and vertical glabellar wrinkles, and the procerus, which is responsible for the transverse wrinkles of the nasal roof.[8] In the glabellar area the procerus and corrugator are tightly bound in a fanlike aponeurotic expansion that intermingles diffusely with the aponeurosis of the frontalis, forming the frontalis-procerus-corrugator aponeurotic expansion.

SURGICAL TECHNIQUE

I usually perform the frontal lift together with a facial and cervical lift, but it could also be carried out as a separate procedure. The operation is routinely performed with the patient under general anesthesia, with fixation of the endotracheal tube to the patient's lower incisor teeth. The incision lines are marked in the area of the shaved scalp.* It is important to carefully mark the midline, which can be scratched for later identification (Fig. 8-4). The coronal incision line, the orbital rims, and the root and dorsum of the nose down to the nasal tip are infiltrated with 0.25% lidocaine hydrochloride (Xylocaine) with epinephrine (1:200,000). The forehead itself is not infiltrated. This procedure can also be carried out with the patient under local anesthesia with sedation.[4,7]

Usually an area approximately 2.5 cm in width is shaved along the coronal line of the scalp. This area is situated about 5 cm behind the hairline. The incision is placed at the posterior border of the trimmed area, approximately parallel with the hairline. It is the natural prolongation of the temporal arched line of the facial rhytidoctomy. The incision is made through the skin and the galea

Text continued on p. 54.

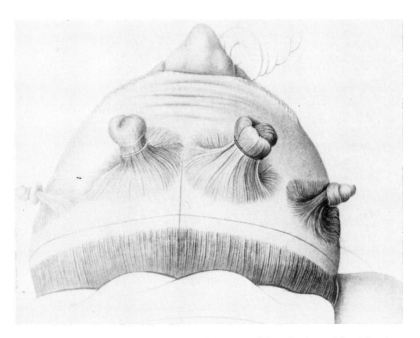

Fig. 8-4. Midline is carefully marked by scratching for later identification.

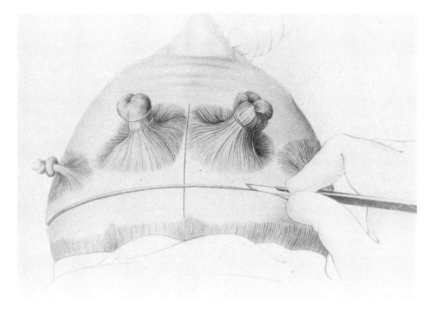

Fig. 8-5. Incision is made through skin and galea aponeurotica.

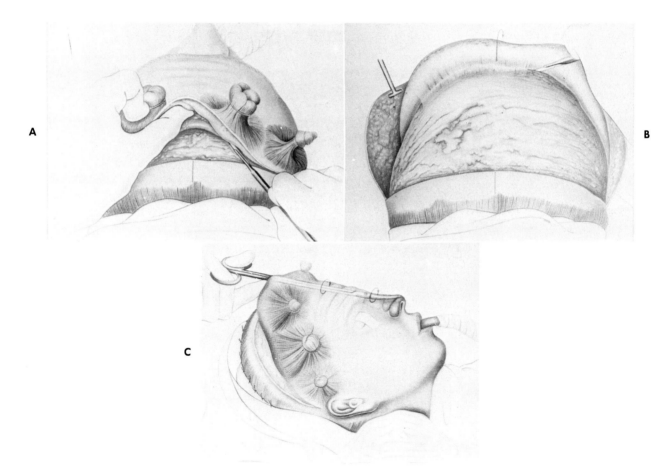

Fig. 8-6. Flap is undermined in subgaleal plane, **A,** to orbital ridges, **B,** to dorsum and tip of nose, **C.**

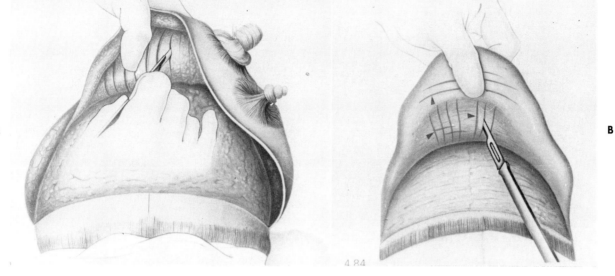

Fig. 8-7. To free aponeurotic expansion, vertical, **A,** and horizontal, **B,** crossing incisions are performed.

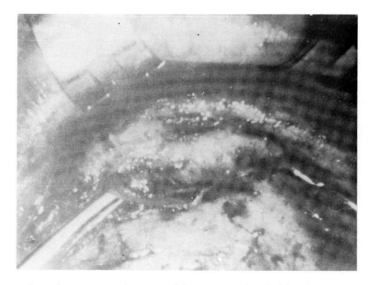

Fig. 8-8. Portion of corrugator is resected in conservative fashion in case of accentuated hypertrophy of glabellar region.

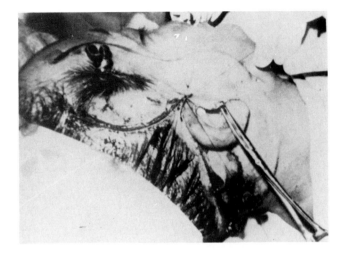

Fig. 8-9. When performed with face-lift, traction of frontal flaps should be done after fixation of facial flaps through key stitches in supraauricular region (blocking technique), preventing excessive traction of forehead in upward direction and imbalance of facial appearance.

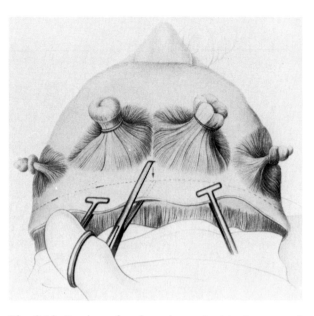

Fig. 8-10. Portion of scalp to be excised is demarcated with Pitanguy small-flap demarcator.

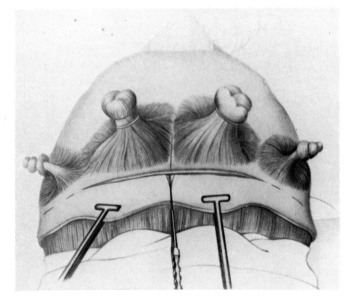

Fig. 8-11. Scalp is incised in midline to marked point and approximated.

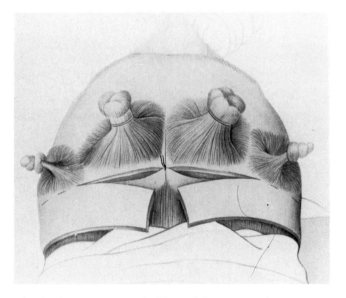

Fig. 8-12. Two symmetrical lateral flaps now exist.

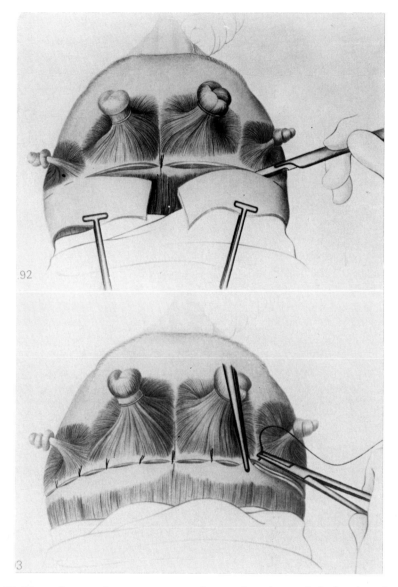

Fig. 8-13. These flaps undergo anteroposterior traction along relatively selected vectors, achieving desired effect on each side of face.

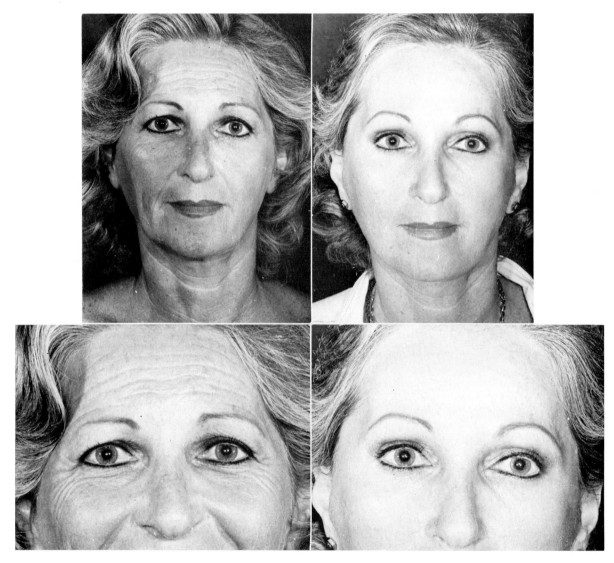

Fig. 8-14. Preoperative and postoperative views showing that this traction improves frontoglabellar and nasal wrinkles and results in moderate lifting of eyebrows and nasal tip.

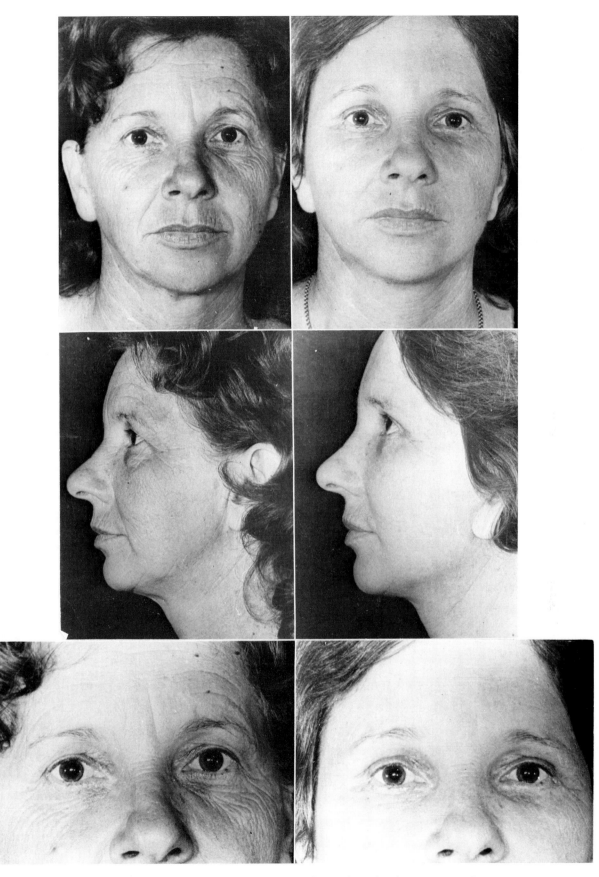

Fig. 8-15. Preoperative and postoperative views of traction in another patient.

aponeurotica (Fig. 8-5). The flap is undermined in the subgaleal plane (Fig. 8-6, *A*) to the orbital ridges (Fig. 8-6, *B*) and the dorsum and tip of the nose (Fig. 8-6, *C*). The latter maneuver allows improvement of a drooped nose tip, a typical sign of aging.[2,3]

As the scalp flap is reflected over the patient's face, the aponeurosis is exposed, and the temporofrontal neurovascular bundle can be seen in the transition area between the two planes of undermining. As a result of detailed studies and postoperative follow-up, I perform vertical and horizontal crossing incisions in the aponeurotic expansion in order to free it (Fig. 8-7). These incisions should not be deepened to the dermis, since they could cause depressions on the frontal area in the late postoperative period. On the other hand, only in cases of accentuated hypertrophy of the glabellar region do I resect a portion of the corrugator, in a very conservative fashion (Fig. 8-8). I believe that major resections can lead to conspicuous depressions on the forehead. When performed with a face-lift, traction on the frontal flap should be done only after fixation of the facial flaps through key stitches in the supraauricular region (blocking technique) (Fig. 8-9), preventing excessive traction of the forehead in an upward direction and imbalance of the facial appearance.

The portion of scalp flap to be excised is demarcated with a Pitanguy small-flap demarcator (Fig. 8-10). The scalp is incised in the midline to the marked point and approximated (Fig. 8-11). There are then two symmetrical lateral flaps (Fig. 8-12) that will undergo anteroposterior traction along relatively selected vectors (Fig. 8-13), achieving the effect desired on each side of the face. This traction, besides improving the frontoglabellar and nasal wrinkles, results in moderate lifting of the eyebrows and nasal tip[2,4] (Figs. 8-14 and 8-15).

In those cases in which blepharoplasty is indicated, the forehead lift is carried out first, because the forehead and eyebrow lift will decrease the excess of palpebral skin to be resected. In case the patient had undergone a previous blepharoplasty, great care should be taken in the resection and superior advancement of the forehead flap, to avoid lagophthalmos and problems due to corneal exposure.* At the end of the procedure, a com-

---

*EDITOR'S NOTE: It is wise to check the adequacy of the upper lid skin preoperatively and again with the patient under sedation or anesthesia. If in doubt, abandon the forehead lift. (B.L.K.)

pressive dressing of wet gauze and cotton pads is held by an elastic bandage. Since the flap lies over a hard surface, such compression helps to decrease the risk of hematomas. (For the same reason, great care must be taken to avoid excessive compression to avoid the risk of creating ischemia in the forehead flap.)

RESULTS

The results of this operation are gratifying to both patient and surgeon (Figs. 18-14 and 18-15).

COMPLICATIONS

The usual postoperative course does not present specific problems.[1,3,4] Possible complications may be due to inappropriate handling of the flap, excessive tension, and deepening of the incision into the dermis, as mentioned above. In my series of 280 cases, no major complications were noted.*

GENERAL COMMENTS

Recently there has been an increase in the percentage of forehead lifts in patients undergoing facelift surgery on my service. Younger patients are also undergoing this surgery more frequently.

The technique described in this chapter avoids placing the incisions on bald areas, thus avoiding the risk of noticeable scarring.

The criss-crossing incisions on the aponeurosis achieve satisfactory treatment of the muscles without the possibility of depressions in the frontal flap, as could happen with more aggressive procedures on the frontalis muscle. The blocking technique, as mentioned before, will avoid excessive lifting of the hairline.[3]

---

*EDITOR'S NOTE: Viñas et al. (Plast. Reconstr. Surg. **57**:452, 1976) reported three cases of slough, the worst of which occurred in a hypertensive patient who had a secondary hematoma and did not return for several days. We believe that the only potentially serious complication is the rare case of severe hematoma. Diagnosis is easy because of its cardinal, unmistakable symptom: severe, excruciating pain refractory to all forms of palliation, including nerve blocks and intravenous analgesics. Treatment, also easy, consists of immediate decompression and evacuation. If carried out promptly, complete, uneventful healing may be expected. (See Chapter 11.) (B.L.K.)

REFERENCES

1. Baker, T.J., and Gordon, H.J.: Complications of rhytidectomy, Plast. Reconstr. Surg. **40**:31, 1967.
2. Patterson, C.N., and Durham, N.C.: Surgery of the aging nose. In Plastic and reconstructive surgery of the face and neck, vol. 1, New York, 1977, Grune & Stratton, Inc.

3. Pitanguy, I.: Aesthetic plastic surgery of head and body, Heildelberg, 1981, Springer-Verlag, p. 202.
4. Pitanguy, I.: Indications for and treatment of frontal and glabellar wrinkles in an analysis of 3,404 consecutive cases of rhytidectomy, Plast. Reconstr. Surg. **67:**157, 1981.
5. Pitanguy, I., and Silviera Ramos, A.: Considerações sobre as variações do ramo frontal do nervo facial, Rev. Bras. Cir. **52**(6):341, 1966.
6. Pitanguy, I., and Silveira Ramos, A.: The frontal branch of the facial nerve: the importance of its variations in face lifting, Plast. Reconstr. Surg. **38:**352, 1966.
7. Pitanguy, I., et al.: Rugas fronto-glabelares: detalhes e importância da ressecção da expansão aponeurótica dos corrugadores e ação sobre os músculos frontais e procerus e tratamento tegumentar e muscular da região fronto-glabelar, Rev. Bras. Cir. **65:**40, 1975.
8. Spalteholz, E.: Atlas de anatomia humana, vol. 2, Barcelona, Spain, 1965, Labor.

SUGGESTED READINGS

Bonavita Paez, E.: Ritidectomia, Rev. Cir. Plast. Urug. **4:**15, 1965.
Castañares, S.: Forehead wrinkles and glabellar frown and ptosis of the eyebrows, Plast. Reconstr. Surg. **34:**406, 1964.
Converse, J.M.: Reconstructive surgery, Philadelphia, 1964, W.B. Saunders Co., pp. 1306-1342.
Conway, H.: The surgical face lifting, Plast. Reconstr. Surg. **45:**124, 1970.
Edwards, S.B.: Bilateral neurotomy for frontalis hypermotility, Plast. Reconstr. Surg. **19:**337, 1957.
Fomon, S.: Cosmetic surgery: principles and practice, Philadelphia, 1960, J.B. Lippincott Co.
Gonzalez-Ulloa, M.: Facial wrinkles, Plast. Reconstr. Surg. **29:**458, 1962.
Gonzalez-Ulloa, M., and Stevens, E.: Senility of the face: basic studies to understand its causes and effects, Plast. Reconstr. Surg. **36:**239, 1965.
Gonzalez-Ulloa, M., and Stevens, E.: Rhytidoplasty and related procedures to correct the case of the appearance of facial senility, Int. Surg. **49:**361, 1968.
Hollander, M.M.: Rhytidectomy: anatomical and surgical considerations, Plast. Reconstr. Surg. **20:**218, 1957.
Kiechlin, H.: Sur la correction des rides intersourciliers, Ann. Chir. Plast. **9:**140, 1964.
Marino, H.: Frontal rhytidectomy, Bol. Soc. Cir. B. Aires **47:**93, 1963.
Marino, H.: Treatment of wrinkles of forehead, Prensa Med. Argent. **51:**1368, 1964.
Passot, R.: La chirurgie esthétique des rides du visage, Presse Med. **27:**258, 1919.
Pitanguy, I.: La ritidoplastica: soluzione eccletica del problema, Minerva Chir. **22**(17):942, 1967.
Pitanguy, I.: Ritidectomia, Trib. Med. **354:**8, 1969.
Pitanguy, I.: Ritidoplastia: considerações em torno de 2.226 casos pessoais, Rev. Bras. Cir. **61:**173, 1971.
Pitanguy, I.: Direção da tração em ritidoplastias, Rev. Bras. Cir. **61:**113, 1971.
Rebello, C., and Franco, T.: Tratamento cirúrgico das rugas da face, Rev. Col. Bras. Cir. **2**(9):10, 1970.
Rees, T.: Cosmetic facial surgery, Philadelphia, 1973, W.B. Saunders Co.
Uchida, J.: A method of frontal rhytidectomy, Plast. Reconstr. Surg. **35:**218, 1965.

Chapter 9

Temple lift

Matthew C. Gleason

The temple lift is an operation designed to correct drooping of the lateral eyebrows and eyelids. The lateral forehead skin, especially that portion designated as the temple, is continuous with the thin, elastic tissues of the cheeks and face, so that with aging it loses its elasticity and follows the gravitational pull downward. This ptosis is especially reflected in the inferior displacement of the lateral eyebrow. In youth, the medial eyebrow begins near the supraorbital rim above the inner canthus and arches gracefully upward to reach its zenith two thirds the distance to the lateral orbit before descending in an increasing trajectory to the level of the supraorbital ridge. Judicious plucking of the eyebrow hairs and eyebrow pencils are commonly used by women to enhance this arch and, in later life, to camouflage its senescent plunge.

The brow skin inferior to the eyebrows is continuous with the eyelid skin, so that as the eyebrows assume a lower position, this brow skin spills over onto the eyelids, presenting as pseudoblepharochalasis. Indeed, the patient usually will present this problem to the surgeon by requesting "eyelid surgery." If the unwary surgeon accedes to the patient's suggestion, both surgeon and patient will be disappointed by the incomplete resolution of the problem. If, on the other hand, the surgeon brings to the patient's attention that there is an anatomical displacement of the eyebrow; that instead of an arch the eyebrow is horizontal in its medial portion and laterally drops below the bony orbital rim, giving a "sad look"; or that the arch of the eyebrow is formed not of hair but of eyebrow pencil, the surgeon can make a preoperative determination as to how much benefit will be obtained from eyelid surgery. The surgeon can further outline the prob-

lem by gently elevating the lateral eyebrow with the thumb and noting the amount of improvement. If the skin and subcutaneous tissues slide easily upward and simultaneously tighten most of the lax lateral eyelid skin, then an accurate diagnosis of ptosis of the lateral forehead skin can be made. It should be clearly explained to the patient that only by correcting the true problem (i.e., the lax forehead and temple skin) can a true correction be made of the eyelid skin (Figs. 9-1 and 9-2). This does not always mean that a temple lift should be done; indeed, where the ptosis is only moderate, a blepharoplasty may be preferred because of its simplicity. However, the shortcomings of the blepharoplasty are now fully recognized and understood.

Various means of correction need to be considered. Excision of an ellipse of skin above the eyebrow will bring the eyebrow and lax skin upward. It is the simplest approach and possibly the surgery of choice in men with deep horizontal furrows in which the surgical scars can be hidden. In women the scars are placed just above the eyebrow hairs, where they can be partially camouflaged. Unfortunately, the incisions must extend beyond the eyebrow to pull up the lateral droop of the eyelid. This extended part of the scar leaves a noticeable scar, and for this reason, I avoid a supra-eyebrow correction if possible. In order to hide the scar, the surgical approach must be in the scalp above the hairline. There are two techniques that use this approach: the forehead lift and the temple lift.[1] The forehead lift, as described by Viñas, Caviglia, and Cortinas,[3] is the operation of choice where deep vertical frown creases and horizontal brow furrows traverse the forehead skin. However, where the forehead is smooth or the hairline high, then a temple lift

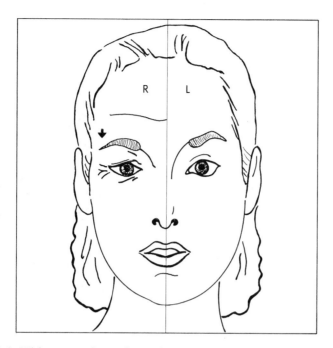

Fig. 9-1. With age, eyebrow descends, producing pseudochalasia on right.

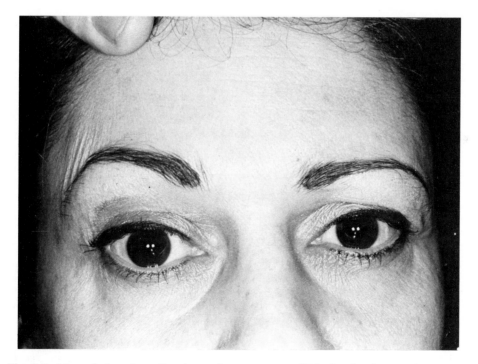

Fig. 9-2. Manual elevation of eyebrow demonstrates relief of redundant eyelid. This is basis of temple lift operation. (From Gleason, M.C.: The temple lift. In Goulian, D.C., and Courtiss, E.H., editors: Symposium of surgery on the aging face, St. Louis, 1978, The C.V. Mosby Co.)

(alone, or in combination with a rhytidectomy) can be considered. The advantage of the temple lift over the forehead lift is that it achieves an easier lateral elevation because the dissection of the forehead portion is superficial to the inelastic galea, rather than deep to it, as in the forehead lift. The temple lift is a natural extension of the rhytidectomy incision, whereas the forehead lift requires either two separate incisions in the temple region or at least a partial lateral transection of the galea in order to pull the rhytidectomy cheek flap upward. However, the superficial dissection that allows the temple flap to provide more lift than the forehead flap also puts the frontal nerve at more risk. This is covered more fully under the section on complications.

TECHNIQUE (Figs. 9-3 and 9-4, *B*)

The patient's hair is shampooed the night before surgery. At the time of surgery a 3 cm strip of scalp is clipped well behind the hairline, beginning in front of the ear and extending cephalad to almost the midline. The face and scalp are prepared and draped, and 0.5% lidocaine hydrochloride (Xylocaine) is injected into the tissues for anesthesia.

The incision begins in front of the root of the helix and continues in the shaved scalp until a point above and in line with the mideyebrow is reached. Undermining starts in front of the ear at the same level as a rhytidectomy. Dissection is above the superficial temporal fascia and continues toward the lateral canthus to separate the orbicularis fibers from the skin and release the crow's-feet. The dissection proceeds superiorly until the frontal branch of the superficial temporal artery is located. This small artery lies superior to the frontal nerve. Occasionally it can be seen pulsating. More often, it can be palpated. Once this landmark has been located, the dissec-

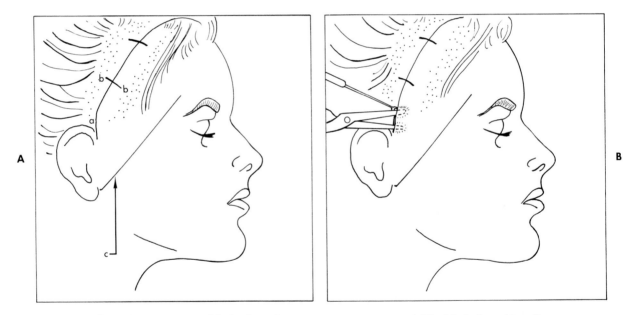

Fig. 9-3. **A,** Temporal hair shaved preparatory to temporal lift. Methylene blue line indicates proposed line of incision *(a)* and transverse line *(b)* for demonstration purposes to indicate amount of elevation that can be achieved. Line from earlobe to 1.5 cm above eyebrow *(c)* indicates course of underlying frontal branch of facial nerve.[2] **B,** Initial undermining begins as in superficial rhytidectomy level. Dissection continues superiorly in superficial plane until hairline and frontal branch of superficial temporal artery are reached, and then becomes deep to galea (see text). **C,** Superficial dissection frees skin of lateral canthus from fibers of orbicularis muscle to aid in alleviating crow's-feet. **D,** Temporal flap has been fully dissected. Frontal branch of superficial temporal artery *(b)* is superior to frontal nerve. Forceps *(d)* holds transected galea. Above forceps *(a)* dissection is deep to galea. Below forceps *(c)* dissection is superficial to frontalis muscle and temporalis fascia (See also Fig. 9-4, *B*). **E,** Undermined temple skin pulled straight upward and secured with single suture. There is no lateral traction. Note elevation of horizontal methylene blue line *(b')*, compared with *b*, both of which were on same level prior to elevation of temple flap. **F,** Overlapping skin to be removed.

tion proceeds medially to the mideyebrow superficial to the frontalis muscle. The frontal nerve is especially vulnerable during this part of the dissection,* so hemostasis should be obtained at the lowest possible setting. The deep dissection may then be done by elevating the scalp incision and galea away from the periosteum of the frontal

bone. The dissection proceeds inferiorly until the level beneath the superficial dissection is reached. The two levels (the deep and the superficial) are joined by transecting the galea and frontalis muscle superior to the superficial temporal artery and the frontal nerve. The lateral brow skin is drawn upward with gentle traction on the temple flap, and it will be found that a 2 cm pull superiorly will elevate the eyebrow approximately 1 cm. The excess scalp skin is excised, and little if any skin is removed laterally. (A lateral pull is not desired

*EDITOR'S NOTE: Indeed. See Correia, P., and Zani, R.: Surgical anatomy of the facial nerve, as related to ancillary operations in rhytidoplasty, Plast. Reconstr. Surg. **52**:551, 1973. (B.L.K.)

Text continued on p. 64.

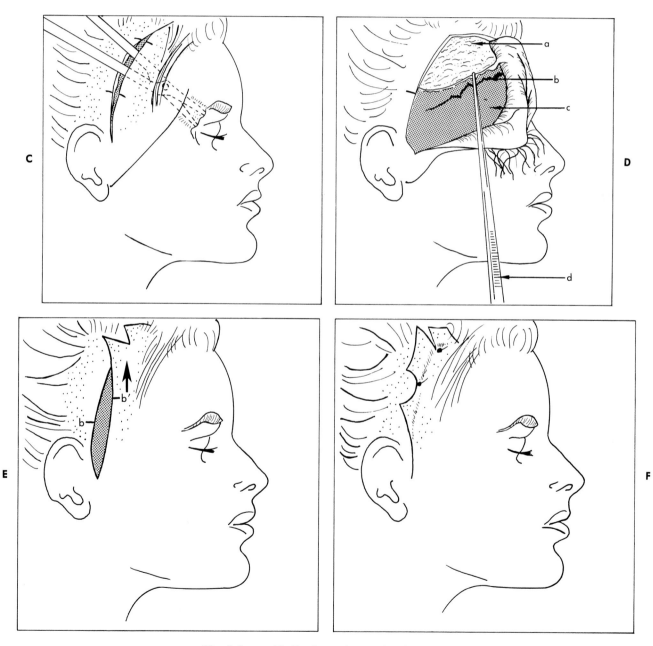

Fig. 9-3, cont'd. For legend see opposite page.

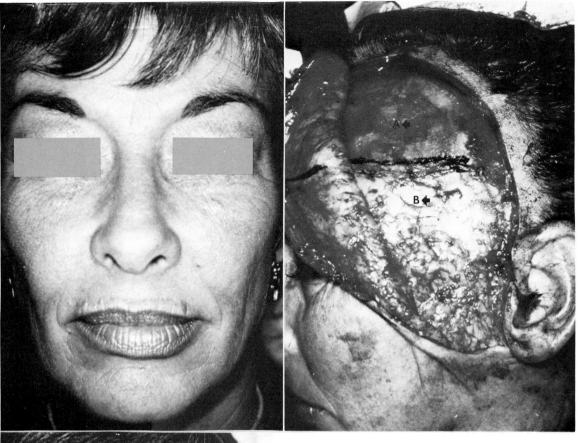

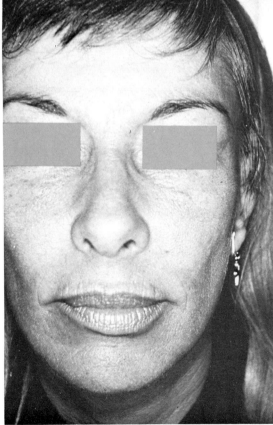

Fig. 9-4. A, Upper eyelids are ptotic and hooded. **B,** Rhytidectomy incision continues into temple lift. Solid line marks junction of dissection superficial to temporalis fascia and frontalis muscle *(B)*, with dissection deep to galea and frontalis muscle *(A)*. Transection at this level protects frontal nerve and hair follicles and allows temple flap to be advanced superiorly with ease. **C,** Postoperative result of rhytidectomy with temple lift and upper blepharoplasty.

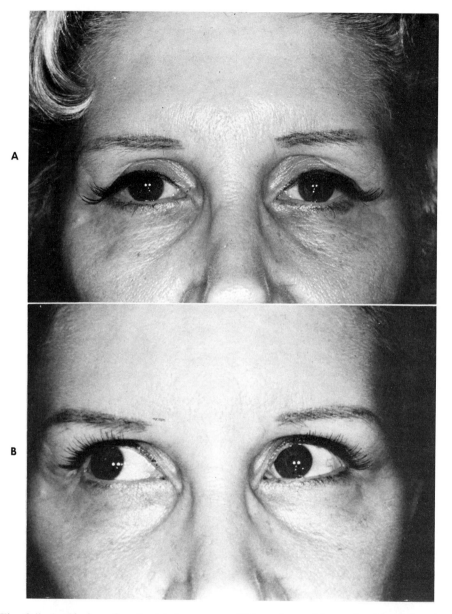

Fig. 9-5. A, Choice of patient is important. This patient with ptosis of lateral eyebrow and eyelid is ideal candidate. Forehead is smooth. **B,** Postoperative result of temple lift. Lateral eyebrow has been elevated and eyebrow arch restored. Lateral eyebrow skin has been tightened without blepharoplasty.

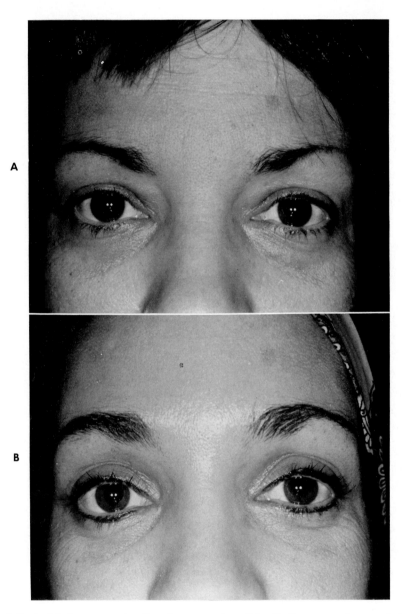

Fig. 9-6. A, Moderate ptosis of eyebrows and eyelids. **B,** Postoperative result is good, but probably blepharoplasty would have given equally good result and is simpler.

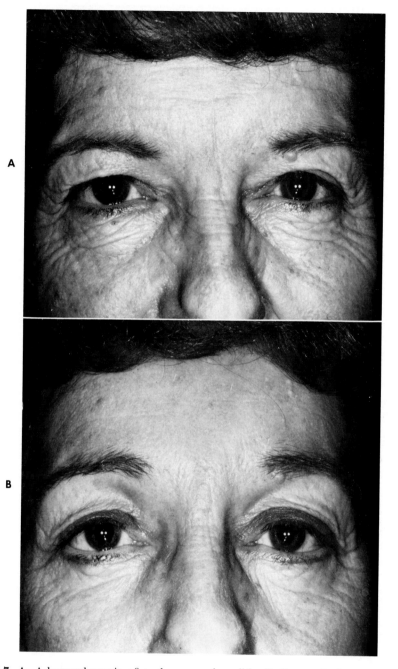

Fig. 9-7. A, Advanced ptosis of eyebrows and eyelids. **B,** Postoperative appearance is much improved but patient will require secondary blepharoplasty. Experience will indicate those patients in whom both temple lift and blepharoplasty are needed.

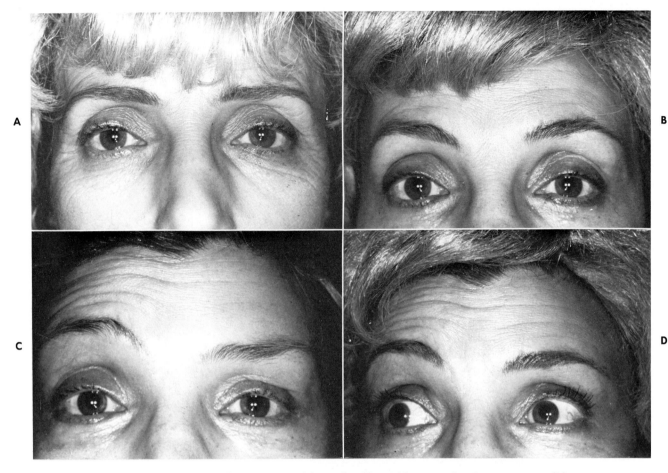

Fig. 9-8. A, Patient before surgery with ptosis of lateral brow, redundant upper eyelids, and crow's-feet. **B,** Good postoperative result with elevation of eyebrows. **C,** However, attempt to wrinkle forehead displays left paresis. **D,** Six months later, spontaneous frontalis function is returning. (From Gleason, M.C.: Forehead and eyebrow lifts. In Courtiss, E.H., editor: Aesthetic surgery: trouble—how to avoid it and how to treat it, St. Louis, 1978, The C.V. Mosby Co.)

and can produce an unwanted pseudo-Oriental expression.) Two tacking sutures are used to hold the temple flap superiorly, and then a running 4-0 nylon suture completes the closure.

If the temple lift is done in conjunction with a rhytidectomy, the temple lift is done last, since it is made technically easier by the increased exposure of the rhytidectomy. Since the upward pull on the temple flap is directly transmitted to the cheek tissue, the lateral canthal creases (crow's-feet) are especially benefited. After the temple flaps have been tacked in place, the remainder of the rhytidectomy tissues are tailored as needed. The temptation to elevate the cheek tissues more than 2 cm should be resisted, since increased tension on the hair-bearing temple may lead to prolonged alopecia. Postoperative care is similar to that of the rhytidectomy. Results have been gratifying (Figs. 9-4 to 9-7).

COMPLICATIONS

Extensive surgical procedures are correspondingly accompanied by increased chances of complications. A frontal nerve palsy is the most common complication, since the nerve traverses the area of surgery (Fig. 9-8).[2] The frontal nerve is rarely if ever seen during the temple lift, and so inadvertent injury is not realized until after the procedure has been completed and the local anesthesia dissipated. Unless the nerve was seen during the original dissection, reexploration is of little benefit. Furthermore, the most probable cause of palsy is injury either from the cautery or from overstretching the nerve. In either case, motion generally returns within 3 months. In my personal experience, 9 patients out of 100 had a unilateral transient palsy with 1 having permanent paresis. While the 9% may seem high, all but 2 cases were in the early phase of my experience.

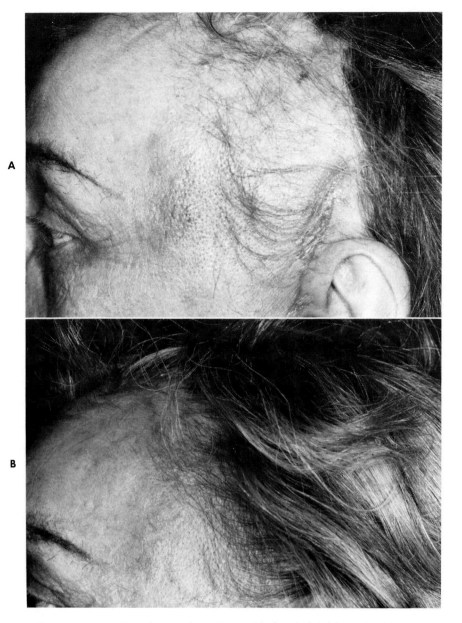

Fig. 9-9. A, Postoperative alopecia in patient with fine hair, thin scalp skin, sparse subcutaneous tissue, and too much tension on skin flap. **B,** One year later there is good regrowth.

Alopecia, correspondingly, lessened when excess flap tension was minimized by removing only 2 cm of scalp. Out of the 100 patients, 1 had temporal alopecia, which required hair plug transplants (Fig. 9-9).

Proper selection of patients reduces complications. The ideal patient has firm skin, a thick layer of subcutaneous tissue, and a vigorous growth of hair. One should avoid the patient who is elderly with thin skin, skeletonized subcutaneous tissue, and sparse hair. Men are not usually suitable candidates because of their high temple hairline and widow's peak. I have encountered no problems secondary to hematoma or skin loss.

REFERENCES

1. Gleason, M.D.: Brow lifting through a temporal scalp approach, Plast. Reconstr. Surg. **52:**141, 1973.
2. Pitanguy, I., and Ramos, A.S.: The frontal branch of the facial nerve: importance of variations in face-lifting, Plast. Reconstr. Surg. **38:**352, 1966.
3. Viñas, J.C., Caviglia, C., and Cortinas, J.L.: Forehead rhytidectomy and brow lifting, Plast. Reconstr. Surg. **57:**445, 1976.

Chapter 10

Modified brow lift

George C. Peck

The problems of achieving a brow lift and correcting crow's-feet have been difficult and complicated. The standard face-lift does little to improve either crow's-feet or lateral upper eyelid hooding. The classic technique of blepharoplasty, as described by Castañares,[1] does not improve either of these problems. In recent years the technique of the forehead lift has become more popular and has often been described as the only means for achieving a brow lift. However, the appearance of many of these patients can be improved with much less surgery. This chapter presents a technique to improve the brow and crow's-feet.

TECHNIQUE

Fig. 10-1 shows the pattern of skin excision that is used. Lateral to the lateral canthus the incision extends upward into the eyebrow area. This produces an elevation of the entire crow's-feet area. It also elevates the skin in this area of the lower eyelid so that much less skin excision is necessary from the lower eyelid. This will help to prevent postoperative ectropion of the lower eyelid. In the center of the upper eyelid the caudal incision is approximately 7 mm from the eyelid margin, which is usually the position of the most caudal crease. In the deep-set eye, however, the

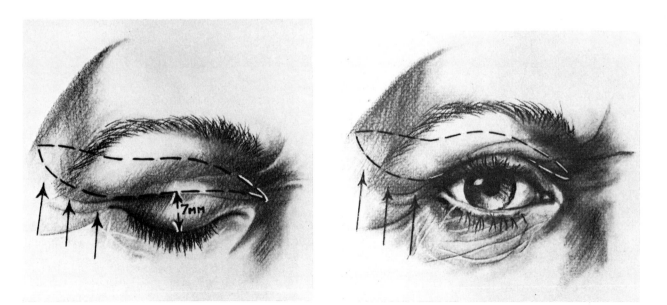

Fig. 10-1. Pattern of skin excision.

Fig. 10-2. Skin pattern in open eye.

incision must be placed more cephalad so that it will be greater than 7 mm.

Fig. 10-2 shows the appearance of the skin pattern in the open eye. Fig. 10-3 shows the lateral view and the area in which there will be skin elevation and tightening. No undermining is done to effect this elevation. Fig. 10-4 shows the usual fat removal from the medial and middle pockets. Fig. 10-5 shows the usual Castañares lower eyelid blepharoplasty, with very little skin removal and fat removal from the medial, middle, and lateral pockets. Fig. 10-6 shows the closure of the incisions using a running 5-0 nylon suture in the upper eyelid and interrupted 5-0 nylon sutures in the lower eyelid. Fig. 10-7 shows preoperative and postoperative views of a 57-year-old woman with hooding and a marked crow's-feet deformity bilaterally. The postoperative views were taken 10 weeks after surgery. We can see the lateral scar and the red line, which will eventually fade. Note how the entire crow's-feet area and upper eyelid have been improved.

Fig. 10-8 shows preoperative and postoperative views of a 61-year-old woman with marked hooding and a minimal crow's-feet deformity. The primary hooding deformity occupies the lateral two thirds of the upper eyelid area. The lower eyelids have also been done. The scars are barely visible after 9 months in the postoperative

pictures. Fig. 10-9 shows a 53-year old woman with hooding and crow's-feet improved by the described technique. The scars are not noticeable after 6 months in the postoperative pictures. Fig. 10-10 shows a 62-year-old woman. The postoperative photographs were taken 2 months after surgery, and we can see the slight red line of the scar that remains. This will fade in time. Fig. 10-11 shows preoperative and postoperative views of a 62-year-old woman with hooding and crow's-feet. This patient has a deep-set eye, and in such cases it is important that little skin is taken from the upper eyelid and that the incision is placed more than 7 mm from the lid margin. In the postoperative views we can barely notice the scar, but we can see how high the incision has been placed.

Fig. 10-12 shows preoperative and postoperative views of a 51-year-old woman with a tired, sad appearance. The aim of this procedure was to give this executive career woman a fresher appearance. *A* and *B* of Fig. 10-12 are frontal views; the combined surgery of face-lifting and central one-third chemical peeling was all done at the same time. *C* and *D* are frontal views with the patient looking serious. *D* was taken 2 months postoperatively, and the scars are barely noticeable. *E* and *F* are frontal views with the patient smiling. Note the improvement of all lines. *G* and *H* are frontal views with the patient's eyes closed *H*

Text continued on p. 76.

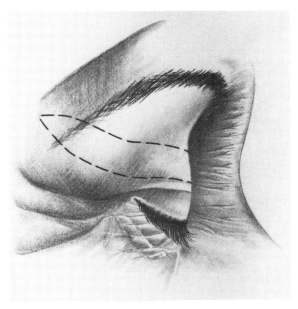

Fig. 10-3. Lateral view.

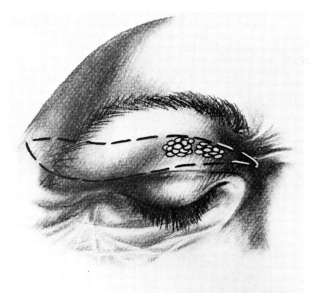

Fig. 10-4. Usual fat removal from medial and middle pockets.

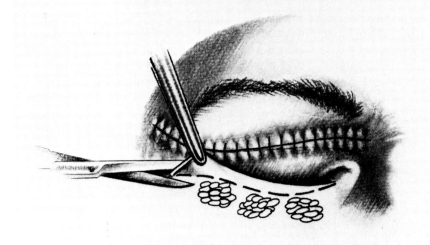

Fig. 10-5. Castañares lower eyelid blepharoplasty.

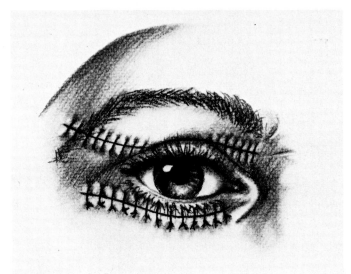

Fig. 10-6. Closure of incisions.

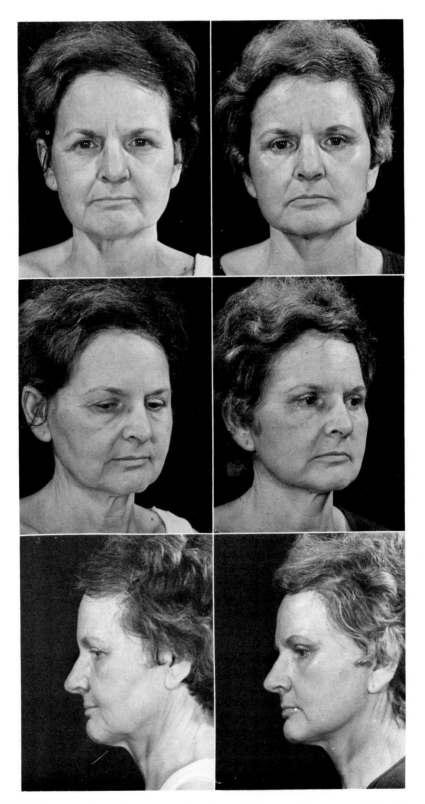

Fig. 10-7. Preoperative and postoperative views of 57-year-old woman with hooding and marked crow's-feet deformity.

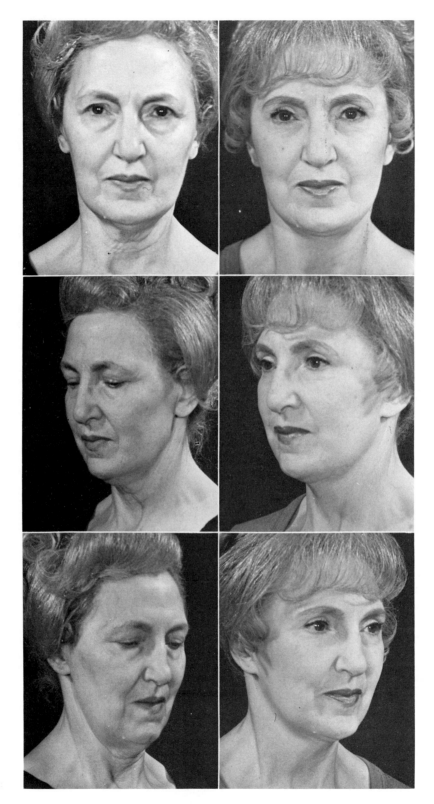

Fig. 10-8. Preoperative and postoperative views of 61-year-old woman with marked hooding and minimal crow's-feet deformity.

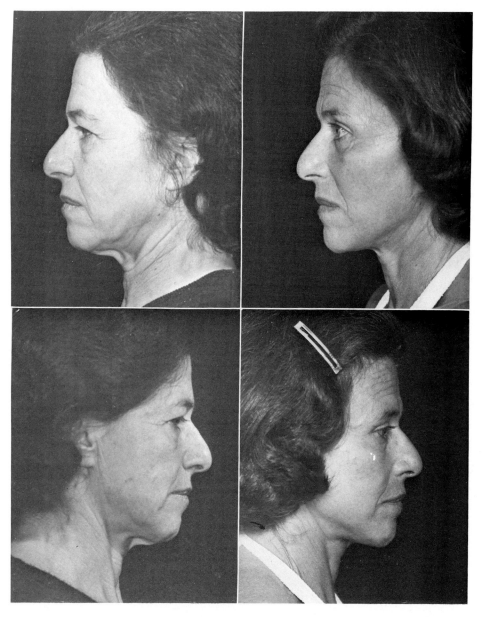

Fig. 10-9. Preoperative and postoperative views of 53-year-old woman with hooding and crow's-feet improved by described technique.

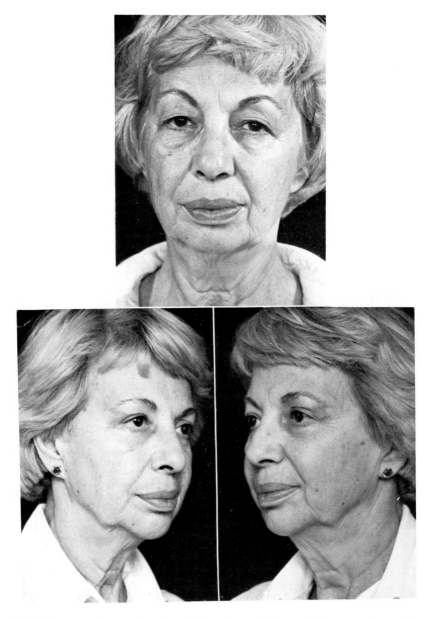

Fig. 10-10. Preoperative and postoperative views of 62-year-old woman 2 months after surgery.

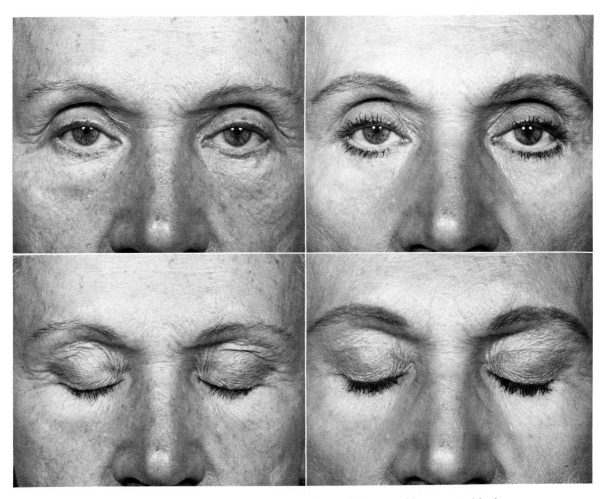

Fig. 10-11. Preoperative and postoperative views of 62-year-old woman with deep-set eye. Note how high incision has been placed.

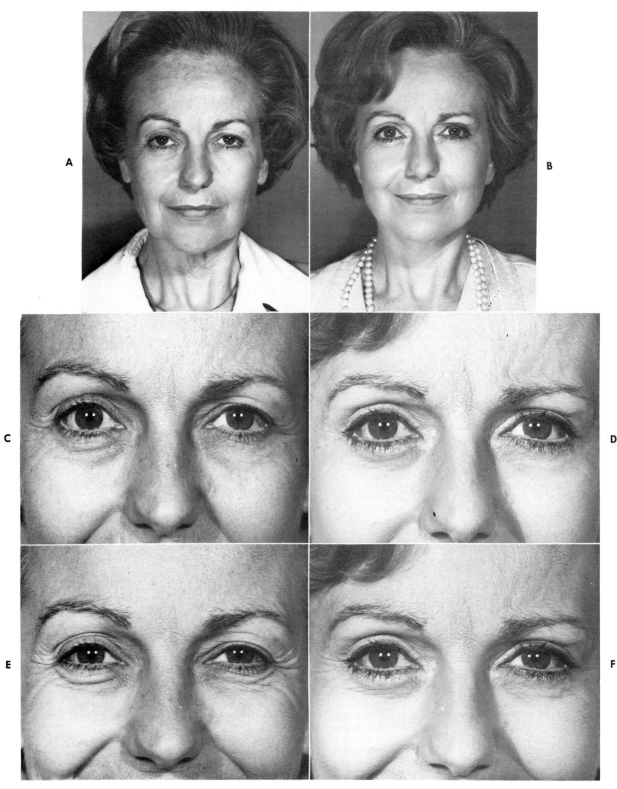

Fig. 10-12. Preoperative and postoperative views of 51-year-old woman with tired, sad appearance. **A** and **B,** Frontal views. **C** and **D,** Frontal views, patient serious. **E** and **F,** Frontal views, patient smiling.

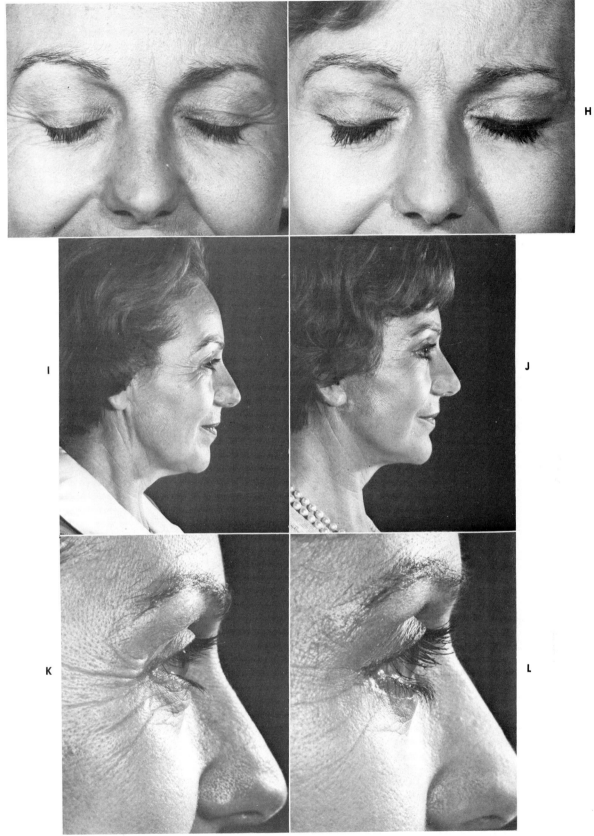

Fig. 10-12, cont'd. G and **H,** Frontal views, patient's eyes closed. **H** shows scar position. **I** and **J,** Right profile views. **K** and **L,** Right profile close-ups. *Continued.*

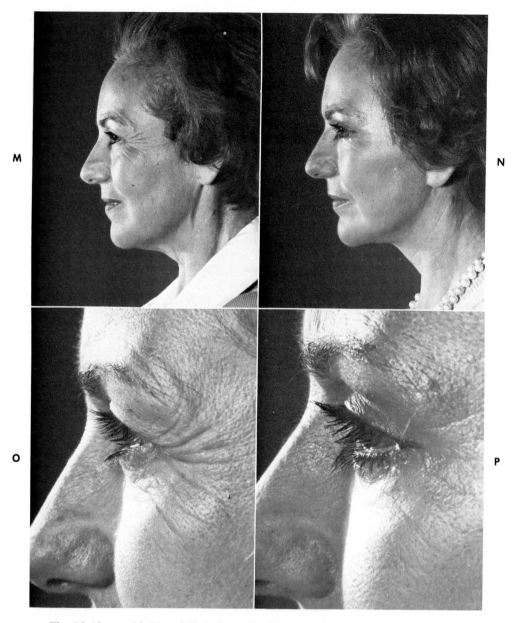

Fig. 10-12, cont'd. M and **N,** Left profile views. **O** and **P,** Left profile close-ups.

shows the scar position. *I* and *J* are right profile views, with *K* and *L* close-ups. *M* and *N* are left profile views, with *O* and *P* close-ups.

CONCLUSION

In conclusion, this technique for upper eyelid blepharoplasty and the brow lift has been used in 93 cases, with good to excellent aesthetic results. The only complication to date has been a noticeable scar in three patients, in the lateral extent of the incision. These were improved by a secondary revision. It must be emphasized that it is not the intention of this chapter to condemn the forehead lift; rather, it is to offer a more conservative approach that will give many patients a satisfactory aesthetic improvement. In some instances a chemical peel of the forehead, combined with this procedure, can offer good improvement.

REFERENCE

1. Castañares, S.: Blepharoplasty for herniated intraorbital fat, Plast. Reconstr. Surg. **8:**46, 1951.

Chapter 11

Problems and complications in the forehead lift

Bernard L. Kaye

The forehead lift, or brow lift, is a surgical procedure that is comparatively free of problems and complications. Most complications are minor and require routine management; serious complications are rare[5] (see outline below). This freedom from significant complications is a boon to both patient and surgeon.

    A. Minor problems (by-products of surgery)
        1. Early postoperative pain
        2. Numbness of the scalp
        3. Itching and paresthesias
        4. Elevation of the frontal hairline
    B. Minor complications
        1. Spot necrosis
        2. Temporary hair loss
        3. Temporary forehead lag
        4. Temporary surface depression
        5. Widened scars
        6. Minor hematoma
    C. Major complications
        1. Massive hematoma
        2. Necrosis
        3. Lagophthalmos
        4. Infection
        5. Changes in facial expression

MINOR PROBLEMS

Some minor problems that arise in the forehead lift are not complications in the usual sense, but normal by-products of the operation. These problems include early postoperative pain, numbness of the scalp, itching and paresthesias, and elevation of the frontal hairline.

Early postoperative pain

Some patients complain of pain in the frontal region, usually beginning within the first few hours after surgery and lasting up to 48 hours. It is often described as a severe frontal headache and is most likely caused by stretching of the supraorbital and supratrochlear nerves as a result of the forehead lift. It is possible to delay the onset and diminish the intensity of the pain by injecting, at the end of the surgery, a long-acting, local anesthetic such as bupivacaine (Marcaine) or etidocaine (Duranest) around the supraorbital and supratrochlear nerves where they emerge from their foramina. This type of pain does not respond well to systemic analgesics, whereas a local anesthetic nerve block is highly effective. Most patients require only a single local block postoperatively.

Numbness of the scalp

Loss of sensation in the anterior scalp region is produced when the coronal incision divides the supraorbital nerves as they cross from the forehead into the scalp. This by-product of surgery should be discussed preoperatively with prospective patients, and they should be informed that, while in the majority of cases most sensation returns, there are instances where the loss of sensation may be permanent.

Limiting the number of levels of divisions of the supraorbital nerves helps maintain sensation. This can be accomplished by interrupting the incisions directly over the courses of the supraorbi-

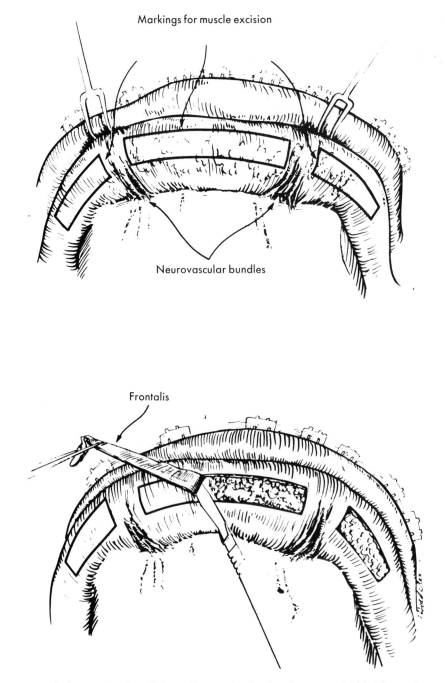

Fig. 11-1. Excision of strips of frontalis muscle, leaving intact vertical bridges of muscle over courses of supraorbital nerves. (Redrawn from Kaye, B.L.: Forehead and brow. In Rees, T.D., editor: Aesthetic plastic surgery, Philadelphia, 1980, W.B. Saunders Co.)

tal nerves when incising or excising a strip of frontalis muscle to reduce the pull of the frontalis on the raised forehead flap, leaving vertical bridges of intact muscle a few millimeters wide over these areas (Fig. 11-1).

Postoperative numbness in the midforehead region has not been a problem in my experience, even though excising the origins of the corrugators (to reduce frowning) undoubtedly divides some of the fine branches of the supratrochlear nerves, which are intertwined within the corrugator muscle fibers. This is probably due to the generous crossover between the supratrochlear and supraorbital areas of sensation in the central forehead region.

Itching and paresthesias

With the return of sensation can come itching and paresthesias, which generally appear a few weeks to several months after surgery. These symptoms rarely require treatment, especially if the patient has been informed preoperatively that these feelings are a normal part of recovery. Severe itching can cause some patients to persist in scratching their scalps, leading to ulcerations (Fig. 11-2). These normally heal after the scratching is stopped. To reduce severe itching, trimeprazine tartrate (Temaril), 2.5 mg four times a day, or cyproheptadine hydrochloride (Periactin), 4 mg four times a day, may be prescribed.

Elevation of the frontal hairline

Some elevation of the hairline is an inevitable by-product of any lifting procedure, whether it be a conventional face-lift, where the elevation occurs at the sideburns and temporal hairline, or a forehead lift, where the frontal hairline is raised. Usually less lifting is done and less skin is removed in the center of the forehead flap than at the lateral portions, restricting the degree of ele-

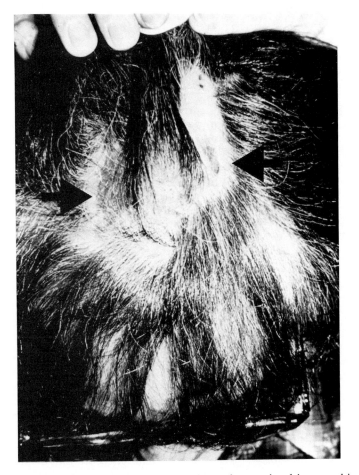

Fig. 11-2. Ulcerations produced in scalp of patient who persisted in scratching because of postoperative itching. These ultimately healed.

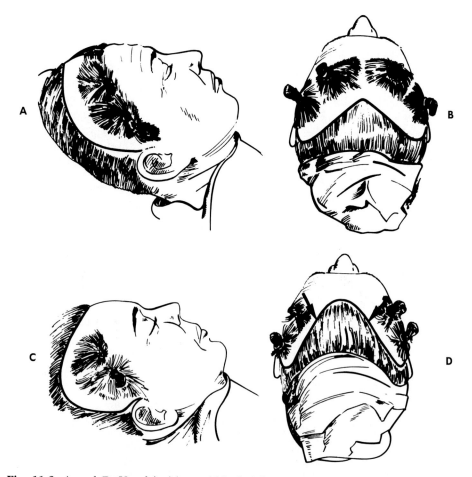

Fig. 11-3. A and **B,** Usual incision, within hairline. **C** and **D,** Alternative incision for patients with high hairlines. Central portion of incision is anterior to hairline *(between arrows).* (Redrawn from Kaye, B.L.: Forehead and brow. In Rees, T.D., editor: Aesthetic plastic surgery, Philadelphia, 1980, W.B. Saunders Co.)

vation in the central portion of the hairline, but some elevation must be accepted as a normal trade-off for having the incision made within the hair-bearing portion of the scalp.

For the patient who already has a high frontal hairline, additional frontal elevation can be avoided by making the central portion of the incision (between the temporal areas) anterior to the hairline[4,5] (Fig. 11-3). Two advantages are gained: the middle third of the frontal hairline on the forehead is not elevated by the procedure, and should a second forehead lift ever be necessary, the central frontal hairline stays at the same level.[5,6] The trade-off is a central incision line located at the edge of the hairline. This is easily covered by a slight overlap of hair, usually without a change in the hairstyle, since many patients with high frontal hairlines already wear their hair slightly lower on their foreheads.

If the incision anterior to the hairline is made with an intervening margin of hairless skin, that strip appearing above the incision line will increase the difficulty of hiding the incision line with hairstyling (Fig. 11-4). Therefore the incision should be made directly at the edge of the hairline, even sacrificing a small segment of hair-bearing skin if necessary.

MINOR COMPLICATIONS
Spot necrosis

Spot necrosis (Fig. 11-5) can occur as a result of tying the initial pilot sutures in the perpendicular pilot incisions too tightly (Fig. 11-6). These pilot incisions are made perpendicular to the coronal incision line, and the forehead flap is trimmed segmentally. The generous vascularity of the flap may cause the pilot incisions to bleed profusely, and the surgeon is naturally tempted to tie

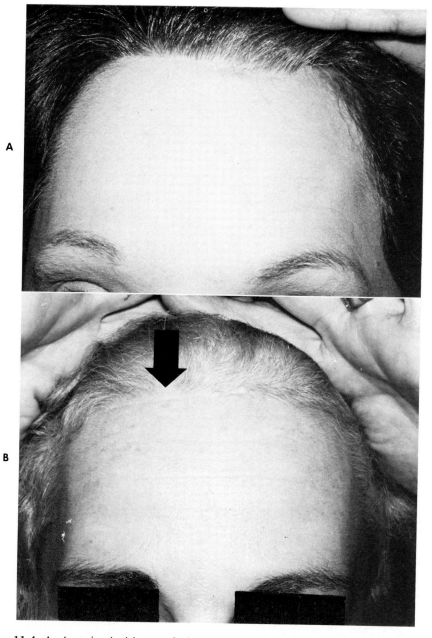

Fig. 11-4. A, Anterior incision made immediately against frontal hairline. **B,** Anterior incision made slightly anterior to frontal hairline, particularly on right. Note small visible strip of intervening forehead skin.

the pilot sutures tightly to stop the bleeding at the depths of the incisions. To avoid necrosis, these sutures should be tied more loosely than is normally done to control bleeding, or, if the pilot sutures are tied tightly, they should be removed after the remainder of the suturing is completed.[2]

If spot necrosis occurs, the crusts should be allowed to separate and secondary healing permitted to take place. It is a simple matter to excise any resulting scars later.

Temporary hair loss

Postoperatively, some of the hair follicles in the flap may enter a resting or telogen phase (possibly due to tension), which results in temporary thinning of hair anterior to the incision starting about 2 weeks after the operation. The patient may be reassured that normal growth will probably return within 2 to 3 months.

To help prevent this problem, the edges of the forehead flap should be trimmed conservatively to

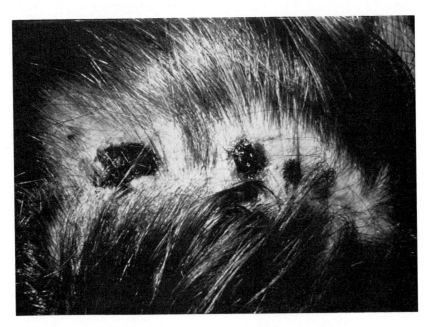

Fig. 11-5. Areas of spot necrosis in suture line.

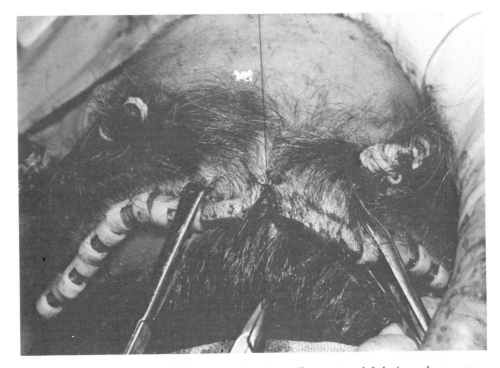

Fig. 11-6. Probable cause of spot necrosis: tying pilot suture tightly in order to stop brisk bleeding often seen at depth of pilot incision.

reduce tension. Avoiding cutting of hair follicles and excisions of the frontalis strip in the temporal hair-bearing portions of the flap will also help avoid hair loss.

Temporary forehead lag

Occasional instances of temporary forehead lag in my series may have been caused by locating the frontalis strip excisions too low in the lateral portions of the flap. To prevent frontal motor nerve injury, it is necessary to keep in mind the location and course of the frontal branches of the facial nerve when excising or incising strips of frontalis muscle in the lateral portions of the forehead flap. In this area the frontal nerve branches are located immediately superficial to the frontalis muscle.[3] They course along a path starting from a point 0.5 cm below the tragus of the ear and passing 1.5 cm superior to the lateral edge of the eyebrow (Fig. 11-7).[10] To avoid injury to the nerve (or nerves), the lateral frontalis strip excisions should be kept at least 3 cm superior to the eyebrow and orbital rim.

In cases where the forehead lift is done in conjunction with a face-lift, it is possible to reconcile the deep plane of the forehead lift with the superficial plane of the face-lift by surgically defining a fascial "web" or pedicle ("mesotemporalis" of Marino[8]) containing the frontal branches of the facial nerve. The definition of this pedicle is done by gentle, blunt dissection with a finger wrapped in a thin gauze sponge, using a peeling motion (Figs. 11-8 and 11-9). Nerve branches are stronger than connective tissue and can tolerate gentle, blunt dissection far better than the onslaught of a knife or scissors. Moreover, the frontal nerve is often made up of multiple branches instead of a single branch (Fig. 11-10), which increases the chance of recovery of motor function following apparent frontal nerve injury.

Forehead lag usually resolves itself without treatment. The recovery period is more tolerable for patients who have had a forehead lift than for those who have had only a face-lift, since there is no annoying droop of the involved eyebrow after a forehead lift.* Electromyography can be done if motion does not return in a reasonable time, but this is mainly for reassurance of patient and surgeon, since full recovery usually takes place.

---

*EDITOR'S NOTE: Some patients like the nerve-injured side better than the intact side, because it does not wrinkle. (B.L.K.)

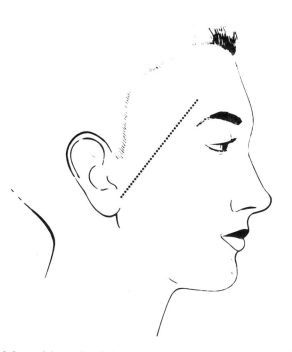

Fig. 11-7. Course of frontal branch of facial nerve, starting 0.5 cm inferior to tragus and passing 1.5 cm superior to lateral end of eyebrow. (Based on data from Pitanguy, I., and Silveira Ramos, A.: The frontal branch of the facial nerve: the importance of its variations in face lifting, Plast. Reconstr. Surg. **38**:352, 1966.)

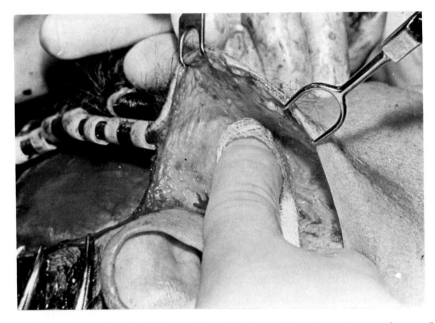

Fig. 11-8. Combined forehead lift and face-lift. Deep dissection above and superficial dissection below was reconciled by creation of pedicle or "web" containing branches of frontal nerve. Dissection was with gauze-wrapped finger. (From Kaye, B.L.: The forehead lift: a useful adjunct to face lift and blepharoplasty, Plast. Reconstr. Surg. **60**:161, 1977.)

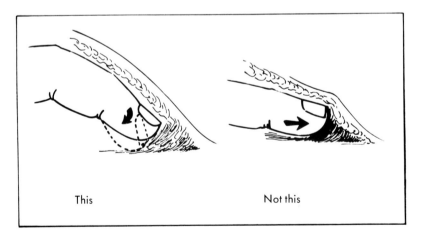

This   Not this

Fig. 11-9. Dissection should be with peeling motion *(left)* rather than pushing motion *(right)*. (Redrawn from Kaye, B.L.: Forehead and brow. In Rees, T.D., editor: Aesthetic plastic surgery, Philadelphia, 1980, W.B. Saunders Co.)

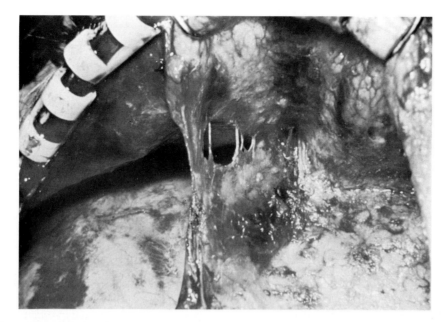

Fig. 11-10. Case in which connective tissue of pedicle parted with blunt dissection, leaving intact multiple branches of frontal nerve. (Patient had full forehead motion immediately postoperatively.)

Temporary surface depression

External depressions in forehead contour due to excision of corrugator origins or strips of frontalis muscle are extremely rare despite initial concern.[9] One of my patients developed a shallow depression approximately 1 cm in diameter in the mid–left forehead several weeks after surgery (Fig. 11-11, *A*). It disappeared a few months later without treatment (Fig. 11-11, *B*).

Glabellar depressions caused by corrugator resections can be avoided by limiting the resections to about 0.5 cm of the origins of the corrugators.[7]

Widened scars

Forehead scars may occasionally widen with the passage of time. In one instance where significant spreading of the scar did occur, the patient exhibited widened scars elsewhere on her body and hyperextensibility of the joints (Fig. 11-12), which suggested the possibility that the cause of the problem could have been a forme fruste of Ehlers-Danlos syndrome.

My neurosurgical colleagues recommend closing the forehead with a double-layered repair in which the galea is repaired as a separate layer and the skin and subcutaneous tissue are then closed with sutures or staples to prevent wide scars. I have started using such a double-layered closure but have not yet determined its efficacy.

Minor hematoma

The relative avascularity of the plane of dissection for the forehead lift reduces the incidence of hematomas. Treatment of the rare minor hematomas that may occur (Fig. 11-13) is simple. The fluid is aspirated every few days, and a light compression bandage is applied overnight. The procedure is repeated until the fluid ceases to accumulate. Instead of aspiration, Stark[11] suggests daily intradermal injections of hyaluronidase over (rather than into) the accumulation of fluid to encourage venous and lymphatic dispersion of the fluid.

MAJOR COMPLICATIONS
Massive hematoma

Fortunately, massive hematoma is a rare complication. The onset is early, during the first few hours postoperatively. Its single outstanding symptom is unremitting, excruciating pain that is unresponsive to all usual methods of treatment. The pain is not reduced by systemic analgesics, even when administered intravenously, and it is even refractory to supraorbital and supratrochlear nerve blocks (Fig. 11-14, *A*). The forehead is swollen, but to a lesser extent than might be expected given the marked severity of the pain. The swelling is limited by the inelasticity of the forehead flap. This inextensibility allows intense pres-

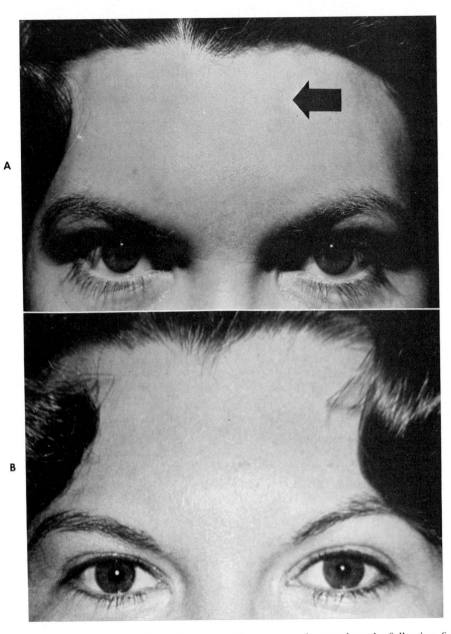

Fig. 11-11. A, Temporary 1 cm depression that appeared several weeks following forehead lift. (This is difficult to demonstrate in photograph.) **B,** Spontaneous disappearance of depression several months later.

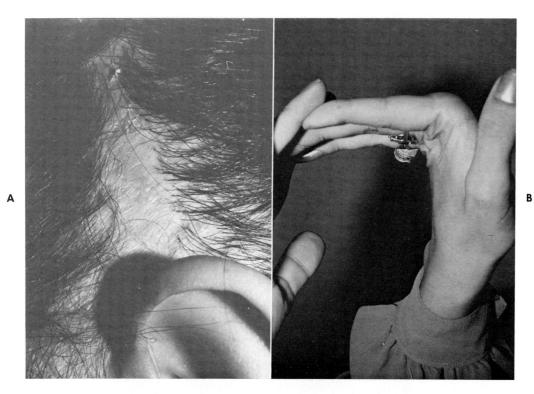

Fig. 11-12. A, Widened temporal portion of forehead lift scar. **B,** Same patient showing hyperextensibility of joints, suggesting possible forme fruste of Ehlers-Danlos syndrome.

sure to build up under the forehead flap thus causing the excruciating pain. Interference with circulation poses a grave threat to the viability of the flap.

Relief can be obtained only by immediate decompression of the hematoma. This is done easily and rapidly by opening the suture line and releasing the great pressure that has built up under the flap. It is necessary to open the suture line only as much as is required to remove any clots and to identify and tie off the bleeding vessels; even a partial opening of the suture line is sufficient to release the pressure and provide immediate relief from pain (Fig. 11-14, *B* and *C*). Prompt treatment can ensure uneventful healing without sequelae.

Necrosis

Three cases of necrosis have been reported by Viñas et al.[12] One of these occurred in a hypertensive patient who suffered a slough of the scalp with a good deal of resulting alopecia. This complication was due to a hematoma that had gone undetected for several days. Another patient developed an infection that produced a small, spontaneously healing slough with transient alopecia. A third patient experienced a slough in the vicinity of an old traumatic scar, but this healed quickly and left only an area of depigmentation. Old scars do not necessarily pose a threat to the circulation of the forehead flap. One of my patients had a 3 cm upper central forehead scar secondary to previous excision of a lesion and experienced no difficulty after undergoing a brow lift. In addition, at least two patients in my series who had previously undergone direct eyebrow lifts by means of skin excision suffered no ill effects to flap circulation subsequent to forehead lifts.

Because of the danger of a tight compression bandage causing necrosis, neither elastic tape nor elastic bandages should be employed for forehead lifts. Instead, a lightly applied, well-padded Kling bandage is recommended.

Lagophthalmos

A brow lift always reduces the apparent amount of excess upper eyelid skin in patients with both excess upper lid overhang and ptosis of

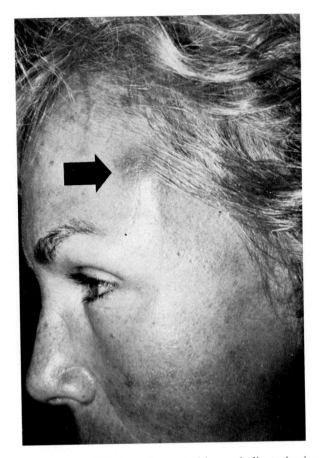

Fig. 11-13. Minor hematoma. This is easily treated by periodic aspiration until it disappears.

the forehead and brows. For this reason, when both a brow lift and an upper lid blepharoplasty are to be done during the same operation, it is usually preferable to do the brow lift first. After the brow lift the leftover excess upper lid skin can be safely determined and excised. In many instances the brow left alone will correct both problems and obviate the need for an upper lid skin excision.

Preoperative evaluation must be done with particular care in candidates for a forehead lift who have previously undergone an upper lid blepharoplasty. As part of the preoperative evaluation, the surgeon should hold up the forehead in the anticipated new position and check to make sure that the patient's eyes will still close adequately without forcing. (A good Bell's phenomenon is a favorable asset.) A second evaluation should be performed immediately before the actual surgery, after the upper lids have relaxed with the patient under sedation or general anesthesia. If, after relaxation, the upper lids are

raised enough to produce significant corneal exposure, the surgeon should consider abandoning the forehead lift or limiting the scalp excision to the most lateral parts of the flap.[5]

Infection

The excellent vascularity of the forehead flap probably explains the very low incidence of infection following forehead lifts. Additional precautions to reduce the chance of infection are the routine preoperative shampooing of the hair with antibacterial soaps such as chlorhexidine gluconate (Hibiclens), povidone iodine (Betadine Surgical Scrub), or hexachlorophene detergent cleanser (pHisoHex) and preventive antibiotics (which I employ empirically) begun preoperatively or intraoperatively and continued briefly postoperatively.

Changes in facial expression

The creation of too much tension in the flap, either in part or in whole, can produce changes in

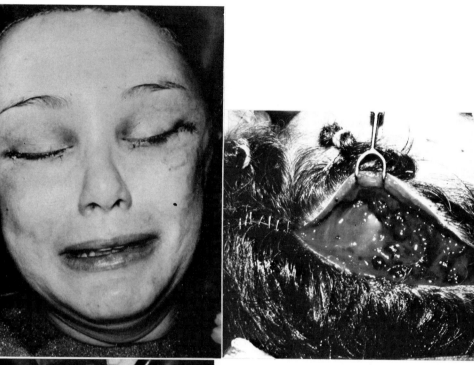

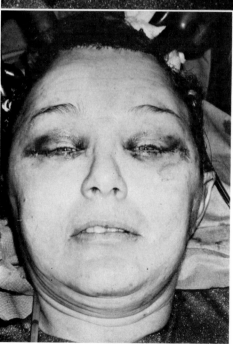

Fig. 11-14. A, Major hematoma appearing early in postoperative period. Patient is expressing excruciating pain that is refractory to treatment. **B,** Decompression of hematoma and removal of clots. **C,** Patient has immediate relief after decompression.

expression. Eyebrows that have been raised too high laterally can cause the patient to look angry. Excessive elevation of the medial portions of the eyebrow, which results in eyebrows that slant downward from medial to lateral, produces a look of sadness. If the eyebrows are raised too high centrally or totally, there will be a surprised or startled expression.[1]

The forehead lift is less likely to cause altered facial expression than is the direct eyebrow lift because the forehead and brows can be elevated as a unit. The brows are raised naturally and maintain normal facial expression. Correction of preexisting facial expression problems is also possible. A slight extra elevation of the central portion of the flap will alter a constant angry expression, and raising the lateral part of the flap will correct a sad look.

Although some surgeons have tried to develop mathematical guides for determining the amount of skin to be excised when trimming the flap to raise the eyebrows, I believe the best approach is one that incorporates an intuitive aesthetic sense, good surgical judgment, and a conservative attitude toward trimming. Usually 1 cm, or less, of scalp is excised at the center of the flap, and not more than 2 cm is excised laterally.

CONCLUSIONS

The forehead lift is a procedure that is relatively free of significant problems and complications. The minor problems that might occur, such as early postoperative pain, numbness, itching, and minor hematomas, are easily managed and should not prevent a final successful outcome. Careful preoperative preparation and sound intraoperative aesthetic and surgical judgment can prevent lagophthalmos and changes in facial expression. Infection may be avoided by following routine antibacterial procedures. Necrosis can be prevented by avoiding pressure bandages, treating massive hematomas promptly, and exercising caution when elevating a flap with old scars.

The most important serious major complication is the massive hematoma. This rare problem is easily identified by its single unmistakable symptom of excruciating pain, which is refractory to treatment. Prompt decompression provides immediate relief from pain and permits normal, uneventful healing.

REFERENCES

1. Connell, B.F: Personal communication, 1980.
2. Connell, B.F.: Personal communication, 1981.
3. Correia, P. de C., and Zani, R.: Surgical anatomy of the facial nerve as related to ancillary operations in rhytidoplasty, Plast. Reconstr. Surg. **52**:549, 1973.
4. Kaye, B.L.: The forehead lift: a useful adjunct to face lift and blepharoplasty, Plast. Reconstr. Surg. **60**:161, 1977.
5. Kaye, B.L.: Forehead and brow. In Rees, T.D., editor: Aesthetic plastic surgery, Philadelphia, 1980, W.B. Saunders Co.
6. Kaye B.L.: The forehead lift. In Goldwyn, R.M., editor: Long-term results in plastic and reconstructive surgery, Boston, 1980, Little, Brown & Co.
7. Kaye, B.L.: Discussion of Pitanguy, I.: Indications for and treatment of frontal and glabellar wrinkles in an analysis of 3,404 consecutive cases of rhytidectomy, Plast. Reconstr. Surg. **67**:167, 1981.
8. Marino, H.: The surgery of facial expression. In Hueston, J.T., editor: Transactions of the Fifth International Congress of Plastic and Reconstructive Surgeons, Melbourne, 1971, Butterworths Pty., Ltd.
9. Pitanguy, I.: Indications for and treatment of frontal and glabellar wrinkles in an analysis of 3,404 consecutive cases of rhytidectomy, Plast. Reconstr. Surg. **67**:157, 1981.
10. Pitanguy, I., and Silveira Ramos, A.: The frontal branch of the facial nerve: the importance of its variations in face lifting, Plast. Reconstr. Surg. **38**:352, 1966.
11. Stark, R.B.: Aesthetic plastic surgery, Boston, 1980, Little, Brown, & Co., p. 140.
12. Viñas, J.C., Caviglia, C., and Cortinas, J.L.: Forehead rhytidoplasty and brow lifting, Plast. Reconstr. Surg. **57**:445, 1976.

Chapter 12

Excision of the buccal fat pad to refine the obese midface

Fernando Ortiz Monasterio
Alvaro Olmedo

The volume of the face is produced by the three-dimensional characteristics of the skeleton, the facial and masticatory musculature, the skin and subcutaneous fat, and the salivary glands. In the midface, some extra volume is provided by the buccal fat pad.

Excision of the fat pad was brought to our attention by Drs. D. Kipp and F. Dunton[5] from Dallas many years ago. They combined this procedure with rhytidectomy to decrease the volume of the cheeks and refine the contour of the obese midface. The buccal fat pad had been used as a flap to close fistulas of the maxillary sinus, but no references could be found involving its surgical excision for aesthetic purposes. During the last 10 years we have removed buccal fat pads from a large number of patients to reduce the fullness of the midface and to enhance the prominence of the malar areas both in young and in older people. This chapter is a report of our experience with this procedure.

ANATOMY AND PHYSIOLOGY

The buccal fat pad was first described in 1732 by Heister[4] and later by Bichat in 1801 in rather vague terms as a mass of fatty tissue located under the masseter muscle and having its greatest volume behind the buccinator muscle. Bichat[1] published his book on anatomy in 1829, and the term *fat pad of Bichat* was generally adopted.

In 1884 Ranke[7] pointed out that this mass of fat persisted during severe conditions of emaciation, even when all the subcutaneous fat had disappeared. He also suggested its possible relation

with suckling because of its large volume in infants. Recent studies by Paturet,[6] Couly and Hureau,[3] and Cadenat and Bouyssou[2] demonstrated the role of the buccal fat pad as part of a complex gliding mechanism of the masticatory muscles that separates the muscles from each other, from the surrounding fascia, and from the ascending ramus of the mandible. The facial fat pad is only the anterior extension of this syssarcosis. It is located immediately under the buccinator and in front of the masseter muscles. It is well encapsulated in its own compartment, separated from the two posterior pads that extend into the temporal and pterygoid spaces (Figs. 12-1 and 12-2).

Loss of facial fat is a sign of aging. This characteristic of advanced age can also be observed in some persons in their early sixties. This change is usually observed in individuals with thin faces.

The permanence of Bichat's fat pad throughout life has been documented by anatomical studies. It is our impression that persons with fat faces in which the buccal fat pad plays a role maintain the round facial shape all their lives. To confirm this impression, we have examined the photographic records of 46 persons—10 men and 36 women—who had round faces with prominent cheeks. The characteristic round face was not associated in any of them with general obesity, although some of them were slightly overweight. The ages of this group are shown in Table 12-1.

The photographic records of all of these persons were examined. Only those having adequate pictorial documentation throughout all their lives were included in this study. Representative pho-

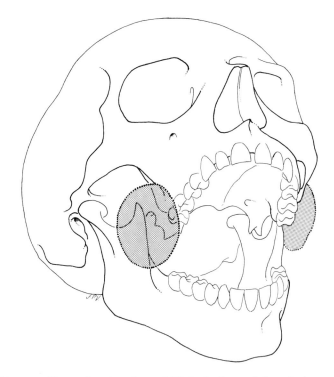

Fig. 12-1. Diagram illustrating location of Bichat's fat pad in relation to mouth and mandible.

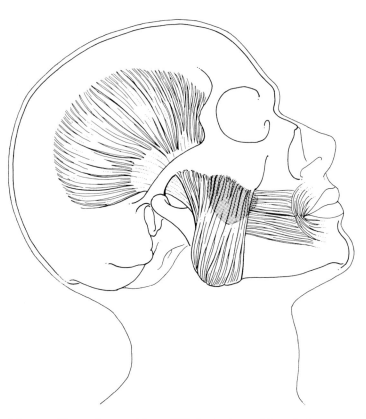

Fig. 12-2. Diagram illustrating position of Bichat's fat pad in relation to muscles. It is located under buccinator and between masses of masseter, temporalis, and pterygoid muscles and is anterior extension of gliding mechanism for masticatory muscles.

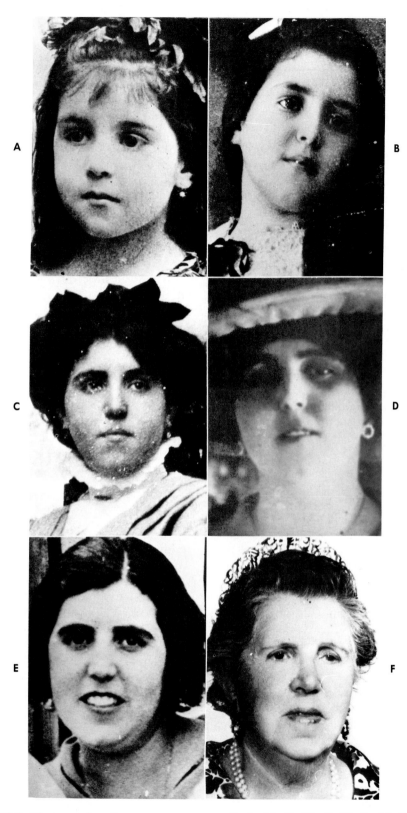

Fig. 12-3. Photographs of same person at age 9, **A,** 13, **B,** 22, **C,** 30, **D,** 50, **E,** and 87, **F.**

Table 12-1. Obese cheeks: retrospective photographic study

Age	Number of persons examined
60 to 70	8
71 to 75	14
76 to 80	15
81 to 85	7
86 to 90	2
TOTAL	46

Table 12-2. Obese cheeks: retrospective photographic study of persistence of the buccal fat pad in 46 persons

Age	Fat pad persisted	Fat pad absorbed
60 to 70	8	—
71 to 75	14	—
76 to 80	13	2
81 to 85	5	2
86 to 90	1	1
TOTAL	41	5

tographs from every decade were selected for analysis (Fig. 12-3).

The study revealed that the round face persisted in the entire group through the seventh decade of life (between 60 and 70 years of age). Two individuals showed a decrease of facial fat in the eighth decade, two in the ninth decade, and one in the tenth decade (Tables 12-1 and 12-2).

From these studies as well as our own observation that the buccal fat pad plays only a limited role in maintaining facial volume, we can assume that its resection will not prematurely produce the changes in facial contour associated with old age.

SURGICAL TECHNIQUES

The buccal fat pad is easily approached through the mouth or through the cheek. For the oral approach, an incision is made about 0.5 cm lateral to the upper sulcus. The incision begins at the level of the first premolar and extends for 2 cm posteriorly, parallel with the buccal sulcus (Fig. 12-4). Several small vessels crossing the incision line transversely may be coagulated if necessary. The thin fibrous layer covering the deep structures is penetrated by blunt dissection. The scissors are introduced in the direction of the temporomandibular joint, and the buccal fat is readily exposed. It can be easily differentiated from the subcutaneous fat of the cheek by its lighter color and its thin capsule, which is similar to a capsule surrounding a well-demarcated lipoma.

By gentle traction the whole fat pad is exteriorized (Fig. 12-5). Minimal blunt dissection is necessary to free the sac from its pedicle. A small vessel is sometimes encountered and may be coagulated at this time. The procedure is repeated on the opposite side. Each cavity is packed with a wet sponge that is removed at the end of the operation or in the recovery room. No sutures are used. Local anesthesia may be used for this procedure, although infiltration with 1:200,000 epi-

nephrine solution is convenient when the operation is done with the patient under general anesthesia.

When the procedure is associated with a facelift, we prefer to approach the fat pad through the cheek. Once the skin flaps have been elevated and hemostasis has been achieved the fascia is opened through a horizontal incision beginning on front of the anterior edge of the masseter muscle, about 1 cm above the level of the angle of the mouth. The fibers of the buccinator muscle are carefully separated by blunt dissection, and the buccal fat pad is found immediately under the muscle (Fig. 12-6). By gentle traction the pad is exteriorized and removed. The small vessels are coagulated. No sutures are used to close the fascia.

RESULTS

In our series of 97 patients in whom this procedure was performed, in 39 cases in combination with a rhytidectomy, the results were evaluated by frontal, lateral, and three-quarter photographs of the face taken preoperatively and postoperatively. In all of these patients a decrease in volume of the cheeks was obtained, producing a depression under the malar prominence. The correction was considered minimal to moderate by the patients and by us. Striking changes were rare, but all patients agreed that excision of the fat pad had improved the facial contour by providing an impression of angularity (Figs. 12-7 to 12-9).

Most patients had moderate trismus postoperatively, with minimal limitation in opening their mouths. This symptom disappeared in a few days without treatment.

COMPLICATIONS

Hematomas formed in the cavity during the immediate postoperative period when the intraoral approach was used. Four such patients re-

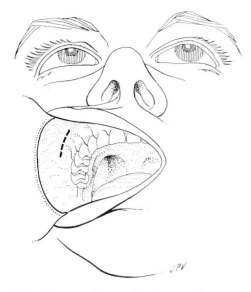

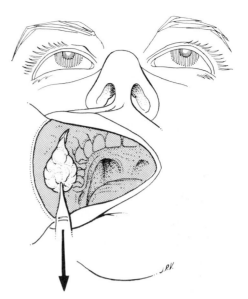

Fig. 12-4. Diagram illustrating intraoral approach to buccal fat pad. Dotted line shows incision slightly lateral to upper sulcus, extending posteriorly 2 cm from level of first premolar.

Fig. 12-5. Blunt dissection allows exposure of well-demarcated fat pad. It is easily exteriorized by gentle traction.

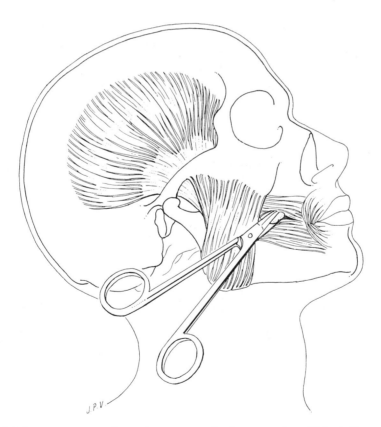

Fig. 12-6. Diagram representing subcutaneous cheek approach to Bichat's fat pad. Once rhytidectomy skin flap has been elevated, pad is exposed by blunt dissection through fibers of buccinator muscle medially to anterior border of masseter muscle.

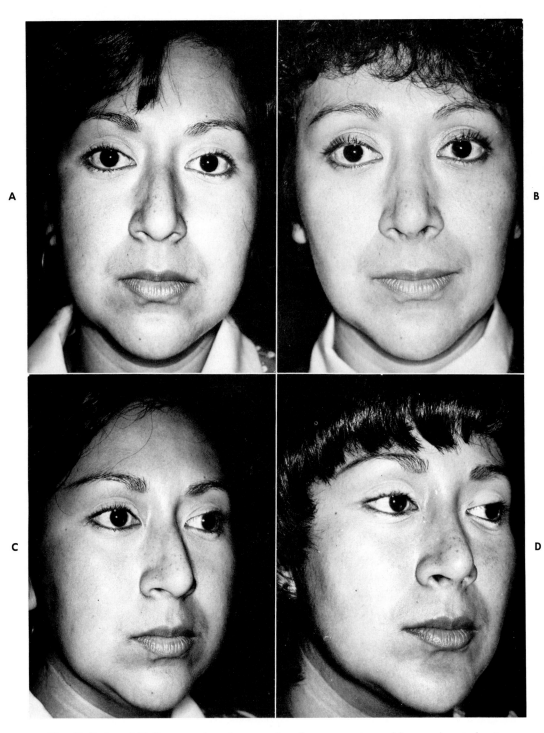

Fig. 12-7. A and **C,** Preoperative photographs of young patient with prominent cheeks. **B** and **D,** Postoperative photographs after removal of buccal fat pad through intraoral approach.

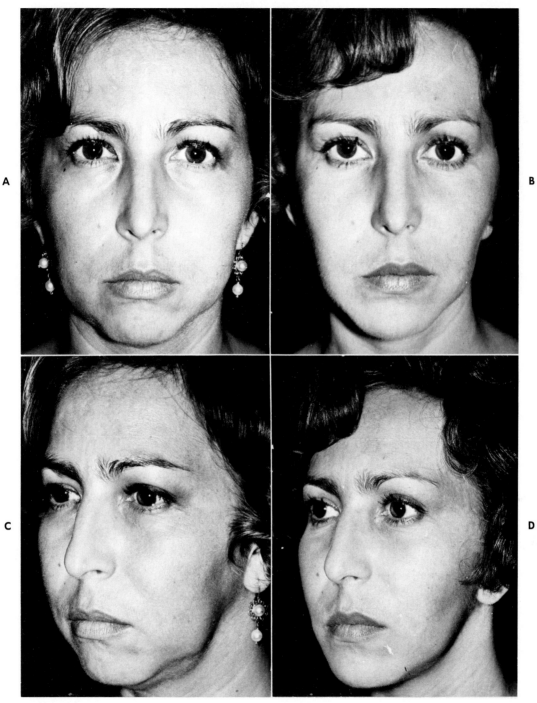

Fig. 12-8. A and **C,** Preoperative photographs of patient with prominent cheeks. **B** and **D,** Postoperative photographs of same patient after rhytidectomy and removal of buccal fat pad.

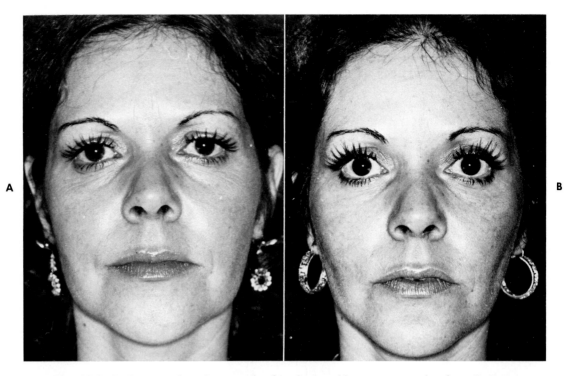

Fig. 12-9. A, Preoperative photograph of patient seeking more angular face. **B,** Postoperative photograph after rhytidectomy and removal of fat pad.

quired drainage and packing at the bedside. Two patients had hematomas that were detected on the third postoperative day. Both of these were drained in the office, and one of them developed an abscess requiring subsequent drainage and antibiotics. No permanent sequelae resulted. In these two patients the fat pads were also removed through the intraoral route. There were no hematomas when the subcutaneous rhytidectomy–cheek approach was used.

Three patients had trismus producing moderate limitation of movement of the mandible, accompanied by some pain. In each of these the symptom followed the formation of a hematoma that required postoperative draining. Local application of heat and mild physiotherapy were used in these patients for a few weeks, and there was complete recovery.

PREVENTION OF HEMATOMAS

Meticulous hemostasis is necessary to prevent postoperative bleeding. All of the hematomas in our series occurred when the intraoral route was used and the field of vision was limited. We now coagulate all the visible vessels as the operation progresses and clamp the pedicle before excising the fat pad. As an added precaution, we pack the cavity with gauze for 1 hour and use no sutures in the oral mucosa. No complications have occurred since we adopted these measures.

REFERENCES

1. Bichat, X.: Anatomie descriptive, Paris, 1829, Gabon-Chaude.
2. Cadenat, H., and Bouyssou, M.: Conditions anatomiques des cellulites de la boule de Bichat, Actual. Odontostomatol. **20:**421, 1952.
3. Couly, G., and Hureau, J.: Les espaces de glissement celluloadipeux de l'appareil manducateur, Arch. Anat. Pathol. **23:**4, 1975.
4. Heister, L.: "Compendium anatomicum" Nuremberg 732. Translated to French in Anatomie, nouv. ed., Paris, 1753, Vincent.
5. Kipp, D., and Dunton, F.: Personal communication.
6. Paturet: Traite d'anatomie humaine, Paris, 1951, Masson.
7. Ranke, F.: Ein Sangpolster der menschlichen Backe, Wirchows Arch. Pathol. Anat. **43:**527, 1884.

Chapter 13

Repair of aging in the male patient

Michael M. Gurdin

Surgery for the repair of the aging face in the male patient was not common prior to 1950. Although male entertainers had requested this work, it was unusual. In the decade of the 1950s and with the advent of commercial television, these requests increased. The drummer at the back of the band saw *his* baggy eyelids, *his* lop ears, or *his* crooked nose and sought relief through plastic surgery.

In the 1960s politicians found television to be the most effective means of reaching the people, and the press began discussing "makeup" used by these politicians before they appeared on television. It was only a short step from makeup and wearing hairpieces to the more convenient and lasting surgical repair.

AGING DEFECTS

When a woman consults a surgeon regarding aging, she seeks a more youthful appearance. When a man consults a surgeon regarding aging, generally he seeks relief from one or more defects incidental to aging, but he is not compulsive about looking younger. He wants relief from these (to him) defects. The following are some of the defects that I have encountered and treated:

1. Male pattern baldness
2. Marked forehead wrinkling
3. Deep vertical frown lines over the central forehead between the eyebrows
4. Drooping eyebrows
5. Redundant skin of the eyelids
6. Herniated fat of the eyelids (baggy eyelids)
7. Crow's-feet lateral to the eyes
8. Prominent alar-facial folds
9. Submental and cervical skin and fat redundancy ("turkey gobbler neck")
10. Redundancy (jowls) over the mandible
11. Drooping nasal tip

In some cases the patient is best served by a face-lift done in combination with one or more of the special ancillary procedures. In other instances a face-lift is contraindicated because of lack of hair, the patient's physical condition, age, socioeconomic status, or because face-lifting would not correct the defect that is distressing the patient.

Repair of the aging face in the male patient is different from that in the female patient. The male patient usually has more redundant skin and subcutaneous fat and more relaxed muscles of the face and neck. He also has less hair to hide the scars of surgery. The skin of the male patient is thicker, and both the beard pattern and the existence or threat of male pattern baldness must be respected. The male patient heals with more noticeable scars. He does not accept these readily and is not able to hide them with abundant hair or cover them with makeup.

During the past few years there have been numerous scientific publications on face-lifting techniques.* These have emphasized the forehead lift for wrinkling of the forehead, drooping eyebrows, and glabellar frown lines; the superficial musculoaponeurotic undermining with tightening techniques for correction of the central portion of the face; and submental lipectomy and platysma muscle operations for the lower face and neck.

I shall not attempt to duplicate these reports but will limit my remarks to personal experiences of what I do and do not do and why.

The ideal rhytidectomy incision in the male patient should:

1. Allow wide exposure of the subcutaneous tissues for surgical repair, shifting of tissues, lipectomy, and careful hemostasis

---

*References 2, 4-7, 9-12, 14.

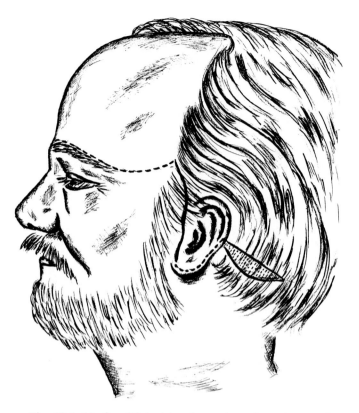

Fig. 13-1. My face-lift incision for male patients (see text).

2. Allow ample excision of redundant skin without distorting the hairline or beard pattern
3. Leave minimal or no visible scars

These ideals are sometimes difficult to attain. Variations and compromise are often necessary.

Fig. 13-1 illustrates my face-lift incision for the male patient. This incision is designed to respect male pattern baldness, the hair pattern, and the beard pattern. In the forehead region the incision can be extended into the suprabrow region, or a direct excision of the redundant forehead skin through a horizontal crease can be done. It provides good exposure of the middle of the face and, with the addition of a submental incision, exposure of the platysma muscle for defatting and operative procedures. It also retains adequate hairless skin anterior to the ear, and the scar is hidden by the sideburn. With this incision the lift can be more vertical than posterior. This is often desirable in men. Adequate skin can be excised without distorting the temporal hair pattern by excising a horizontal wedge of sideburn below the temporal hair. This excision merely elevates the

beard pattern and leaves enough sideburn to hide the vertical scar in front of the ear. It also allows the preservation of hairless skin in front of the ear. Posteriorly the scar is well hidden behind the ear and in the occipital scalp.

Fig. 13-2 illustrates another type of male face-lift incision. I do not recommend this incision in male patients because:

1. It will alter the temporal hair area and remove hair-bearing scalp. This can be an early site for male pattern baldness.
2. It removes the hairless skin anterior to the ear and may alter the beard pattern.
3. It gives a more posterior and less vertical lift.
4. It leaves a visible scar below the occipital hair scalp.
5. If it is carried anterior to the sideburn or temporal hair, a visible scar will remain.

FOREHEAD WRINKLES AND FROWN LINES

Male pattern baldness or the possibility of it developing makes the coronal scalp approach haz-

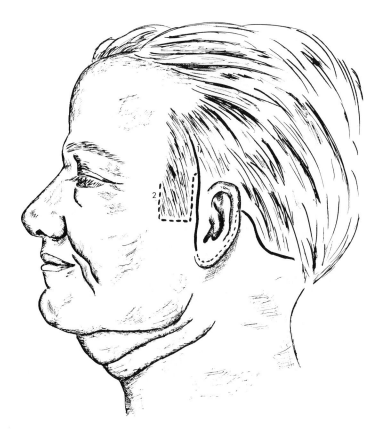

Fig. 13-2. Another male face-lift incision, which I do not advocate (see text).

ardous in the male patient, and I do not recommend it.*

My face-lift incision (Fig. 13-1) allows extension into either the suprabrow area or a vertical crease in the forehead (Fig. 13-3). These incisions allow excision of skin, wide undermining of the forehead skin, and resection of the frontalis muscle above and of the procerus and corrugator muscles in the glabella region. This operation may be done separately or in combination with a rhytidectomy. Placement of scars and wound closure must be meticulous, or residual scars will remain (Fig. 13-4).

NECK REPAIR

In the neck region a submental incision can be added if submental lipectomy and platysma muscle surgery are to be done. The submental lipectomy done at the time of the rhytidectomy has been described in numerous publications,[2,6,9] as

has the submental lipectomy alone.[1,3,7,8,13] Fig. 13-5 shows a method used by me and published[7] but later abandoned because of prominent and visible scarring on the front of the neck. In my experience, a better method has been the "H" or "I" excision, or the "Z" excision without crossing the upper crease at the level of the thyroid cartilage (Figs. 13-6 and 13-7).

PROBLEMS

In addition to male pattern baldness and the beard pattern that should be preserved, male patients have more skin, more subcutaneous fat, and more skin of poor quality. In the patient shown in Fig. 13-8, the result of surgery was not satisfactory. The patient should not have been operated on for cosmetic reasons.

COMPLICATIONS

Male patients have more complications, and they are more severe. The most common complication is postoperative bleeding. Scarring in the male patient's skin is apt to be heavier and more apparent than that in the female patient. Ectro-

*EDITOR'S NOTE: In my opinion, it is less hazardous in middle-aged or older men with adequate hair coverage, because by that time hair loss patterns have stabilized. (B.L.K.)

Text continued on p. 109.

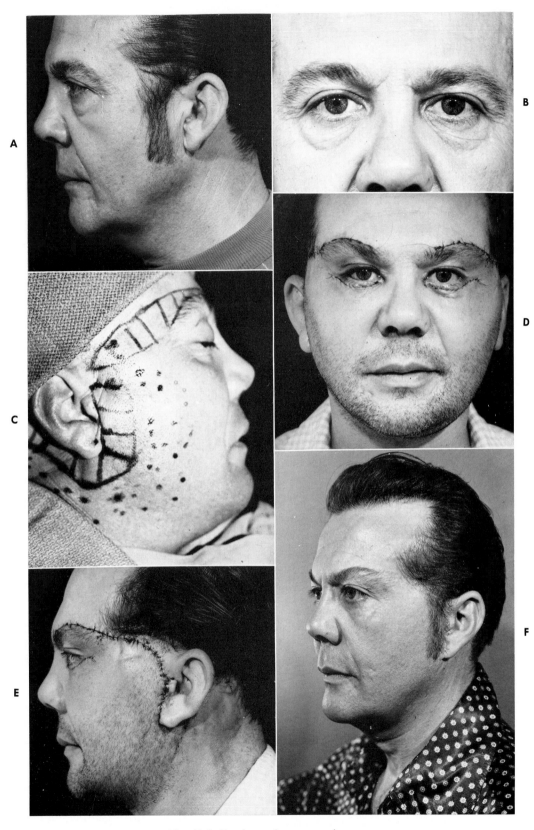

Fig. 13-3. For legend see opposite page.

Fig. 13-3. A, Preoperative profile showing drooping brows, jowls, and submental droop. **B,** Close-up of eyelid region showing drooping eyebrows and fat pads, lower eyelids. **C,** Rhytidectomy incision outlined showing amount of skin to be excised. **D,** Three days postoperative full-face view showing placement of incisions and beard pattern. **E,** Three days postoperative profile showing placement of incisions and beard pattern. **F,** Three months postoperative photograph showing absence of visible scars. NOTE: Fullness of lower neck is old tracheostomy scar.

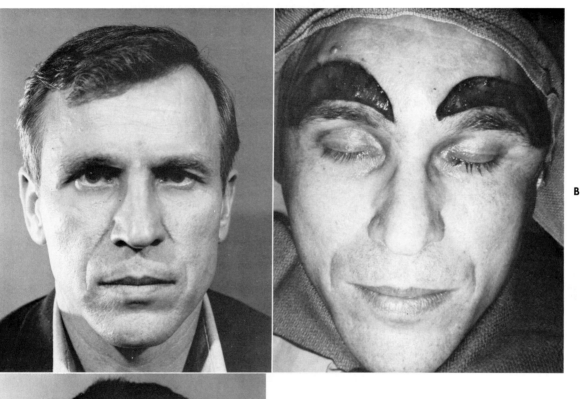

A

B

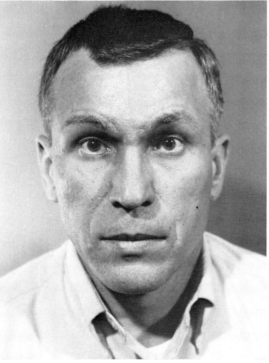

C

Fig. 13-4. A, Preoperative photograph of patient with drooping eyebrows. High forehead precludes coronal incision. **B,** Operative excision showing amount of skin removed and access to frown muscles as well as elevation of eyebrows. **C,** One month postoperative photograph showing visible scars due to poor placement of incisions. Scar revision was required in this patient.

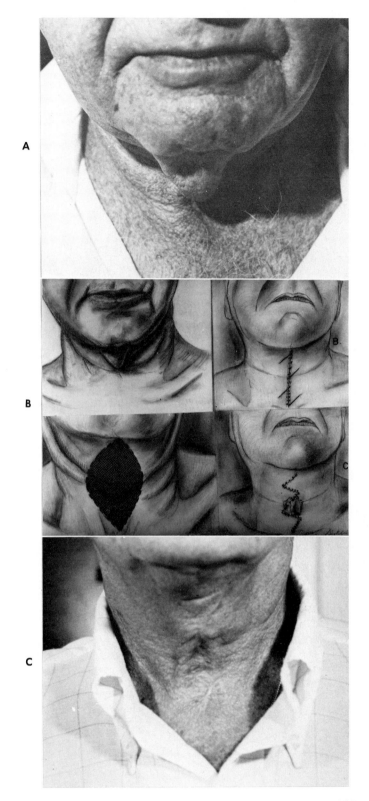

Fig. 13-5. A, Preoperative photograph of patient showing turkey gobbler deformity. **B,** Illustration of vertical elliptical excision and closure with multiple Z-plasties. **C,** Resulting scar on front of neck. This method was subsequently abandoned for incision not extending below level of thyroid cartilage.

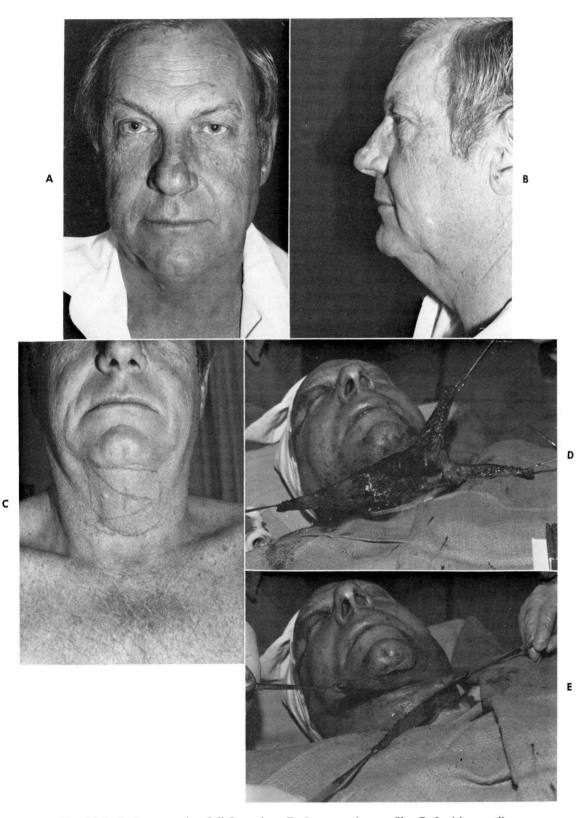

Fig. 13-6. A, Preoperative full-face view. **B,** Preoperative profile. **C,** Incision outline. NOTE: Lowest incision is in middle crease of neck. **D,** Incisions are elevated, neck defatted, and platysma sutured in midline. **E,** Flaps are replaced after defatting and prior to reduction to about one fourth of their original size and length. NOTE: Flaps are replaced into their original position. *Continued.*

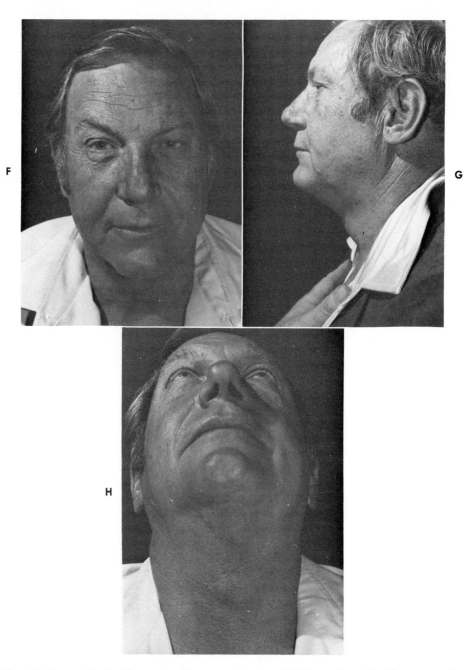

Fig. 13-6, cont'd. F, Three months postoperative full-face view. **G,** Three months postoperative profile. **H,** Head extended showing submental scars—3 months postoperatively.

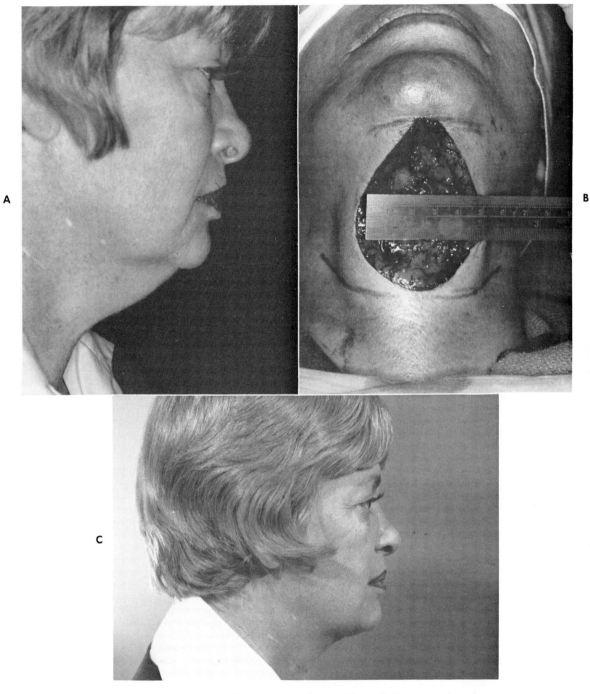

Fig. 13-7. A, Preoperative profile. **B,** Operative excision. **C,** Postoperative view. NOTE: This figure is included to show that this method is applicable to female as well as male patients.

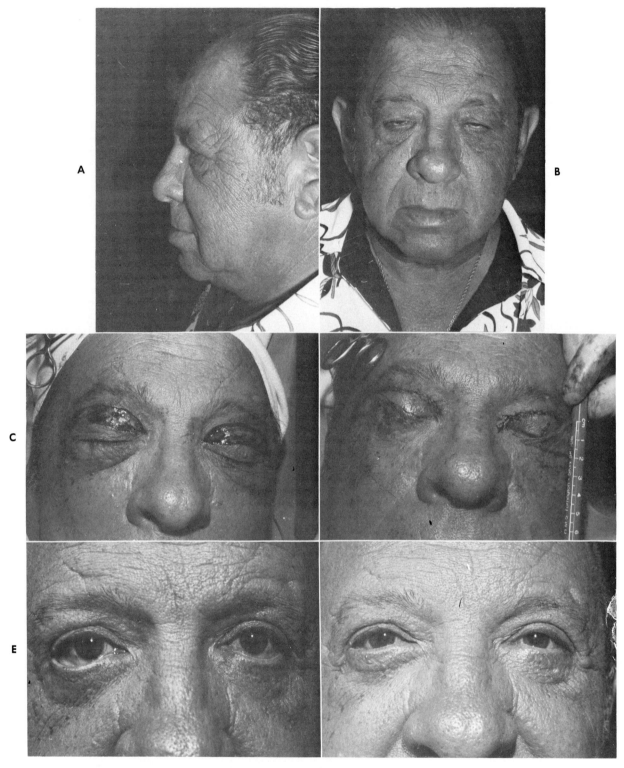

Fig. 13-8. A, Patient with too much skin that is thick, elastic, and cystic. **B,** Photograph showing patient's inability to close his eyes completely preoperatively. This is indication of problems postoperatively. **C** and **D,** Operative photographs showing excision of approximately 2 cm of skin from both upper and lower lids, along with usual defatting procedures. **E,** Immediate postoperative result with bilateral ectropion of lower lids. **F,** Patient five months later with conservative treatment only.

pion of the lower lids has occurred more often.

On the "good news" side, male patients are more satisfied with results and have enjoyed this satisfaction for longer periods of time.

SUMMARY

Rhytidectomy in the male patient is different and more difficult than in the female patient. Everything is done more frequently and more extensively in the male patient. Scarring is less acceptable. The hair and beard patterns must be respected.

Male patients generally enjoy more pleasing and longer-lasting results than do female patients.

REFERENCES

1. Adamson, J.E., Horton, C.E., and Crawford, H.H.: Surgical correction of the "turkey gobbler" deformity, Plast. Reconstr. Surg. **34:**598, 1964.
2. Connell, B.F.: Eyebrow, face and neck lifts for males, Clin. Plas. Sur. **5**(1):15, 1978.
3. Cronin, T.D., and Bigg, T.M.: T-Z plasty for the male "turkey gobbler neck," Plast. Reconstr. Surg. **47:**534, 1971.
4. Gonzalez-Ulloa, M.: History of rhytidectomy, Aesth. Plast. Surg. **4**(1):1, 1980.
5. Gordon, H.L.: Rhytidectomy, Clin. Plast. Surg. **5**(1):97, 1978.
6. Guerrerosantos, J.: The role of the platysma muscle in rhytidoplasty, Clin. Plast. Surg. **5**(1):29, 1978.
7. Gurdin, M.M., and Carlin, G.A.: Aging defects in the male: a regional approach to treatment. In Masters, F.W., and Lewis, J.R., editors: Symposium on aesthetic surgery of the face, eyelid, and breast, St. Louis, 1972, The C.V. Mosby Co.
8. Millard, D.R., Piggott, R.W., and Hedo, A.: Submandibular lipectomy, Plast. Reconstr. Surg. **41:**513, 1968.
9. Millard, D.R., et al.: Submental and submandibular lipectomy in conjunction with face lifts in the male or female, Plast. Reconstr. Surg. **49:**385, 1972.
10. Owsley, J.Q., Jr.: Platysmal-fascial rhytidectomy, Plast. Reconstr. Surg. **60:**843, 1977.
11. Rees, T.L., and Wood-Smith, D.: Cosmetic facial surgery, Philadelphia, 1973, W.B. Saunders Co., p. 134.
12. Skoog, T.: Plastic surgery: new methods and refinements, Philadelphia, 1974, W.B. Saunders Co., p. 300.
13. Viñas, J., Caviglia, C., and Cortinos, J.: Surgical treatment of double chin, Plast. Reconstr. Surg. **50:**119, 1972.
14. Viñas, J., Caviglia, C., and Cortinos, J.: Forehead rhytidoplasty and brow lifting, Plast. Reconstr. Surg. **57:**445, 1976.

Editorial comments
Chapter 13

Dr. Gurdin has pointed out something that is extremely important. "When a man consults a surgeon regarding aging, generally he seeks relief from one or more defects incidental to aging, but he is not compulsive about looking younger." This is so very true.

The obtuse neck can be handled in any number of ways, as described by Dr. Gurdin in his technique as well as in the extensive references he has provided. In addition, a simple vertical incision from the submental region to the hyoid bone combined with fat resection, simple Z-plasty of the leading edges of the platysma, minimal skin resection, and a small Z-plasty of the skin that will serve to form the new angle between the horizontal and vertical portion of the neck skin can give a pleasing improvement (Fig. 1) without involving the patient in an extensive procedure, such as rhytidectomy.

Rhytidectomy in the male patient is more difficult than in the female patient, and complications are more difficult to conceal (Fig. 2).

G.P.G.

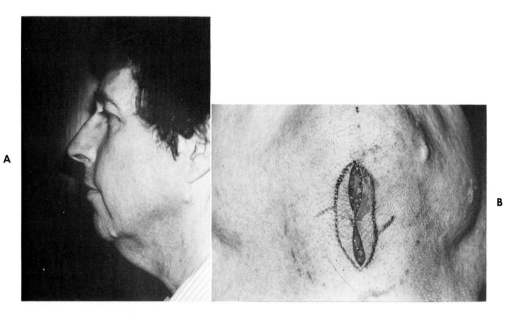

Fig. 1. A, Preoperative profile. **B,** Planned skin excision and Z-plasty (chin at top of photo).

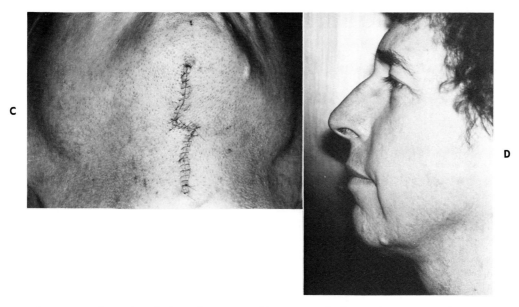

Fig. 1, cont'd. C, Conclusion of surgery (chin at top of photo). **D,** Postoperative profile.

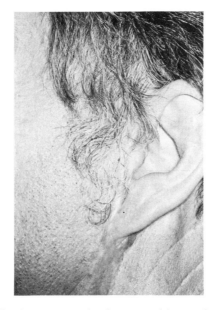

Fig. 2. Postoperative hypertrophic scarring.

Chapter 14

Face-lift in the male patient

Salvador Castañares

Looking old and being old are two entirely different things, for many faces age prematurely. Wrinkles are popularly accepted as symbols of age, but often they do not mean that. The rapid pace of our present life, tension, feelings of insecurity, overstimulation, and, in some geographical areas, overexposure to the sun or to the elements definitely age facial skin prematurely. The psychological, sociological, and economic factors involved in this visible process of aging are important; often they will affect a person's self-image and ability to succeed.

In the past those seeking the help of the plastic surgeon for the rejuvenative and beneficial results of a face-lift were mostly women, but, for a number of years now, more and more men from all walks of life have been resorting to this important surgical aid for the same economic, social, and psychological reasons.

TECHNIQUE

The surgical technique for the face-lift in the male patient is identical in execution to that in the female patient, with one very important exception: allowance for hair distribution about the scalp and face of the male patient. Because of the distribution of scalp hair, which is less to varying degrees in the male patient, modification of the superior and anterior incision sites must be made.

For approximately 25 years I have divided the prospective male face-lift patient into three categories:
1. The patient with a full growth of hair
2. The patient with thinning hair and diminished hair growth above the temples
3. The patient with actual baldness and very little hair above the temples

Regarding the distribution of facial hair, the patient must always be advised that a fine scar will result approximately 6 mm anterior to the ear. This is necessary to prevent having hair-growing skin too close to the ear itself. With this explanation and the benefits obtained, the patient readily accepts the fine and ultimately inconspicuous scar as a small penalty for the rejuvenating improvement.

Fig. 14-1 shows the three sites of the anterior incisions for a face-lift in the male patient. Please note that below the level of the superior third of the ear, the lower and posterior incisions are exactly the same for all patients, male or female. Only the upper anterior incision varies in the male patient, as will be explained.

Posteriorly the incision is carried out on the ear skin, approximately 1 cm above the sulcus to a level in the upper third of the ear (Fig. 14-2). The incision then extends posteriorly into the scalp well above the hairline in an inverted U shape to provide a wide skin-scalp flap for adequate circulation and to prevent distortion of the hairline with a resulting visible scar.

Anterior to the ear the curving incision is placed approximately 6 mm away from it to prevent having hair-growing skin too close to the ear itself.

For the patient with a full growth of hair, the entire operation, including the incision lines (Figs. 14-3 to 14-6), is identical to that for the female patient.

For the patient with a relatively good growth of hair but early thinning at the temples, the upper anterior incision is begun 2 cm above the ear, close to its center (Fig. 14-7).

In this type of patient (Figs. 14-8 and 14-9) the operation is essentially the same as in the female patient or the male patient with a full growth of hair, except for the reduced upper anterior incision.

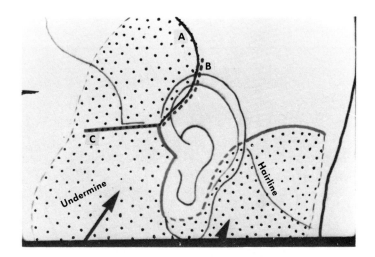

Fig. 14-1. Incision sites for three types of face-lifts for male patients. Fine interrupted lines anteriorly and posteriorly indicate extent of undermining. Arrows show direction of two supporting sutures. *A,* Incision lines for patient with full growth of hair, similar to those for female face-lift. *B,* Incision lines for patient with less hair, but not bald. Incision starts approximately 1 to 2 cm above ear, near its center, and continues downward around ear, as in all cases. *C,* Incision lines for bald patient with marked diminution of hair about temples.

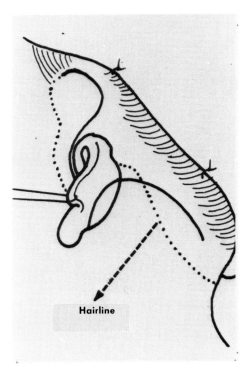

Fig. 14-2. Posterior incision 1 cm lateral to postauricular sulcus and inverted U prolongation into scalp.

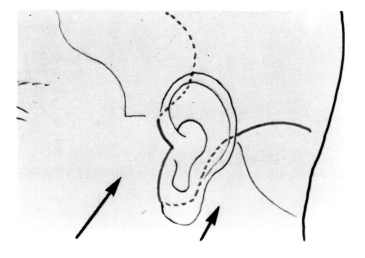

Fig. 14-3. Incision lines for male patient with full growth of hair (similar to incisions for female face-lift).

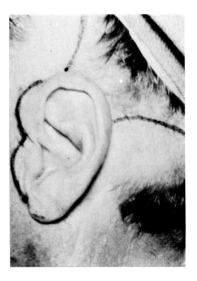

Fig. 14-4. Close-up view of incision lines, taken in operating room, in male patient with full growth of hair. Hair has been only partially trimmed.

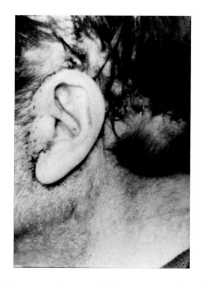

Fig. 14-5. Same patient on fifth postoperative day. Note diminution of space between markings in operating room and after suturing within scalp.

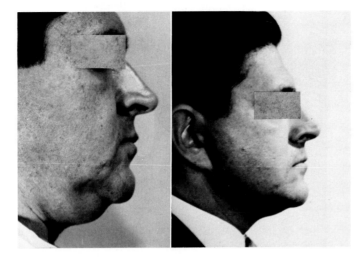

Fig. 14-6. Example of patient with full growth of hair before and after face-lift. Entire operation was done exactly as in female patient.

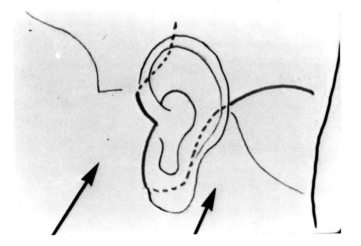

Fig. 14-7. Markings for patient with thinning hair at temples. Superiormost incision starts approximately 2 cm above ear, near its center.

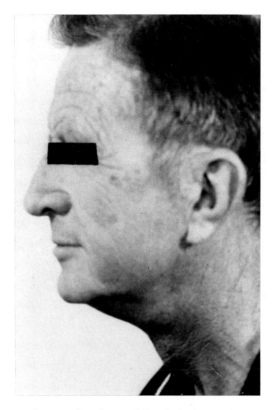

Fig. 14-8. This is second type of patient, with relatively good growth of hair but thinning at temples.

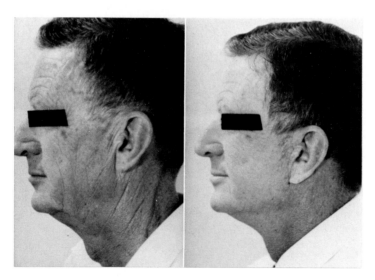

Fig. 14-9. Same patient before and 6 weeks postoperatively.

For the patient with baldness and thin hair about and above the temples (Fig. 14-10), in 1958 I began using a simplified technique that, in my hands, has given satisfactory results. The markings for the incision are shown in Fig. 14-11. Note that the upper anterior aspect of the face and scalp are devoid of incision lines. The rest of the incisions below the sideburn area are exactly the same as in the other two types of face-lifts in the male patient.

It may be noted that with this incision modification the temple hairline is left intact by placing the uppermost incision horizontally at the base of the normal sideburn.

Fig. 14-12 illustrates a typical case in the operating room. I do all my rhytidectomies with the patient under local anesthesia. They can, of course, be done with the patient under general anesthesia, but I prefer local anesthesia (0.5% lidocaine hydrochloride [Xylocaine] with epinephrine) for its simplicity and to minimize complications.

For all male face-lifts the incision in front of the ear is done in a double-curved manner, the arcs joining at a point anterior to the tragus, thus avoiding a straight scar.

For the balding patient the upper curving incision is short, since it starts at the sideburn, where there is a horizontal prolongation.

In the past, in a group of male and female patients, I tried to place the incision behind or on the border of the tragus, but found that in some cases the scar flattened the tragus itself, causing deformity. Also, in the male patient this approach frequently brought hair-bearing skin to the ear itself, causing obvious inconveniences.

In the modified technique for the balding patient, the uppermost incision starts slightly above the tragus, approximately at the level of the external canthus of the eye, descending in a curving manner to the undersurface of the earlobe, where it continues posteriorly as in all other face-lifts, male or female. The important variation is the horizontal incision that extends anteriorly at the base of the sideburn for approximately 5 to 6 cm (Fig. 14-11).

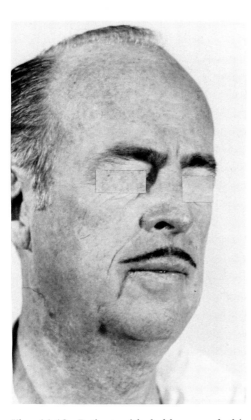

Fig. 14-10. Patient with baldness and thin hair about temples.

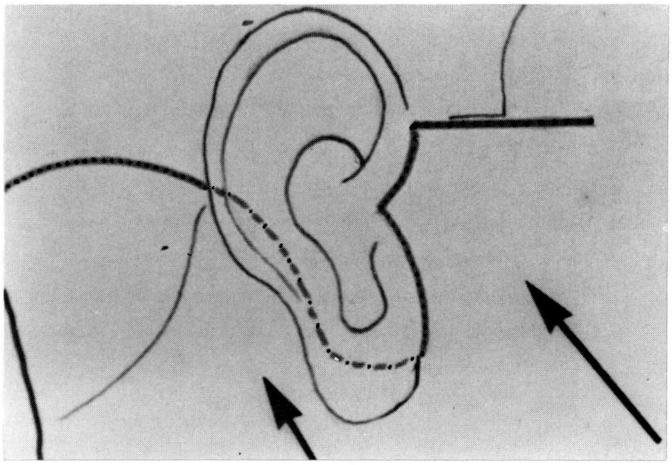

Fig. 14-11. Modification of anterior upper incisions for balding patient with thinning hair about temples. Horizontal incision approximately 5 to 6 cm in length is made at base of sideburn, above tragus. It then descends in double-curving fashion, as in all other male patients.

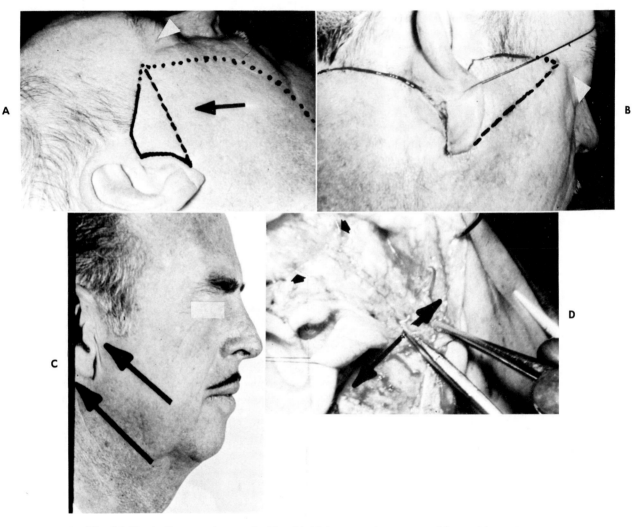

Fig. 14-12. A, Same patient as in Fig. 14-10 in operating room with markings. Arrow points to elevation of undermined skin flap, which will be rotated upward, resulting in triangle of skin that will be resected. Anterior interrupted line indicates extent of undermining. **B,** Horizontal and posterior incisions have been started. Note that posterior incision is made in ear skin. **C,** Arrows indicate directions of elevation of subcutaneous tissues from near center of cheek and submental area with two nonabsorbable sutures. **D,** Upper small arrows point to suture pulling subcutaneous tissues near center of cheek, which will be anchored at malar bone fascia. Longer, lower arrows indicate lower suture anchoring submandibular platysma, fat, and fascia to mastoid bone fascia.

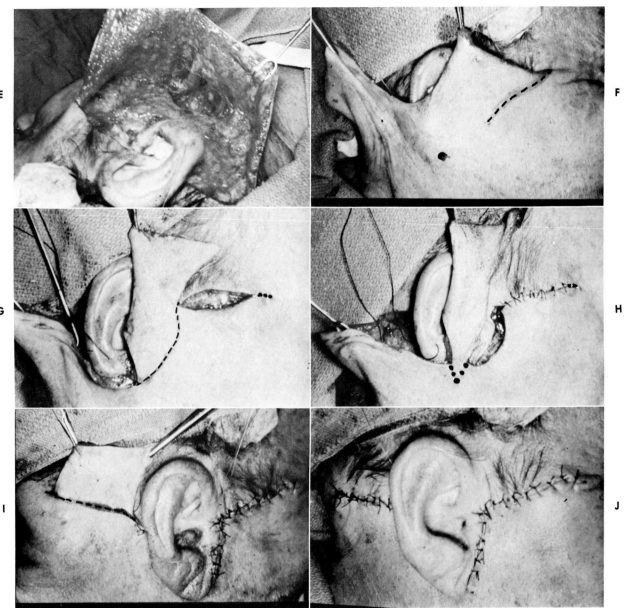

Fig. 14-12, cont'd. E, Extent of undermining in this patient. **F,** Elevation of skin flap. Dot represents point to which skin will be incised and tucked under earlobe. This point corresponds to center of earlobe. **G,** Skin flap has been split to dot and is being tucked under earlobe. Horizontal upper incision at base of sideburn has been made, resulting in triangle of skin that will be resected after flap has been shifted upward and backward. **H,** Horizontal incision is sutured first, starting at its anterior extreme to prevent dog-ear. Anterior excessive skin is being excised, tailoring it to anterior auricular marks. **I,** All anterior suturing has been completed. Excessive posterior skin has been marked for resection. **J,** Completion of operation. *Continued.*

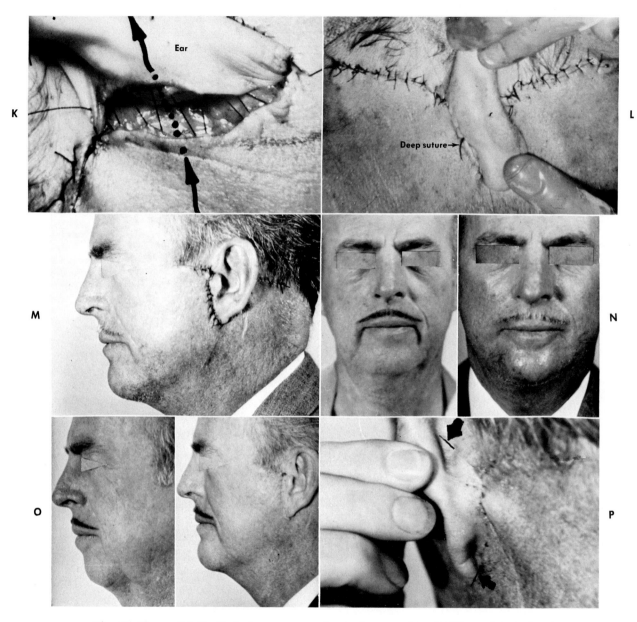

Fig. 14-12, cont'd. K, Posterior manner of suturing ear skin. **L,** View of completed posterior suturing. **M,** Patient on fifth postoperative day, when all anterior sutures are removed. Chin implant was placed during face-lift. **N,** Frontal views of patient before surgery and 5 days postoperatively. Note appearanace of chin. **O,** Profile views before surgery and 8 days postoperatively. **P,** Close-up view of posterior incision lines on eighth postoperative day. Arrow points to subcuticular suture, which is removed 8 to 10 days after surgery.

For many years I have made the posterior incision on the ear skin rather than in the mastoid skin (Figs. 14-2 and 14-12, *B*). Many surgeons are using this approach for the posterior incision, and I feel that it is an excellent maneuver. I urge those who have not used it to try doing so in a few cases; I think they will be gratified. It should be placed approximately 1 cm lateral to the auricular sulcus. Ultimately the scar will fall exactly in the sulcus itself and thus become inconspicuous.

The undermining is carried out in the usual manner. The extent of undermining (Fig. 14-12, *E*) varies according to the need: in heavier individuals it is more extensive, whereas in thinner ones the undermining does ot have to be too extensive. It also varies with the type of skin (e.g., thick, leathery skin requires more undermining than smooth and thin skin). This, of course, is also the case in the female face-lift.

The posterior scalp incision is extended as far back as is necessary (Figs. 14-11 and 14-12, *B*) to provide a good closure and to prevent a posterior vertical neck wrinkle or band of skin in the neck, as is often seen when the incision is not extended enough posteriorly.

I always start the undermining posteriorly and inferiorly, since this approach offers several advantages. For the undermining I use a simple blunt, short, snubbed but strong scissors, which was made for me many years ago by Padgett Instruments Company (Fig. 14-13). With the scissors I can immediately find the line of cleavage. The scissor dissection follows this cleavage plane. Much time and effort in the dissection are saved with this simple instrument, which also leaves intact an adequate pad of subcutaneous fat, preventing possible sloughs and avoiding injury to the hair roots, thus preventing loss of hair. He-

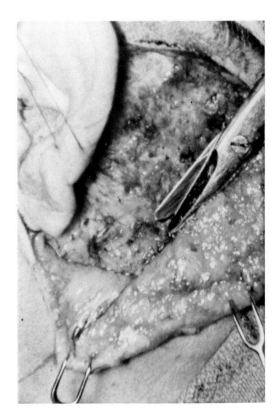

Fig. 14-13. Special scissors for undermining. This instrument easily finds normal line of cleavage and minimizes time and effort in this important maneuver. Note that undermining is started inferiorly and posteriorly. This approach has many advantages.

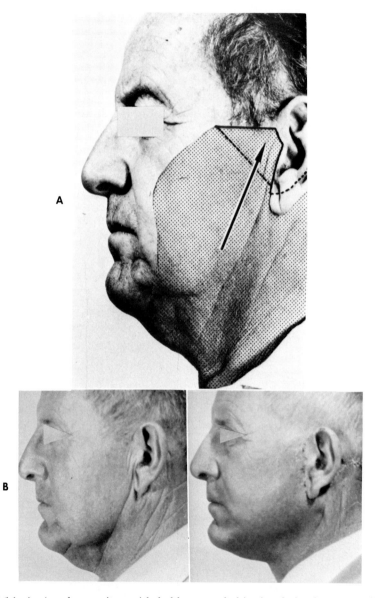

Fig. 14-14. A, Another patient with baldness and thinning hair about temples before surgery. Anterior incision line is shown, starting at base of sideburn. Dark area denotes extent of undermining. Arrow represents direction of anterior nonabsorbable supporting suture. **B,** Profile views of same patient before surgery and 10 days postoperatively.

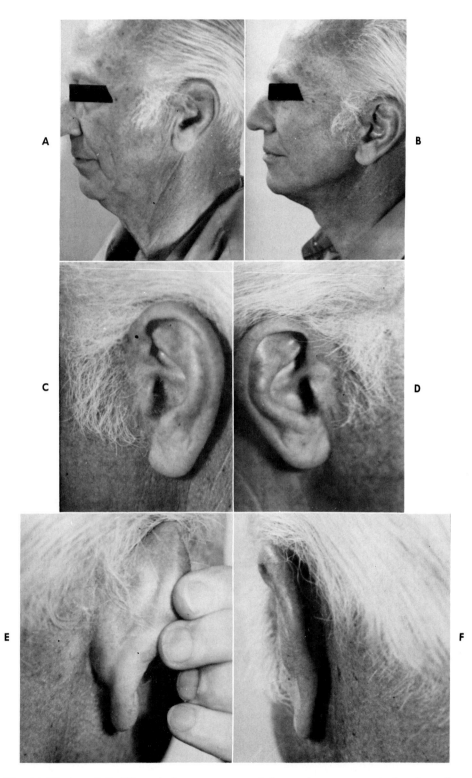

Fig. 14-15. A and **B,** Views before surgery and 6 months postoperatively of another patient with baldness and thinning hair about temples. This patient favored long sideburns. **C** and **D,** Close-up views of same patient 6 months postoperatively showing minimally visible scars and normal regrowth of long sideburns. **E** and **F,** Minimally visible scars posteriorly. Temporooccipital hair covers high inverted U scar nicely.

mostasis is almost always totally controlled by electrocoagulation. I use only a few ligatures, usually at the external temporal artery area.

In years past I used to undermine almost routinely to the nasolabial sulcus, but I later abandoned this practice. It is not necessary; actually, it is better not to extend the undermining that far. I feel that it should stop 2 or 2.5 cm from the nasolabial sulcus so that the skin remains attached to the prominence of the cheek near the sulcus, thus allowing the cheek to be elevated along with the skin when it is shifted upward and posteriorly.

In the past I have used many methods to lift the sagging subcutaneous tissues, platysma, and fascia. For many years now I have simplified this important step through the use of two buried sutures of nonabsorbable material in the direction of the arrows (Fig. 14-12, *C*).

The first, in the direction of the small arrows shown in Fig. 14-12, *D*, elevates the center of the cheek (and thus the corner of the mouth) toward the malar bone, where it is anchored to the thick fascia over it.

The second buried suture starts under the side of the neck below the mandible and close to the midline, suturing and elevating the fat with platysma and fascia and anchoring it to the thick fascia over the mastoid bone, as illustrated by the longer arrows shown in Fig. 14-12, *D*. It should be obvious that these nonabsorbable sutures will sustain the elevation of subcutaneous tissues for 3 or 4 weeks only, which will be enough time for the shifted undermined skin to become attached to the elevated subcutaneous tissues by fibrosis.

In all face-lifts the posterior suturing is important (Fig. 14-12, *K*). It is started at the posterior extreme of the incision line in the neck region, rather than anteriorly, to avoid a posterior dog-ear. The sutures may be interrupted or continuous until the mastoid area is reached, where two or three half-mattress sutures, knotted in the scalp region above, will prevent visible stitch marks in this bare area.

The ear skin is closed with a subcuticular suture of 3-0 or 4-0 Dermalon, which may be removed in 7 to 10 days. The arrow in Fig. 14-12, *K*, points to a single deep suture at the center of the auricular sulcus. This will prevent a dead space here.

On the fifth postoperative day all anterior auricular sutures are removed. Fig. 14-12, *M*, shows the patient on the fifth day, and some of the anterior horizontal sutures have already been removed. Note that a chin implant was placed. This is an excellent ancillary procedure in many face-lifts, male or female.

Figs. 14-14 and 14-15 show the results of surgery in two other patients with baldness and thinning hair about the temples.

SUMMARY

The surgical technique for the male face-lift has been presented with modifications according to the type of hair distribution about the scalp and face of the patient, based on more than 25 years of experience.

As is the case with female patients, I feel that in properly selected male patients the face-lift is one of the most gratifying cosmetic plastic operations to the patient and to the surgeon alike.

SUGGESTED READINGS

Baker, T.J., and Gordon, T.J.: Rhytidectomy in males, Plast. Reconstr. Surg. **44:**219, 1969.

Carlin, A., and Gurdin, M.M.: Ancillary procedures for the aging face and neck, Surg. Clin. North Am. **51:**371, 1971.

Cook, T.E.: Rhytidectomy, Dallas Med. J. **30:**60, 1944.

Edgerton, M.T., et al.: Surgical results and psychosocial changes following rhytidectomy: an evaluation of face lifting, Plast. Reconstr. Surg. **33:**503, 1964.

Gonzalez-Ulloa, M.: Winkle correction: ear-island method, J. Int. Coll. Surg. **25:**620, 1956.

Gonzalez-Ulloa, M. and Stevens, E.: Sectional rhytidectomy, including a description of rhytidectomy in the male, Presented at the thirty-seventh meeting of the American Society for Plastic and Reconstructive Surgery, New Orleans, 1968.

Lewis, J.R., Jr.: Atlas of aesthetic plastic surgery, Boston, 1973, Little, Brown & Co.

Malbec, E.F.: Arrugas de la cara: técnica operatoria, Semana Med. **3:**517, 1957.

Marcus, H.: Rhytidectomy: useful considerations, Boll. Arg. Soc. Plast. Surg. **2:**50, 1959.

Pangman, W.J., and Wallace, R.M.: Cosmetic surgery of the face and neck, Plast. Reconstr. Surg. **27:**544, 1961.

Seltzer, A.P.: Reconstructive surgery for the elderly, Geriatrics **7:**185, 1952.

Skoog, T.: Plastic surgery: new methods and refinements, Philadelphia, 1974, W.B. Saunders Co.

Stark, R.B.: A variation in rhytidectomy incision at the front of the ear, Plast. Reconstr. Surg. **54:**369, 1974.

Sturman, M.J.: Sideburn relationship in the male face lift, Plast. Reconstr. Surg. **57:**248, 1976.

Chapter 15

Rhinoplasty in the older patient: a useful adjunct to rhytidectomy

Bernard L. Kaye

One of the problems of the aging face involves the changes that take place in the nose with time.[2] The nasal cartilages become larger and more bulky, making the tip more bulbous. The tip gradually descends so that the nasolabial angle may approach 90 degrees or less. The nasolabial angle itself becomes more acute as the columella-labial junction retrudes and loses its gentle, obtuse, filletlike shape of youth.

The dorsum of the nose becomes more prominent with increasing age. Mild to moderate hump deformities may become more severe. Noses that did not have hump deformities may show increased lateral dorsal bony ridging or may even develop hump deformities that were not present previously.

The nose may become wider at the dorsum, and the nostrils may flare more with time. The nasal skin, particularly of the lower dorsum and tip, becomes thicker, with more prominent pores, and may even develop mild or extensive rhinophymatous changes.

The surgeon who wishes to effect a more complete facial rejuvenation is obligated to include the nose in an evaluation of aging problems in the middle third of the face. Admittedly, many patients seeking rejuvenative surgery may be totally unaware of the aging changes that have taken place in their own noses. On the other hand, if such patients were shown photographs of people revealing just the middle third of the face, the very same patients would probably guess the approximate ages of the people in the photographs through their own unconscious awareness of changes that take place in the nose with age.

Two types of rhinoplasties may be carried out with rhytidectomy: partial rhinoplasty or complete rhinoplasty.

PARTIAL RHINOPLASTY

The partial rhinoplasty is a particularly useful ancillary procedure with face-lift surgery because it can be done reasonably rapidly and will not prolong the operation unduly. Also, by omitting the steps of complete osteocartilaginous hump removal and infracture, one avoids those elements of the nasal procedure that some surgeons believe cause the most morbidity.

Often a partial rhinoplasty may be an adequate operation to correct most of the aging changes in the nose when it is carried out concomitantly with rhytidectomy or other ancillary rejuvenative procedures (Fig. 15-1). Partial rhinoplasty may include any or all of the following steps:

1. Reduction of nasal tip bulk may be accomplished by removing the cephalic portions of the alar cartilages (a step that in itself may also raise the tip adequately without any further procedures).
2. Bony ridging may be reduced by rasping, or one can achieve a conservative reduction of a bony hump by rasping each side at a slight angle, so as to maintain the shape of the dorsum.
3. In the patient who exhibits a sharp, retruded columella-labial angle, insertion of a retrolabial cartilage graft just posterior to that angle can fill out and round out the sharp angle (Fig. 15-2). The graft may be

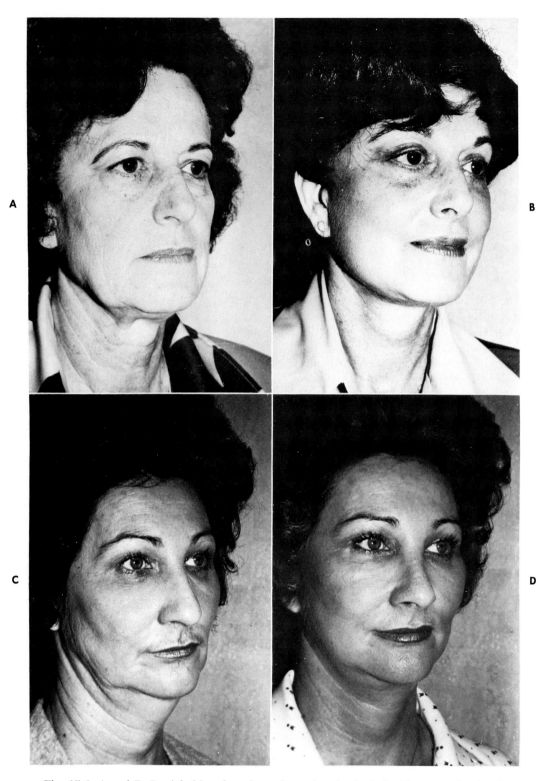

Fig. 15-1. A and **B,** Partial rhinoplasty in patient who also had rhytidectomy, forehead lift, blepharoplasty, and perioral peel-abrasion. **C** and **D,** Partial rhinoplasty in patient who also had rhytidectomy and ancillary procedures.

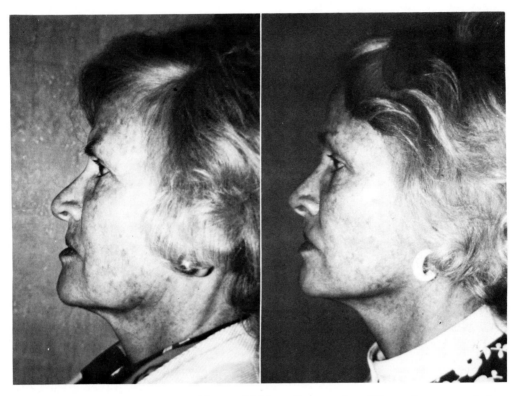

Fig. 15-2. Partial rhinoplasty with retrolabial cartilage graft to fill out sharp, retruded columella-labial angle. Graft contributes to tip elevation and projection. Patient also had face-lift and forehead lift.

inserted either through the transfixion incision or, if there is just a partial transfixion incision, through a separate stab incision at the inner base of the columella. The graft may be made up of two layers of alar cartilage, previously removed with the tip reduction procedure and sutured together to give added bulk. Note that this step also adds projection to a retruded tip and can also raise a drooping tip.

4. If neither tip reduction nor insertion of a retrolabial cartilage graft is sufficient to raise a drooping tip, one may also trim conservatively the anterior portion of the caudal edge of the septal cartilage with its accompanying mucosal lining. Because the membranous septum has a tendency to stretch in the older patient, it may be helpful to trim just a little more lining than one would ordinarily take in the younger individual— perhaps 1 mm more. On the other hand, those patients who are reluctant to have their nostrils showing, even temporarily, should be informed that they may benefit from a secondary raising of their tips some months later. Interestingly, many patients report that they breathe better after their tips have been elevated,[4] and it is easy to anticipate this improvement preoperatively by manually lifting the nasal tip slightly.

5. For those patients whose nostrils have become overly wide and are now revealed when their drooping tips are raised to a more normal level, alaplasties are helpful to narrow the nostrils.

COMPLETE RHINOPLASTY

There can be situations, either due to anatomical deformity or because of the patient's wishes, where a complete rhinoplasty may be the most desirable operation (Fig. 15-3). In addition to the steps described for the partial rhinoplasty, the complete rhinoplasty involves removal of the osteocartilaginous hump and infracture of the nasal bones. This operation can be done at the same stage as a face-lift or at another stage, depending on the surgeon's preference and individual rate of operating. If it can be done reasonably expeditiously without sacrificing safety or quality of the operation, I believe there is no reason why it cannot be done along with a face-lift. I do not believe that the taping and splinting of the nose interferes with the results of the face-lift operation.

Adding the partial or complete rhinoplasty to the rejuvenative procedures does not prolong the patient's total recovery time, which is governed by recovery from the face-lift operation itself rather than just the rhinoplasty.

RHINOPLASTY IN THE OLDER PATIENT

Rhinoplasty can be a useful procedure in the older patient,[2,6] either as an adjunct ancillary rejuvenative procedure or by itself. Some observant older patients will seek rhinoplasty because they noticed changes directly related to age, including increased lengthening of the nose accompanied by increased bulbousness of the tip, drooping of the tip and columella, and increased prominence of the dorsum. Other older patients may come to the plastic surgeon to correct long-standing nasal deformities that they always wanted to have improved but, for one reason or another, were not able to do so.[2] They may not have had the financial means nor the available time for the surgery and its postoperative recovery period. Many older persons, no longer employed, may have felt threatened by their fear of criticism from former colleagues. They may also have experienced or expected family criticism or derision. Some, who may have experienced a life-long desire for rhinoplasty, may have had their desire maligned as ridiculous, perhaps because their particular nose configuration has been the family's most prominent and notable feature for generations.

Whether rhinoplasty is done in the older patient as a partial or complete procedure, and whether it is done as a single operation or in conjunction with a face-lift, there are several special considerations to keep in mind about it. There is as great a need (or an even greater one) for artistic judgment in performing rhinoplasty on the older patient as there is in the younger individual. Although rhinoplasties tend to be more conservative now then they were some years ago,[5] there is an even greater need for conservatism in surgery for the older patient, who does not want to feel conspicuous or look "nose bobbed".[1] Reduction rhinoplasty is "all take and no give,"[3] and in the older patient one should usually take less. The older patient usually wants little or no dorsal concavity, and many will request a relatively straight nose. Also, many are terrified at the thought of a piglike look with elevated, flaring nostrils.

Health problems frequently associated with increasing age, including hypertension, arteriosclerosis, and cardiopulmonary disease, call for more

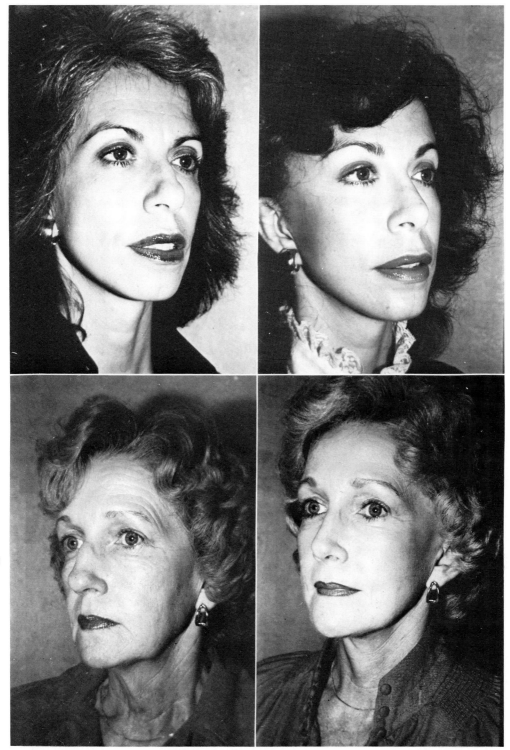

Fig. 15-3. A and **B,** Complete rhinoplasty in patient who had rhytidectomy, forehead lift, blepharoplasty, and perioral peel-abrasion. **C** and **D,** Complete rhinoplasty with rhytidectomy, forehead lift, and chin augmentation.

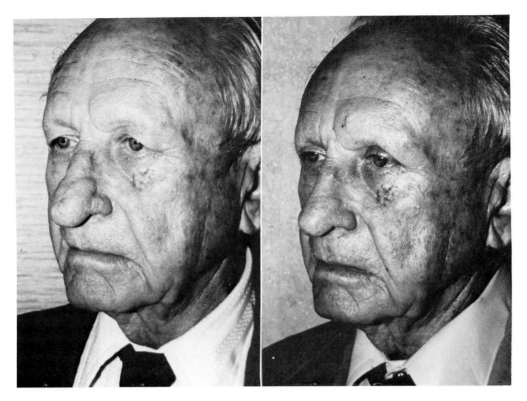

Fig. 15-4. Bulbous drooping tip and rhinophyma in older patient treated by combination of shaving, lower rhinoplasty, and external transverse skin excision. Patient also had upper lid blepharoplasty. (From Kaye, B.L.: Rhinoplasty in the older patient, Aesth. Plast. Surg. **3**:57, 1979.)

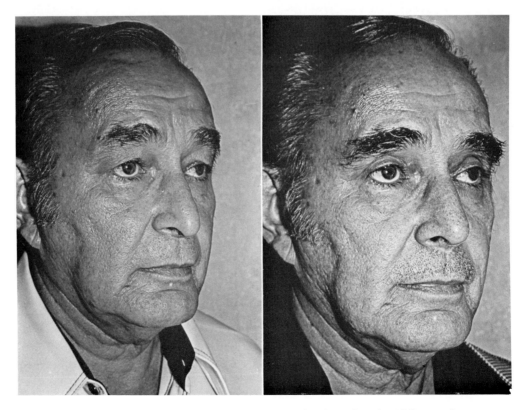

Fig. 15-5. Partial rhinoplasty in older patient to raise drooping tip. (Often patients report improvement in breathing after this operation.) Patient also had upper lid blepharoplasty.

detailed and thorough preoperative medical evaluation. The presence of such conditions, however, is not in itself a contraindication to rhinoplasty, provided the patient is judged to be able to safely tolerate the surgery and anesthesia.

In the older patient one should be more concerned about the coronary vasoconstrictive pressor effects of epinephrine. I recommend that the epinephrine concentration in the local anesthetic solution be more dilute, between 1:200,000 and 1:400,000. Experience demonstrates clearly that the more dilute solution can achieve the desired degree of vasoconstriction, provided one waits long enough for the dilute epinephrine solution to provide its vasoconstrictive effect.

There are tissue differences in older patients as compared with younger individuals. Cartilage may be tougher or more brittle. It is more difficult to shave the cartilaginous dorsum, and the septum is harder to cut. Alar cartilages are more likely to fracture as they are being removed. Bone is more brittle and may comminute more during osteotomy. On the other hand, it may be easier to achieve a complete fracture in the older individual without fear of getting a green-stick fracture. As mentioned above, the membranous septum tends to stretch more, and, in shortening the anterior caudal septum, it is worthwhile to take just a bit more mucosa than one would remove in a younger patient.

The skin tends to shrink down less over the newly formed skeletal framework than it would in a younger patient. Nevertheless, it is rarely necessary to resect external skin except in some cases of rhinophyma (Fig. 15-4). Moreover, if external incisions are required, they may be expected to heal better than they would in the younger patient, in keeping with the tendency for older patients' scars to heal less visibly.

SUMMARY

Nasal changes can constitute one of the problems that must be considered in planning facial rejuvenative surgery, and these can be treated by partial or complete rhinoplasty, either with face-lift surgery or independently. Rhinoplasty is an operation that can be done in older as well as younger patients. Although there are some differences in approach, procedure, and tissues in the older patient, these do not detract from the fact that rhinoplasty can be an effective, worthwhile procedure in the older age group (Fig. 15-5).

REFERENCES

1. Brown, J.B., and McDowell, F.: Plastic surgery of the nose, St. Louis, 1951, The C.V. Mosby Co.
2. Kaye, B.L.: Rhinoplasty in the older patient, Aesth. Plast. Surg. **3**:57, 1979.
3. Millard, D.R.: Adjuncts in augmentation mentoplasty and corrective rhinoplasty, Plast. Reconstr. Surg. **36**:56, 1965.
4. Patterson, C.N.: Surgery of the anatomically weak and aging nose, N.C. Med. J. **33**:692, 1972.
5. Rees, T.D.: Current concepts in rhinoplasty, Clin. Plast. Surg. **4**:131, 1977.
6. Rees, T.D.: Rhinoplasty in the older adult, Ann. Plast. Surg. **1**:27, 1978.

Chapter 16

Problems and complications in platysma-SMAS cervicofacial rhytidectomy

Sherrell J. Aston

Conventional face-lift techniques by facial and cervical skin undermining, skin flap elevation and rotation, and excision of excess skin often fall short in providing the result anticipated by the patient and desired by the surgeon. This is not surprising when one considers that only a small percentage of patients requesting face-lift operations have laxity of the cervical and facial skin as their only deformity. The majority of patients have facial, jawline, and neck deformities caused by a combination of factors, the most common of which are (1) the effect of the generalized aging process on all the facial and cervical tissues, (2) localized or generalized fat deposits in the cheeks, along the jaw line, or in the submental and submandibular areas, and, (3) anatomical deformities genetically determined (i.e., an obtuse cervicomental angle). Individual patients sometimes have specific deformities that are peculiar to their anatomy. The platysma muscle frequently contributes to neck deformities and is often the most obvious component of the deformity.

Surgical techniques that permit (1) tightening the superficial musculoaponeurotic system (SMAS) over the cheeks, (2) extensive resection of fat deposits from the cheeks, jawline, and submandibular and submental areas, and (3) alteration of the platysma muscle anatomy in the neck have improved the results in many patients undergoing cervicofacial rhytidectomy. In fact, current techniques permit the surgeon to selectively design a surgical procedure for an individual patient's deformity so as to correct problems insufficiently improved by conventional face-lifting procedures. A number of authors have made contributions to these recent surgical techniques.*

The purpose of this chapter is to discuss problems, complications, and their solutions as related to the more extensive procedures for cervicofacial rhytidectomy. It should be noted at the outset that in my experience, there has been no higher incidence of surgical complications with the more extensive procedures than that anticipated for conventional face-lifting techniques. Therefore this chapter primarily deals with (1) pitfalls to avoid by adapting the appropriate surgical procedure to the anatomical deformity of a given patient and (2) pitfalls to avoid in the excecution of the indicated surgical procedure.

SMAS AND PLATYSMA MUSCLE ANATOMY
SMAS anatomy

The SMAS is a single layer of superficial fascia of the face most easily defined over the parotid gland and cheek area[3] (Fig. 16-1). The SMAS is thickest in the preauricular area over the surface of the parotid fascia. Superiorly, the SMAS passes superficial to the zygomatic arch and is in continuity with the posterior portion of the frontalis muscle, adhering to the periosteum in the tem-

---

*References 6-10, 13-19, 21-26.

132

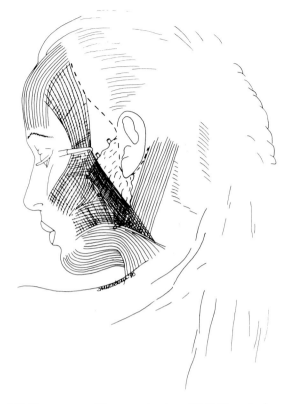

Fig. 16-1. SMAS anatomy. Note continuity of SMAS and platysma muscle.

porozygomatic arch by thin expansions. Inferiorly, the SMAS is in continuity with the platysma muscle along the jawline and in the upper neck. Although thin, the SMAS extends throughout the cheek area and medially to the nasolabial fold. A thin layer of subcutaneous fat is located between the SMAS and dermis. The SMAS is a continuous fibrous network beneath the dermis; it covers the muscles of facial expression and comprises all the attachments of the superficial muscles of facial expression to the dermis.

Medial to the anterior border of the parotid gland, the SMAS becomes significantly thinner and provides only a thin layer of protection to the facial nerve branches. Because of the thinness of the SMAS anterior to the parotid gland, surgical dissection of the SMAS in this area is difficult and dangerous. The only nerves that pass through the SMAS are sensory nerves.

Dissection and elevation of the SMAS in the preauricular area, beginning at the zygomatic arch, extending medially to the anterior border of the parotid gland, and continuing inferiorly below the mandibular border, in continuity with the platysma muscle, produces a lifting effect on the jaw-

line and cheeks and in some patients transmits pull to the nasolabial fold region. Thus SMAS dissection and elevation in the cheek provides a deep-layer support system analogous to platysma muscle surgery in the neck.

Platysma muscle anatomy

The platysma muscle is a thin, flat muscle that lies just beneath the skin of the anterior and lateral surfaces of the neck and belongs to the facial expression muscle group (Fig. 16-2). Deep to the platysma muscle lies the superficial layer of the deep cervical fascia. The plane between the platysma and the superficial layer of the deep cervical fascia is relatively avascular and easily dissected.

The platysma muscle varies in shape, thickness, and elasticity from patient to patient (Fig. 16-3). In general, it is thicker in men than in women. The medial borders of the right and left platysma muscles are separated below the level of the hyoid bone in most patients.[26] In 30% to 40% of patients there is a decussation of platysma fibers from each side across the midline near the level of the hyoid bone and up to the inferior bor-

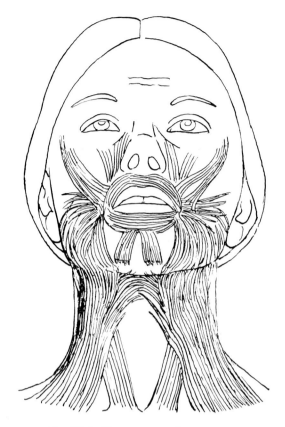

Fig. 16-2. Platysma muscle anatomy.

der of the mandible. The platysma inserts along the lower border of the mandible, attaches to the overlying skin, and is contiguous with the SMAS over the cheeks. Inferiorly, the platysma extends below the clavicles and attaches to the skin over the upper portion of the pectoralis and deltoid muscles. The platysma muscle receives its motor innervation through the cervical branch of the seventh cranial nerve.

The platysma muscle interdigitates with the depressor muscles of the lower lip (depressor anguli oris, depressor labii inferioris) and in some patients functions synchronously in depressing the lateral lower lip (Fig. 16-4). Loss of platysma muscle function produces no permanent effect on facial muscle function. Theoretically, when the platysma muscle is denervated, a transient decrease in lateral lower lip depression may occur until full depressor function is taken over by the lip depressor muscles. However, it is difficult to document a platysma muscle procedure as causing a decrease in lip depression when other causes are possible with the more extensive facial procedures.

PITFALLS AND COMPLICATIONS

The most frequently performed extended cervicofacial procedures are (1) elevation, rotation, and advancement of the SMAS (most often in continuity with the platysma muscle); (2) complete transverse division of the platysma muscle; (3) partial division of the platysma muscle medially and/or laterally; (4) suture approximation of medial platysma borders; and (5) appropriate resection of fat from the cheeks, jawline, and neck. Variations of these techniques must be adapted for the specific anatomical deformities of each individual patient.

The major pitfalls and problems of cervicofacial defatting and platysma-SMAS surgical techniques are (1) recurrent platysma bands, (2) inappropriate level of platysma muscle transection, (3) inadequate cervicofacial defatting, and (4) cervical depressions and irregularities. Significant problems and pitfalls are possible with SMAS dissection procedures, but I have not experienced such in more than 300 patients (600 SMAS dissections). Theoretical problems following SMAS dissection, rotation, and advancement could include (1) facial

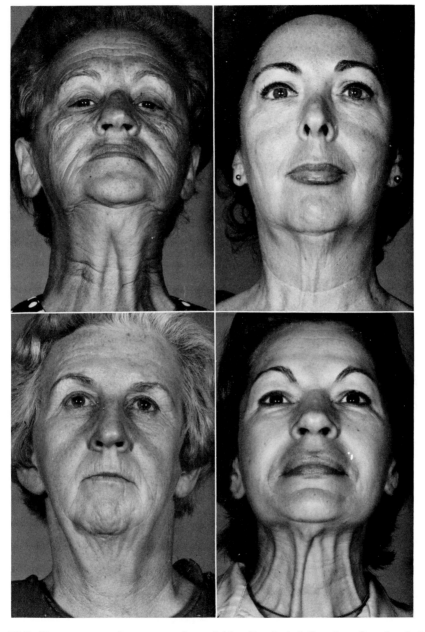

Fig. 16-3. Platysma muscle anatomy is variable. Cervical deformity of each of these patients is in part due to platysma muscle.

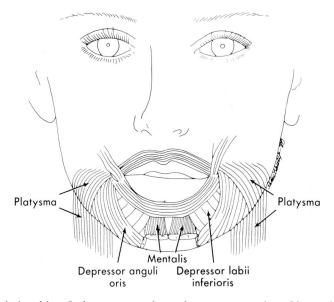

Platysma   Platysma

Mentalis
Depressor anguli   Depressor labii
oris   inferioris

Fig. 16-4. Relationship of platysma muscle to depressor muscles of lower lip. Platysma muscle helps depress corners of lower lip in some patients.

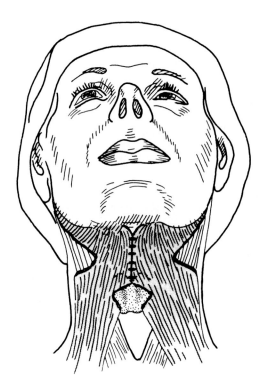

Fig. 16-5. Wedge resection of medial borders of platysma muscle below level of midline approximation interrupts continuity of vertical platysma bands. In addition, lateral borders of platysma are altered as indicated.

nerve (or branch) injury if dissection were carried too deep, (2) parotid cyst formation if the parotid fascia were violated and the gland injured, and (3) surface irregularities in the cheek if SMAS dissection, contouring, and suturing were inadequately performed.

Recurrent platysma muscle bands

Vertical platysma muscle bands appear most often near the midline of the neck. These vertical platysma bands result from the medial borders of the right and left platysma muscle becoming lax as a result of generalized aging of tissues in the neck and accompanying medial descent of the platysma muscles under the force of gravity. Vertical platysma bands situated more laterally in the neck are not uncommon.

Vertical platysma bands without significant muscle redundancy are corrected by midline suturing of the medial platysma muscle borders and a procedure that breaks the continuity of the vertical band (i.e., full-width platysma muscle transection or anterior wedge resection of the muscle border). Redundant medial platysma borders require vertical excision of excess muscle and approximation of the free, cut medial edges in order to reduce anterior neck bulk and give a snug sling effect when lateral muscle flaps are advanced.[4,17] Vertical excision of redundant medial platysma borders and midline approximation of the edges should be done prior to advancing lateral platysma flaps in a cephaloposterior direction. Patients with thin necks and vertical platysma bands can have their appearance improved by midline approximation of the medial platysma borders and resection of a wedge of platysma muscle below the level of platysma approximation (Fig. 16-5). In most patients cephaloposterior advancement of the lateral edge of the platysma muscle in continuity with the SMAS helps secure the desired sling effect on the anterior surface of the neck along the jawline.

Recurrent platysma bands frequently occur in the early postoperative period following conventional face-lifting techniques, which do nothing specifically aimed at eliminating bands. Likewise, recurrent bands can compromise the results of more extensive procedures. When such recurrent bands appear, the cause is likely to be one of the following:

1. Failure to approximate the medial platysma borders in the midline. Full-width or partial-width platysma muscle transection and lateral platysma flap rotation without midline suturing permits the recurrence of medial bands more laterally placed in the neck (Fig. 16-6). Midline suture approximation stabilizes the muscle sling as the lateral platysma borders are retracted laterally.

2. Failure to interrupt the continuity of the band. Midline muscle suturing without muscle band transection and flap rotation does not interrupt vertical muscle bands and may not correct muscle laxity. Prominent midline vertical bands are particularly apt to recur following lateral L-shaped platysma flaps if nothing is done to interrupt the continuity of the medial muscle bands (Fig. 16-7). In fact, with L-shaped platysma flaps, anterior neck bands may recur even when the muscles are approximated in the midline. In such cases the bands may be visible from the inferior limit of muscle approximation down to the clavicles. When full transverse width muscle transection is performed, care must be taken to ensure that the muscle transection is actually complete. It is easy to leave the medial-most portion of the muscle intact when transection is made from lateral to medial. The medial muscle edge must be examined through an anterior neck or submental incision.

3. Excess tension placed on sutures approximating the medial platysma borders, such that the sutures cut through the muscle in the early postoperative period (Fig. 16-8). There are two primary reasons why the sutures may cut through the muscles. First, if sutures approximating the medial platysma borders are tied too tightly, the muscle within the suture loop will rapidly necrose, and the suture will become ineffective, regardless of whether or not lateral platysma flaps are made. One must keep in mind that the platysma is muscle (90% water) and is covered with a thin layer of fascia.

The second cause of recurrent bands caused by excess tension has to do with the relationship between medial muscle approximation and lateral platysma flaps. Suture approximation of the medial platysma borders prior to the creation of platysma flaps laterally stabilizes the midline and produces a secure sling effect when the platysma flaps are advanced in the cephaloposterior direction. Suture approximation of the medial platysma borders after cephaloposterior advancement of the lateral edges of the platysma muscle

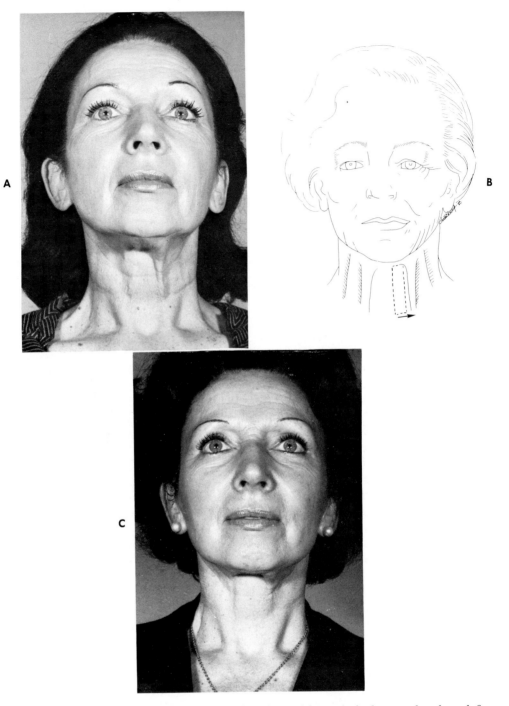

Fig. 16-6. A, Preoperative appearance of patient with vertical platysma band on left side. **B,** Vertical resection of muscle band from left medial platysma border. **C,** Appearance 12 months following vertical resection of portion of left platysma band and full transverse width platysma muscle flap. Medial borders of platysma were not sutured together. Vertical platysma band has moved more laterally. Level of platysma muscle transection is obvious.

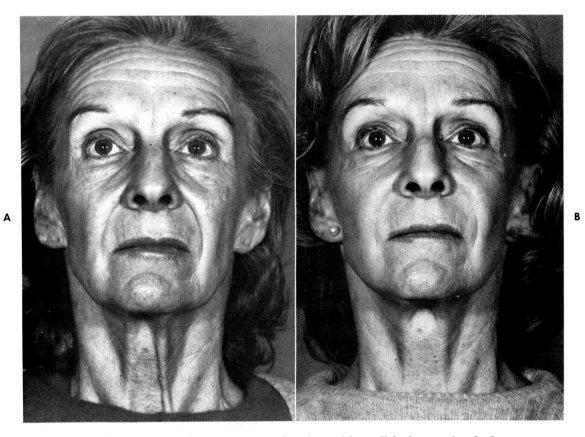

Fig. 16-7. A, Preoperative appearance of patient with medial platysma bands due to redundancy and laxity. **B,** Appearance 13 months following vertical excision of portion of platysma bands and partial-width platysma muscle flap. Medial borders of platysma were not sutured together.

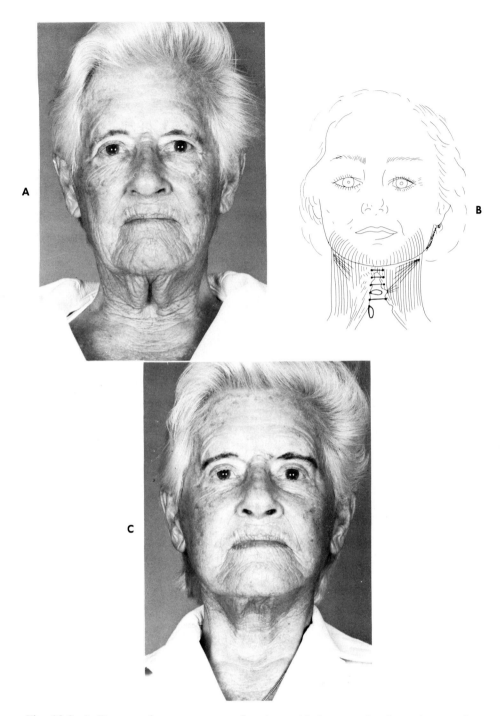

Fig. 16-8. A, Preoperative appearance of patient with large, redundant platysma borders. **B,** Depiction of midline sutures cutting through medial muscle border. **C,** Appearance 7 months following bilateral vertical muscle excision, full-width platysma muscle flaps, and midline muscle suturing as final step in surgical procedure. Midline muscle approximation was under tension. Disruption of midline sutures explains recurrent bands.

may produce excessive tension on the platysma muscle sutures medially. The sutures may "cut through" the medial muscle borders in the early postoperative period, resulting in recurrent platysma bands. In addition, excessive tension on the medial platysma borders for midline approximation may be associated with a great deal of postoperative discomfort, producing a restrictive "band around the neck" or a "feeling of being choked." While neck tightness due to platysma muscle surgery usually subsides after a few weeks, uncomfortable tightness may persist for many months. Platysma and SMAS flaps should be snug but not tight.

Inappropriate level of platysma muscle transection

The platysma muscle surgical technique for each individual patient depends on (1) individual platysma muscle anatomy, which varies in shape, thickness, and elasticity; (2) the skeletal anatomy of the mandible and neck, including hyoid position and size of the thyroid cartilage; and (3) the amount of submental and submandibular fat and occasional subplatysmal fat deposits. The specific anatomy of the patient's deformity determines whether the platysma muscle should be transected full width across its belly, partially transected, or not transected at all. Female patients with vertical bands in a thin neck are best cut and sutured below the upper level of the thyroid cartilage to prevent accentuation of the thyroid cartilage. An overly prominent Adam's apple can be unsightly in a female patient. Some patients with an obtuse cervicomental angle will get a greater deepening of the cervicomental angle and better definition of the neck and jawline if the platysma is transected just at the upper level of the thyroid cartilage, so that the cut muscle contracts above the cartilage. The low-neck fullness of the thyroid cartilage then suggests a smaller neck above and a deeper cervicomental angle.

Transection of the platysma too high in the neck can cause a platysma muscle "roll" in the submandibular area (Fig. 16-9). In patients in whom the platysma muscle is thick, such as

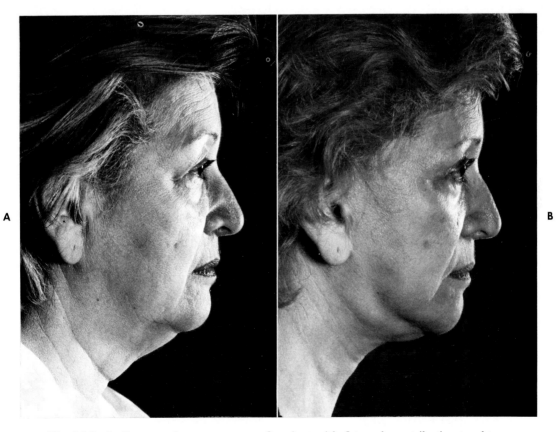

Fig. 16-9. A, Preoperative appearance of patient with fat neck contributing to obtuse cervicomental angle. **B,** Appearance 10 months following lipectomy of neck and full-width transection of platysma muscle too near border of mandible.

women with masculine-type necks, and in men, where the platysma is usually thicker,[7] this problem can be significant and almost impossible to correct. It is difficult to state specific numerical measurements for the level of the platysma muscle transection, since this is part of the surgical judgment that must be made based on a given patient's anatomy. However, I usually begin platysma transection at least 5 to 6 cm below the angle of the mandible. Transection of the platysma at or below this level reduces the chance of marginal mandibular nerve injury. Dingman and Grabb[11] reported that the marginal mandibular nerve is always within 1 cm of the border of the mandible in 100 dissections of cadaverous specimens. Baker and Conley[5] reported finding the marginal mandibular nerve as low as 4 cm below the mandibular border in live surgical dissections. The direction and level of the lateral-to-medial interruption of the platysma is determined by what one is attempting to accomplish in each individual patient.

Inadequate cervicofacial defatting

Platysma-SMAS surgery has stimulated a more aggressive approach to face and neck undermining and to more extensive fat excision. Appropriate cervicofacial fat resection is often more important than platysma-SMAS surgery in obtaining the best possible result in patients with fat faces and necks.

The appearance of the patient with a poorly defined cervicomental angle and a fat face and neck is best improved with lower facial, submental, and submandibular lipectomy, medial platysma muscle suturing, and full-width platysma flaps (Fig. 16-10). If the platysma is found to be thin or attenuated after fat is removed from its surface, complete muscle transection is not necessary. Lateral advancement of the uninterrupted lateral platysma borders or partial-width flaps help form the cervical sling if the midline is stabilized by suturing together the medial platysma borders.

Inadequate cervicofacial fat excision will leave

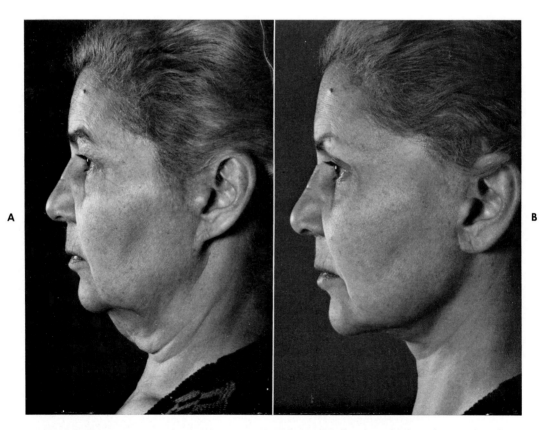

A   B

Fig. 16-10. A, Preoperative appearance of patient with fat deposits in submental and submandibular areas, along jawline, and in cheeks. There is no distinction between cheeks, jawline, and neck as they blend together. **B,** Appearance following lipectomy of neck along jawline and in cheeks, midline muscle suturing, and full-width platysma muscle flaps.

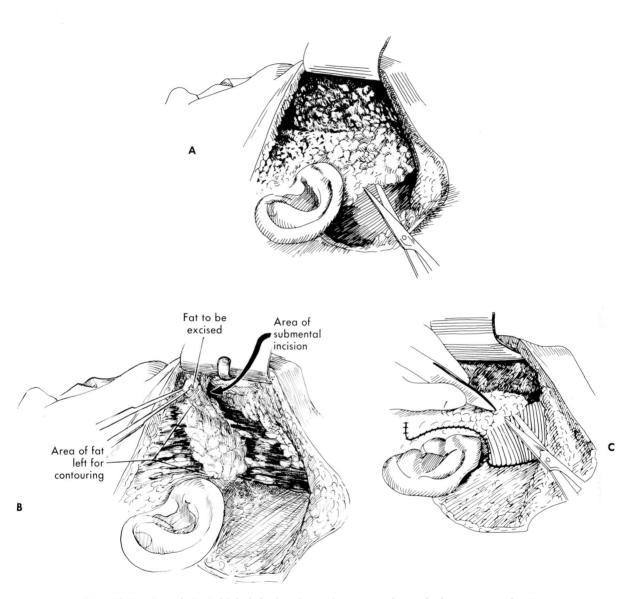

Fig. 16-11. A and **B,** Initial defatting in neck over surface of platysma muscle. Fat immediately adjacent to mandibular border is not resected at this time. **C,** Final jawline contouring after platysma-SMAS flaps have been sutured into position.

deforming bulges along the mandibular border and in the submental and submandibular areas. Residual fat on the surface of the platysma muscle near the mandibular border may be obvious as a bulge in the upper neck after the platysma muscle is transected, producing a smaller neck at the level of the muscle. A major portion of fat excision in the neck along the jawline is performed prior to cutting and rotating platysma and SMAS flaps. The platysma muscle just below the mandibular border is not completely defatted nor final jawline contouring attempted until the platysma-SMAS flap has been sutured into its new position[2,4] (Fig. 16-11). This precaution prevents elevation at defatted muscle above the mandibular border, which would produce an abnormal appearance in the face at the junction of the facial fat and defatted muscle.

The most difficult area of fat resection is beneath the mandibular border just proximal to the medial-most extension of the submaxillary gland. Access to fat in this area is obtained by the combined use of the lateral facial skin flaps and the submental incision.

Cervical contour irregularities

Surface depressions and irregularities may occur following extensive cervicofacial defatting and platysma-modifying procedures. It is particularly important to resect fat evenly across the neck and jawline in order to leave a constant thickness of fat on the skin flap. When the platysma muscle is transected, the superior and inferior cut edges must be beveled to prevent ridges across the neck (Fig. 16-12). This is especially true in men and in women in whom the platysma muscle is thick.

The likelihood of irregularities and neck depressions is significantly diminished if the superficial layer of the deep cervical fascia, which lies just beneath the platysma, is not incised at the time of platysma transection.[1] This layer of fascia provides a smooth subplatysmal surface when it is not violated. Opening the superficial layer of the deep cervical fascia can produce a deep depression just anterior to the sternocleidomastoid muscle, below the angle of the mandible.

Skinny necks with a thick platysma muscle have the potential for a skeletonized appearance if the small amount of existing fat is removed and

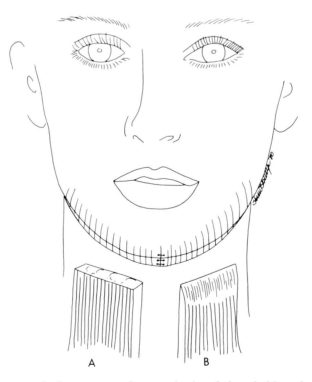

Fig. 16-12. Transected platysma muscle must be beveled and thinned, *A*, to prevent ridges and irregularities in cervical area, *B*.

the platysma muscle is completely transected. This is even more likely to occur in thin necks with prominent sternocleidomastoid muscles. The problem is further accentuated if the superficial layer of the deep cervical fascia is violated.

Ptosis of the submandibular gland is not uncommon. Preoperative examination shows bulges in the digastric triangles due to the submandibular glands in many patients. This is particularly true of patients with short mandibles. A ptotic submandibular gland can be accentuated by extensive cervical defatting. If the platysma is transected too high in the neck, the gland can "fall" from under the muscle and be particularly obvious, spoiling the neck contour. Guerrerosantos[16] reported success in handling this problem by suturing the platysma, cervical fascia, capsule of the submandibular gland, and anterior and posterior bellies of the digastric muscles toward the mastoid fascia so as to lift the gland and the two muscle bellies.

REFERENCES

1. Aston, S.J.: Platysma muscle in rhytidoplasty, Ann. Plast. Surg. **3:**529, 1979.
2. Aston, S.J.: Platysma/SMAS cervicofacial rhytidoplasty, Video Tape Film Library, Educational Foundation, American Society of Plastic and Reconstructive Surgeons, 1980.
3. Aston, S.J.: Male cervicofacial rhytidoplasty. In Courtiss, E., editor: Male aesthetic surgery, Boston, Little, Brown & Co. (In press.)
4. Aston, S.J.: Platysma of SMAS Cervicofacial Rhytidectomy. In Lewis, J.R., editor: Textbook of aesthetic plastic surgery, Boston, Little, Brown & Co., (In press.)
5. Baker, D.C., and Conley, J.: Avoiding facial nerve injuries in rhytidectomy: anatomical variations and pitfalls, Plast. Reconstr. Surg. **64:**781, 1979.
6. Baker, T.J., and Gordon, H.L.: Rhytidectomy in males, Plast. Reconstr. Surg. **44:**219, 1969.
7. Baker, T.J., Gordon, H.L., and Whitlow, D.R.: Our present technique for rhytidectomy, Plast. Reconstr. Surg. **52:**232, 1973.
8. Connell, B.: Cervical lifts—surgical correction of fat contour problems combined with full-width platysma muscle flap, Aesth. Plast. Surg. **1:**355, 1978.
9. Connell, B.: Cervical lifts: the value of platysma muscle flaps, Ann. Plast. Surg. **1:**32, 1978.
10. Connell, B.: Contouring the neck in rhytidectomy by lipectomy and a muscle sling, Plast. Reconstr. Surg. **61:**376, 1978.
11. Dingman, R.O., and Grabb, W.C.: Surgical anatomy of the mandibular ramus of the facial nerve based on the dissection of 100 facial halves, Plast. Reconstr. Surg. **29:**266, 1962.
12. Ellenbogen, R.: Pseudo-paralysis of the mandibular branch of the facial nerve after platysmal face-lift operation, Plast. Reconstr. Surg. **63:**364, 1979.
13. Flowers, R.: Facelift for fat ladies: the extended rhytidectomy, Film presented at the annual meeting of the American Society of Plastic and Reconstructive Surgeons, San Francisco, October 1977.
14. Guerrerosantos, J.: Muscular lift in cervical rhytidoplasty, Plast. Reconstr. Surg. **54:**127, 1974.
15. Guerrerosantos, J.: The role of the platysma muscle in rhytideplasty, Clin. Plast. Surg. **5:**29, 1978.
16. Guerrerosantos, J.: Surgical correction of the fatty fallen neck, Ann. Plast. Surg. **2:**389, 1979.
17. Kaye, B.L.: The extended facelift with ancillary procedures, Ann. Plast. Surg. **6:**335, 1980.
18. Millard, D.R., Jr., Garst, W.P., and Beck, R.L.: Submental and submandibular lipectomy in conjunction with a facelift in the male or female, Plast. Reconstr. Surg. **49:**385, 1972.
19. Millard, D.R., Jr., Pigott, R.W., and Hedo, A.: Submandibular lipectomy, Plast. Reconstr. Surg. **41:**513, 1968.
20. Mitz, V., and Peyronie, M.: Superficial musculoaponeurotic system (SMAS) in the parotid and cheek area, Plast. Reconstr. Surg. **58:**80, 1976.
21. Owsley, J.Q., Jr.: Platysma-fascial rhytidectomy: a preliminary report, Plast. Reconstr. Surg. **60:**843, 1977.
22. Peterson, R.: Cervical-rhytidoplasty—a personal approach, Presented at the Annual Symposium of Aesthetic Plastic Surgery, Guadalajara, Mexico, 1974.
23. Peterson, R.: The role of the platysma muscle in cervical lifts. In Goulian, D., and Courtiss, E.H., editors: Symposium on surgery of the aging face, St. Louis, 1978, The C.V. Mosby Co.
24. Rees, T.D.: Cosmetic facial surgery, Philadelphia, 1973, W.B. Saunders Co.
25. Skoog, T.: Rhytidoplasty—a personal experience and technique, Presented at the Seventh Annual Symposium on Cosmetic Surgery, Miami, February 1973.
26. Skoog, T.: Plastic surgery: new methods and refinements, Philadelphia, 1974, W.B. Saunders Co.
27. Vistnes, L.M., and Souther, S.G.: The anatomical basis for common cosmetic anterior neck deformities, Ann. Plast. Surg. **2:**381, 1979.

Chapter 17

Platysma-SMAS rhytidectomy: a 4-year experience with 273 patients

John Q. Owsley, Jr.

I first used the technique of platysma-SMAS rhytidectomy, which is an extension and modification of the Skoog rhytidectomy, in January 1976.[6,9] A preliminary report on the procedure, published in December 1977,[7] includes a description of my personal experience with 80 patients in whom the Skoog technique was used and 65 patients in whom the platysma-SMAS technique was performed.

The significant difference between the platysma-SMAS technique and the Skoog procedure is that in the platysma-SMAS rhytidectomy the entire superficial musculoaponeurotic system (SMAS), starting in the immediate pretragal region of the face, is elevated in continuity with the platysma muscle from the level of the zygomatic arch to the lower neck. The lifting effect in the cheek and labiomandibular area is effected by advancing the entire SMAS upward and laterally. After resection of the redundant SMAS and muscle tissue, this deep flap is fixed with buried sutures along the zygomatic arch and from the pretragal area down to the midneck level. Since the cheek and neck skin and the subcutaneous tissues are intimately adherent to the deeper platysma-SMAS flap, the lifting effect is attained from the tissues deep to the skin with less extensive superficial dissection. The major advantage of this technique over the Skoog procedure is that the fascial flap, which is elevated from the parotid region, is more substantial than the SMAS tissue, which thins out anterior to the masseter border. The preparotid SMAS will hold sutures with greater tension, and suturing in the pretragal region is not associated with dimpling or puckering, as is frequently encountered in the anterior cheek skin when the Skoog fixation is used.

In the preliminary report on the platysma-SMAS technique, several advantages of the procedure are suggested. These include the benefits of undermining in an avascular plane with minimal separation of the skin from its underlying subcutaneous bed, as well as more rapid healing of the skin incisions, since the major tension of the lift is taken on the deeper fascial layer. Potential disadvantages, including longer operating time and the possibility of injury to the major veins in the neck as well as the branches of the facial and cervical plexus nerves, are acknowledged. At the suggestion of the editor of *Plastic and Reconstructive Surgery*, a cautionary paragraph indicates that this technique requires careful and detailed knowledge of the anatomy of the face and neck and is probably not an appropriate operation to be performed by the novice surgeon.

RESULTS

With this in mind, it seems appropriate to review my experience with the platysma-SMAS rhytidectomy technique over a 4-year period to assess the nature of complications encountered with this operation. During the 4-year period from July 1, 1976, through June 30, 1980, I performed a platysma-SMAS rhytidectomy on 273 patients (Table 17-1). In each instance, I performed the entire operation, including closure of the incisions on both sides. In most instances assistance was provided by an operating room nurse or technician. Approximately two thirds of the patients underwent simultaneous blepharoplasty, and 25 pa-

146

tients in the last 2-year period underwent simultaneous coronal brow lift. A small number of selected patients with extensive cervical fatty deposits had additional subcutaneous undermining of the neck skin and extensive submandibular and submental lipectomies performed.

The charts of the 273 patients were reviewed, and the complications that occurred are listed in Table 17-2. Hematoma was found to be the most common complication, as has been reported in other publications regarding face-lift complications.[1,5,8,10] Intraoperative hematoma, requiring reopening of the initially closed first side, occurred in four patients and was associated in each instance with the acute onset of intraoperative hypertension.[2] The use of intravenous prochlorperazine (Compazine) has been helpful in lowering the elevated blood pressure in such situations, and recently I have also used droperidol for the same effect with good success.

Six patients developed postoperative expanding hematomas that required secondary reoperation within 12 to 24 hours after the face-lift. The 2.2% occurrence of expanding hematoma in this group of patients compares favorably with other published statistics of face-lift complications. I have not done a statistical evaluation of the occurrence of expanding hematoma in my practice prior to using the platysma-SMAS technique, but it remains my impression that expanding hematoma occurred less frequently in this series than in my experience with the standard subcutaneous rhytidectomy. Twenty-four patients had small, localized hematomas requiring needle aspiration during follow-up office care.

The occurrence of five infections was distressing. In three instances the infection occurred in a small, unrecognized hematoma in the area around or behind the earlobe. Patients undergoing platysma-SMAS rhytidectomy normally exhibit more swelling in this area because of the deep suture placement in the platysma muscle flap, and the clinical differentiation between edema in the fatty muscle flap and a small hematoma is sometimes uncertain until fluctuation in the liquefying clot becomes apparent. In three patients infection was diagnosed only after aspiration or drainage through the postauricular incision revealed purulent blood. Appropriate culture and antibiotic therapy was instituted and resulted in rapid resolution of the infection and primary healing.

Table 17-1. Platysma-SMAS rhytidectomy: July 1, 1976, to June 30, 1980

	Rhytidectomy	Simultaneous blepharoplasty	Simultaneous coronal brow lift
1976-1977	57	40	0
1977-1978	51	38	0
1978-1797	80	47	10
1979-1980	85	57	15
TOTALS	273	182	25

Table 17-2. Platysma-SMAS rhytidectomy: 273 operations

Complications	Number of patients	Percentage
Intraoperative hematoma incision reopened	4	1.5
Postoperative expanding hematoma requiring reoperation within 24 hours	6	2.2
Small, localized hematoma requiring needle aspiration during office care	24	8.9
Infection		
Purulent small hematoma responding to office drainage or aspiration plus oral antibiotics	3	1.2
Major infection requiring hospitalization	2	0.7
Facial motor nerve injury		
Frontal	0	0
Buccal	0	0
Cervicomandibular	9	3.3
Motor function recovery within 3 months	8	3.0
Motor function recovery within 6 months	1	0.3
Permanent motor deficit	0	0
Superficial skin incision necrosis	5	1.8
Major skin necrosis	0	0
Temporal hair loss		
Temporary with regrowth in 3 to 4 months	5	1.8
Permanent	0	0
Laceration of external jugular vein requiring ligation	1	0.3
Laceration of greater auricular nerve requiring suture repair	1	0.3

There were two instances of more severe problems with infection requiring hospitalization. One woman developed a high fever and evidence of rapidly developing cellulitis of the left cheek 5 days after her operation. She was treated empirically initially with cephalexin monohydrate (Keflex) and then with intravenous penicillin after hospitalization. Twenty-four hours after hospital admission the left preauricular incision was probed, resulting in drainage of several ml of purulent blood. Culture revealed *Staphylococcus epidermidis* sensitive to erythromycin. There was rapid resolution of the cellulitis with continuing specific antibotic therapy, and the patient made an uneventful recovery without skin loss. Ultimately she had a good aesthetic result.

The second patient, a man who lived some distance away, had an unusual course. A small hematoma in the midregion of the left side of the neck was aspirated approximately a week after surgery, drawing off 4 ml of noninfected liquefied clot. This area appeared to resolve satisfactorily, but several months later the patient returned with recurrence of swelling in the left neck area. A fluctuant mass was present in the region of the previous hematoma aspiration. With the patient under local anesthesia, a 1 cm incision was made in an overlying skin crease and a collection of several ml of purulent material was drained. A Penrose drain was placed and left in position for 5 days. Following removal of the drain, the skin incision healed. Unfortunately, the abcess recurred approximately a month later, and at this time surgical exploration of the area was performed with the patient under general anesthesia.

Through a direct incision over the abcess, a chronic, thick-wall granulating cavity overlying the sternocleidomastoid muscle was exposed and dissected out with some difficulty. The cavity was approximately 5 cm in diameter. The incision was closed primarily with suction drainage, which was left in place for several days. The wound cultured *Staphylococcus epidermidis,* and with appropriate antibiotic therapy for 10 days, the defect healed per primam, and there has been no further recurrence of difficulty in the area.

The risk of facial nerve injury has been a source of major concern in the performance of either the Skoog procedure or platysma-SMAS rhytidctomy.[5] In my initial cautious experience with 80 cases involving the Skoog procedure and in 65 platysma-fascial rhytidectomies, there were no facial nerve injuries.[7] With increasing familiarity with the procedure, I explored the limits of dissection more boldly. In this group of 273 patients, 9 exhibited some disturbance in the motor function of the lower lip. In most instances it was primarily related to the depressor action of the corner of the mouth. Retention of pursing and whistling ability suggested that the deficit was chiefly in the platysma-depressor and related to a cervical branch injury.[4] In two instances there was a greater degree of elevation of the lateral corner and loss of lip function, suggesting that the marginal mandibular branch was not functioning.

There were no permanent motor nerve disturbances; all nine patients who showed initial weakness of the corner of the mouth made a complete recovery of motor function within 3 to 6 months following surgery. There were no instances of temporal or buccal-branch nerve injuries. In an analysis of the occurrence of nerve injuries, it was apparent that these cases ocurred in clusters. In 1978 I introduced the use of a narrow, deep retractor in the performance of the subplatysmal neck dissection and attempted to perform a more extensive separation of the muscle from the underlying deep cervical fascia. This extension in the dissection of all of the fibrous adhesions between the muscle and deep fascia was associated in a short period with four patients who exhibited weakness of the lower lip on one side. I subsequently eliminated the use of the deep retractor and simply relied on hook retraction of the lateral edge of the platysma-SMAS flap. Also, the cutting of the fascial attachments was reduced again to a more blunt and spreading type of dissection, leaving multiple fibrous adhesions.* There were no additional patients with nerve weakness during the following year.

In late 1979 I began to divide the platysma muscle along the lower line of dissection from the lateral border to the anterior midline by approaching the muscle with blunt scissors from beneath the dissected platysma flap. The separation of the platysma was done with minimal superficial dissection of the skin overlying the lower portion of the platysma. I did this platysma muscle division in an attempt to reduce the recurrence of cervical platysma cords, similar to the technique advocated by other surgeons who divide the platysma flap.[3] Three cases of mouth weakness occurred among approximately 50 patients in whom

---

*EDITOR'S NOTE: This is a safer type of dissection. Significant large nerves are strong and will not part with gentle, blunt dissection. However, no nerve can withstand the onslaught of a scissors or knife. (B.L.K.)

this technique was used. All retained pursing and whistling mobility of the lips, so that the deficit appeared to be primarily related to the function of the platysma muscle. All recovered depressor action of the mouth corner within 3 months. Presently I limit platysma muscle division to patients in whom preexisting cervical cords are a prominent problem and take great care to make the transection of the muscle at a level below the superior cervical crease.

The skin incisions healed per primam in all but five patients, who developed small areas of superficial incisional necrosis in the areas of maximum tension above the root of the ear or in the mastoid region. All of these areas healed secondarily with minimal scarring and did not require scar revision. There were no major skin losses in this series, which I feel is a significant substantiation of the value of the technique. Five patients developed partial hair loss in the temple scalp flap adjacent to the scar line, but there was gradual regrowth of the hair within 3 to 4 months following the operation. There were no permanent areas of hair loss.

The external jugular vein was lacerated during the subplatysmal dissection in 1 patient, requiring ligation of the vein. In a second instance there was a partial laceration of the greater auricular nerve, which was repaired with fine sutures. Both of these incidents occurred during my early experience with the procedure, and no major vein or sensory nerve injury in the neck has occurred in the last 3 years. It is worthwhile to point out that the greater auricular nerve and the external jugular vein are almost routinely visualized during the dissection.

As noted in the earlier report on this technique, a longer operating time is a significant factor in the performance of the the sub-SMAS and platysma muscle dissection. With increasing experience, I have reduced my operating time for face-lifting from 3 to 2 hours in most cases, eliminating one of the disadvantages initially cited. This improved facility is, of course, based entirely on encountering an average amount of bleeding during the dissection.

From this present review, it is apparent that hematoma and injury of the facial motor nerve are the most common and significant complications occurring with the platysma-SMAS rhytidectomy. The statistical frequency of hematoma appears to be comparable to that occurring with any type of face-lift procedure.

Facial nerve injuries occurring in this series were all temporary in nature, from which we can conclude that no motor nerves were cut in this series of patients. It is important to note that extensive, elevation of the SMAS flap was performed on both sides in the 273 patients without a single instance of frontal or buccal-branch nerve injury, suggesting that the SMAS dissection is a safe technique. The frequency of injury to the lower branches of the facial nerve in the neck appears comparable to that in other reported series. Careful, gentle spreading dissection in the course of the marginal mandibular nerve branch should ensure its safety. I take care to limit dissection along the border of the mandible to that area posterior to the anterior facial artery where the marginal branch commonly passes below the mandible. It is possible to preserve the cervical branch of the facial nerve by using gentle spreading dissection beneath the platysma without cutting across the multiple fibrous adhesions that do not really limit upward advancement of the platysma-SMAS flap. Transection of the platysma muscle, when indicated, must be performed at a low level in order to reduce the occurrence of loss of function of the platysma in the upper neck and mandibular region.

REFERENCES

1. Baker, D.C., and Conley, J.: Avoiding facial nerve injuries in rhytidectomy: anatomical variations and pitfalls, Plast. Reconstr. Surg. **64:**781, 1979.
2. Berner, R.E., Morain, W.D., and Noe, J.M.: Postoperative hypertension as an etiological factor in hematoma after rhytidectomy: prevention with chlorpromazine, Plast. Reconstr. Surg. **57:**314, 1976.
3. Connell, B.: Contouring the neck in rhytidectomy by lipectomy with a muscle sling, Plast. Reconstr. Surg. **61:**376, 1978.
4. Ellenbogen, R.: Pseudo-paralysis of the mandibular branch of the facial nerve after platysmal face-lift operation, Plast. Reconstr. Surg. **63:**364, 1979.
5. Lemmon, M.L., and Hamra, S.T.: Skoog rhytidectomy: a five year experience with 577 patients, Plast. Reconstr. Surg. **65:**283, 1980.
6. Mitz, V., and Peyronie, M.: Superficial musculoaponeurotic system (SMAS) in the parotid and cheek area, Plast. Reconstr. Surg. **58:**80, 1976.
7. Owsley, J.Q., Jr.: Platysma-fascial rhytidectomy: a preliminary report, Plast. Reconstr. Surg. **60:**843, 1977.
8. Rees, T.D., Lee, Y.C., and Coburn, R.J.: Expanding hematoma after rhytidectomy: a retrospective study, Plast. Reconstr. Surg. **51:**149, 1973.
9. Skoog, T.: Plastic surgery: new methods and refinements, Philadelphia, 1974, W.B. Saunders Co.
10. Thompson, D.P., and Ashley, F.L.: Face-lift complications: a study of 922 cases performed in a 6-year period, Plast. Reconstr. Surg. **61:**40, 1978.

Chapter 18

Anatomy and injuries of the facial nerve in cervicofacial rhytidectomy

Daniel C. Baker

Recently, because the improvement in appearance of the aging or fatty neck from a standard face-lift was sometimes disappointing to both the patient and the surgeon, more extensive and deeper techniques have been developed.[5,12,16,25,29] With the more aggressive methods in which the surgeon elevates the superficial musculoaponeurotic system (SMAS), including platysma muscle and subplatysmal flaps, the dissection is deeper in the face and neck, and this increases the risk of facial nerve injury, especially when the surgeon is inexperienced.

ANATOMY OF THE FACIAL NERVE

Although many dissections have been done to establish the usual pattern, position, and variations,[9] these are relative and cannot be relied on for the specific anatomy of the nerve in the patient at hand. The significance of this is obvious in any operation where a dissection is done in certain levels and the nerve is never specifically visualized.

From clinical experience with parotidectomies, I have found that each facial nerve has its own complex and varied, individual pattern.[1] The main trunk is the most consistent portion of the nerve, usually with a bifurcation inside the parotid gland.

Mandibular branch

The popularization of the techniques for resection of submental and submandibular fat external to the platysma muscle and the transection of this muscle to create a flap require the surgeon

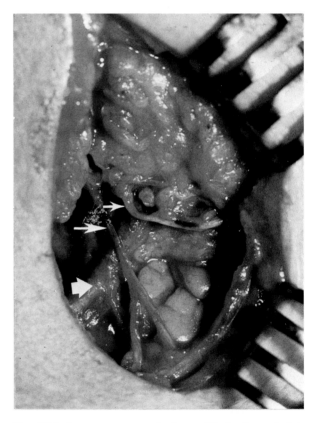

Fig. 18-1. Lowermost marginal mandibular branch *(upper arrow)* and cervical branch *(middle arrow)* passing over facial vein *(lower arrow)* and beneath platysma. (From Baker, D.C., and Conley, J.: Avoiding facial nerve injuries in rhytidectomy, Plast. Reconstr. Surg. **64:**781, 1979.)

using them to be careful to avoid injury to the mandibular division of the facial nerve and its branches (Fig. 18-1).

In 1962 Dingham and Grabb[10] presented an excellent study of the mandibular ramus of the facial nerve, based on the dissection of 100 facial halves. They found that the posterior to the facial artery the mandibular ramus ran above the inferior border of the mandible in 81% of their specimens. In the other 19% the nerve or one or more of its branches ran in an arc, the lowest point of which was 1 cm or less below the inferior border of the mandible. Anterior to the facial artery, all of the branches of the mandibular rami were superior to the inferior border of the mandible. However, they also noted that in many specimens fine branches could be seen running along the lower border of the mandible, some up to 2 cm below it, and that every one of these branches terminated in the platysma.

The above-mentioned study has been a great aid to the surgeon. However, it is important to remember that these dissections were done on cadavers, and that in fixed specimens the tissues are stiff, contracted, less mobile, and shrunken. In clinical experiences with parotidectomies and radical neck dissections, the mandibular branch of the facial nerve was located 1 to 2 cm below the lower border of the mandible in almost every instance.[1,24] In some individuals with lax and atrophic tissues, the branches were as much as 3 to 4 cm below the inferior border of the mandible. It is also important to remember that on the operating table when one extends the neck of the patient, this draws the nerve even lower.

Although the descending cervical division innervates the main body of the platysma muscle at a much lower level, the mandibular division also innervates the upper and anterior portion of this muscle in at least half the cases. Any surgical intervention in this region, or any surgical intervention deep to the platysma muscle for the removal of fat, can put this nerve in jeopardy. Approximately 15% of patients have a connection between the mandibular division and the buccal division (from the upper segment of the facial nerve); in these, the functions of the mandibular nerve may return to a certain degree after it is cut. In the remainder of the cases, however, injury to this nerve may leave a permanent deficit; the latter may be a subtle one if only the platysma muscle branches are affected, but it will be a conspicuous deficit if the entire mandibular division is involved.

Midfacial branches

In his technique for a face-lift, Skoog[29] used blunt dissection between the superficial fascia and the underlying buccinator fat pad, and he tightened the anterior cheek and nasolabial area by pulling the buccal fascia back and suturing it to the masseteric fascia. According to him, the buccal fat pad "covers the parotid duct and facial nerves and vessels on the external surface of the buccinator." However, in my clinical experience in parotidectomies, I have found that the facial nerve lies on the external surface of the fat pad and its thin fascia, and that delicate nerve branches also lie just under the fascia of the masseter muscle at this level (Fig. 18-2) Obviously, dissection in this area must be done cautiously, and plication sutures through the masseteric fascia carry a risk of injury to facial nerve branches.

Studies by Mitz and Peyronie[22] on the SMAS have demonstrated that anatomical dissection in a plane deep to the SMAS over the parotid can be efficacious in a rhytidectomy. In this region the facial nerve is well protected by the overlying gland. They stress, however, that anterior to the parotid area the SMAS is thin, and surgical dissection of the SMAS in this area may be dangerous and difficult. Patients with scant subcutaneous tissue or small parotid glands do not have much protection of the nerve branches here.

Owsley[25] agrees with Mitz and Peyronie[22] that the SMAS becomes thin in the anterior part of the cheek and that suture fixation of the SMAS anterior to the border of the masseter muscle and parotid gland has not been satisfactory.

Mitz and Peyronie emphasize that in the pretragal area and over the parotid gland dissection of the SMAS is relatively safe, but anterior to the parotid such dissection becomes difficult and dangerous. They stress that injury to the facial nerve branches may occur (1) when the SMAS is thin, (2) when the retrofascial dissection is carried too far forward (beyond the anterior edge of the parotid gland), and (3) when the superficial parotid lobe is short, leaving the nerves unprotected.

Facial muscles

Any surgeon using the platysma muscle and subplatysmal techniques should understand the musculature about the mouth, lower lip (Fig. 18-3), and neck and its innervation. The marginal mandibular branch innervates the depressor anguli oris, the depressor labii inferioris, the mentalis, part of the orbicularis oris, and the risorius.[14,15]

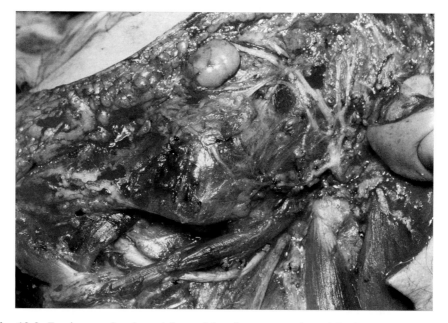

Fig. 18-2. Fascia covering buccal fat pad has been opened, and fat is seen protruding between branches of facial nerve. Note fine branches lying just on top of masseter muscle. (Cervical and marginal mandibular branches have been sacrificed in total parotidectomy for melanoma.) (From Baker, D.C., and Conley, J.: Avoiding facial nerve injuries in rhytidectomy, Plast. Reconstr. Surg. **64:**781, 1979.)

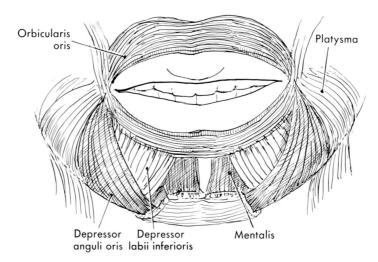

Fig. 18-3. Circumoral and depressor muscles of lower lip. (From Baker, D.C., and Conley, J.: Avoiding facial nerve injuries in rhytidectomy, Plast. Reconstr. Surg. **64:**781, 1979.)

Rubin[28] has categorized three basic types of human smile, each dependent on the relative strength of the individual muscle groups about the mouth.

Ellenbogen[11] has emphasized that the platysma muscle is important in the "full-denture" smile, in which the lower teeth are exposed and the vermilion is everted. He has correctly noted that severing one or all cervical branches of the facial nerve in cutting a platysma flap can give the appearance of a palsy of the marginal mandibular branch. The deformity is not as severe, of course, as that resulting from cutting the entire mandibular division (with a paresis of all of the depressors of the lower lip).

PREVENTING FACIAL NERVE INJURY IN RHYTIDECTOMY

Castañares[3] has reviewed some of the possible causes of facial nerve injury during a rhytidectomy, including the following (Fig. 18-4):

1. Preoperative palsy, coincident Bell's palsy, other concomitant neuropathology, or "normal" facial asymmetry
2. Trauma from the heat of electrocoagulation
3. Local anesthesia injected in the immediate nerve area
4. Deep ligatures or plication sutures
5. Crushing by forceps or clamps
6. Excessive traction and undue stretching
7. Transection of a nerve during deep dissection
8. Hematoma or edema within the nerve sheath
9. Inflammation and infection
10. Distortion of the normal anatomy by adhesions from previous face-lifts or surgery

In the preoperative consultation and evaluation, it may be advisable for the surgeon to inquire about the patient's past history of facial nerve problems such as Bell's palsy. Castañares[3] reported the recurrence of this problem during the postoperative period, and a complete facial paralysis postoperatively warrants a neurological evaluation. A careful notation of facial asymmetries or muscular weakness is essential in the preoperative visit, and these should be pointed out to the patient, who is rarely aware of their presence.

Following the infiltration of the face with a local anesthetic solution, it is not uncommon for a temporary paralysis to occur. As the drug is diffused and metabolized, complete recovery occurs.

It is essential that care be taken in placing any plication sutures, especially about the eye and the buccal region, to avoid compressing and catching small branches of the nerve. This could produce a more lasting paralysis.

Preventing nerve injury during electrocoagulation

Hemostasis with the electrocautery must be done with care, and the current must be low—especially in the vulnerable areas, such as the temporal region—to avoid heat injury to the nerve branches. Contraction of the frontalis or orbicularis muscles during electrocoagulation should be a warning that the nerve is nearby. Similarly, pressure by coagulation forceps on bleeders may pinch an adjacent nerve branch and thus cause damage.

Preventing nerve injury during the raising of fascial or muscle flaps

Extreme caution is mandatory during any raising of the SMAS or a platysma muscle flap. In patients with atrophy or hypoplasia of the platysma muscle, there is very little muscle or fascia over the marginal mandibular branch of the facial nerve. In secondary or tertiary face-lifts, there may be extensive subcutaneous fibrosis, with adhesions of the skin to the underlying platysma muscle, distorting the normal anatomy and making penetration of the muscle by scissors easy and a real danger to the underlying facial nerve branches. Extensive undermining in these patients must be done cautiously, and preferably under direct vision.*

The variations in the anatomy of the marginal mandibular branch have been stressed. Therefore any platysma muscle transection should begin at least 5 cm below the lower mandibular border and be kept in line with the thyroid cartilage. Extra caution should be taken in those patients with very lax skin and atrophic tissue. In removing fat from over the platysma muscle, one should gently taper the excision, rather than picking up a lump and cutting. Removal of fat from over the mandible should always be done under direct vision, using good lighting with constant identification of the level of the platysma muscle. If the muscle is not discernible, removal of fat carries an obvious added risk.

---

*EDITOR'S NOTE: Under these circumstances, undermining should be done with gentle, blunt dissection, such as by spreading with small scissors, or with a finger, wherever possible. (B.L.K.)

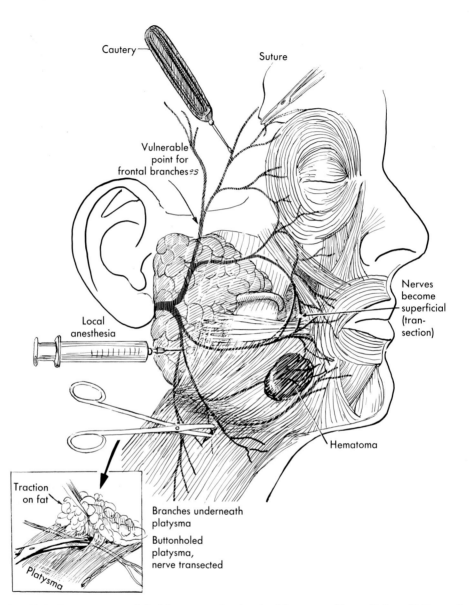

Cautery

Suture

Vulnerable
point for
frontal branches

Local
anesthesia

Nerves
become
superficial
(tran-
section)

Hematoma

Traction
on fat

Platysma

Branches underneath
platysma

Buttonholed
platysma,
nerve transected

Fig. 18-4. Some causes of facial nerve palsy in rhytidectomy. (From Baker, D.C., and Conley, J.: Avoiding facial nerve injuries in rhytidectomy, Plast. Reconstr. Surg. **64:**781, 1979.)

Preventing injury to the temporal division

The frontal branch of the facial nerve is vulnerable to injury in its rather superficial position as it crosses the midpoint of the zygomatic arch. Several authors have studied its anatomy in relation to the face-lift.[9,19,26-28] The temporal branches of the nerve run along the superficial surface of the temporalis fascia. Any operation in which one enters this level or goes beneath it, in the area of the temple, places the motor nerve branches in jeopardy.[8]

After the zygomatic nerve branch exits from the superior part of the parotid gland, it passes over the zygomatic arch beneath the superficial fascia and a thin layer of fibrofatty tissue prior to piercing more deeply into the superficial level of the temporalis fascia (which attaches to the upper portion of the zygoma). This nerve is under jeopardy in this area in face-lift patients who are thin and who have little soft tissue covering the zygomatic arch. Hydrodissection of the superficial layer, by infiltration with local anesthetic solution, is a protective measure.

In a deeper (subfascial) approach in the frontal region, it is imperative to appreciate that the branches of the facial nerve are lateral (superficial) to the dissection at this level in the forehead, whereas in the face they are medial (deep) to the plane of dissection.[8] (This is in accordance with the embryonic derivation of these muscles from the superficial myomere. Peripheral muscle migration separates the superficial myomere from the interlacing derivation of the deep myomere in the middle third of the face.) The connection of these two planes is at the zygomatic arch, and this is where injury may be inflicted on the frontal branch going to the forehead. This branch is superficial as it passes over the zygoma. The deeper technique should therefore be limited at this point, preserving this fascial pedicle and the nerve branch by a two-plane development.[16] (This technical problem does not exist when all planes of dissection are carried out in the superficial fascia.)

If the frontal branch is only stretched or lightly traumatized, it will usually recover within 6 months. Complete transection, however, will result in permanent paralysis or incomplete recovery of forehead movement, because fewer than 15% of these nerve fibers in the brow have any connection with other branches of the same or opposite facial nerve. On the other hand, because of the multiple connections between the facial nerve branches to the orbicularis oculi, paralysis of the eyelids is more unusual after one of them is cut.

(Converse and Coburn[6] reported one such case, in which the patient recovered completely within 1 year.)

Preventing injury to the buccal division

Injury to the buccal branch occurs most often in the loose areolar tissue anterior to the parotid gland, where the nerve becomes superficial to innervate the muscles about the commissure, mouth, and cheek. When an SMAS dissection is carried anterior to the parotid gland, care must be taken to avoid injury to these fine filaments; gentle blunt dissection under direct vision is advised.[16] In this region any plication to the masseteric fascia carries the risk of catching the nerve where it passes over the muscle. Such an injury can usually cause paralysis of a portion of the cheek, upper lip, nasal lobule, commissure of the mouth, and (occasionally) the lower eyelid. However, the fortuitous branching connection system, involving 90% of the nerve filaments in the buccal and zygomatic regions, greatly favors spontaneous return of movement within 3 to 6 months. Sometimes this return of movement may be associated with a slight lag or imbalance; worse, it may result in the development of a spontaneous tic. (Converse and Coburn[6] reported the case of a celebrated South American actress who developed facial twitching after a face-lift, consisting of spasmodic elevations of the upper lip when she was under emotional stress.)

Deformity of marginal mandibular palsy

It is a common misconception that damage to the marginal mandibular branch of the facial nerve results in a drooping of the corner of the mouth. Actually, the opposite occurs—an inability to draw the lower lip downward and laterally or to evert the vermilion border[1,23] (Figs. 18-5 and 18-6). When the patient smiles, that side of the lower lip remains up and becomes flattened and inwardly rotated from the pull of the opposite side and the decreased movement on the paralyzed side (Fig. 18-7).

The deformity is not apparent with the face in repose, because the other depressors are not functioning at that time. Because the orbicularis oris is supplied also by the buccal branch, it may be involved only to a minor extent (or not at all). The deformity results from the failure of the depressor anguli oris and depressor labii inferioris on that side to draw that half of the lower lip downward and laterally. The antagonists to these muscles are then free to exert their pulls unopposed.

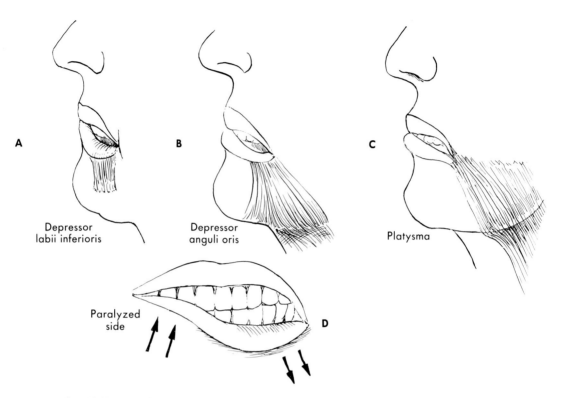

Fig. 18-5. A, Action of depressor labii inferioris is to evert vermilion border and also move lower lip downward and laterally. **B,** Action of depressor anguli oris moves lower lip downward and laterally. **C,** Action of platysma also moves lower lip downward and laterally. **D,** Deformity produced by marginal mandibular palsy primarily results from inaction of the two depressor muscles. Elevators may accentuate this deformity by pulling inert lower lip upward and laterally. Platysma is significant active depressor in only a small percentage of individuals. (From Baker, D.C., and Conley, J.: Avoiding facial nerve injuries in rhytidectomy, Plast. Reconstr. Surg. **64:**781, 1979.)

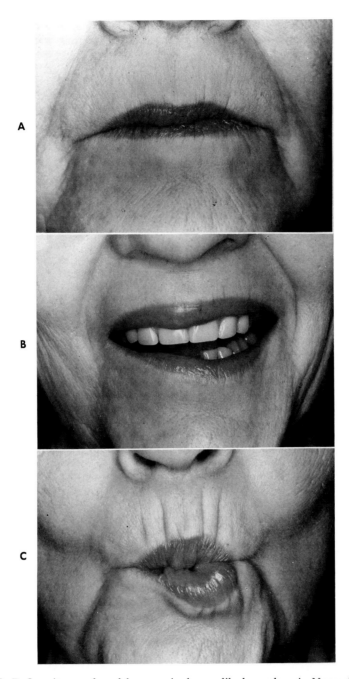

Fig. 18-6. Deformity produced by marginal mandibular palsy. **A,** Normal appearance in repose except for slight loss of bulk in right lower lip. **B,** Inability to draw paralyzed right lower lip downward and laterally as well as inability to evert vermilion border. **C,** Portion of orbicularis oris is involved in this patient. Because this muscle is also supplied by buccal branch, it may only be involved to a variable extent or not at all. (From Baker, D.C., and Conley, J.: Avoiding facial nerve injuries in rhytidectomy, Plast. Reconstr. Surg. **64:**781, 1979.)

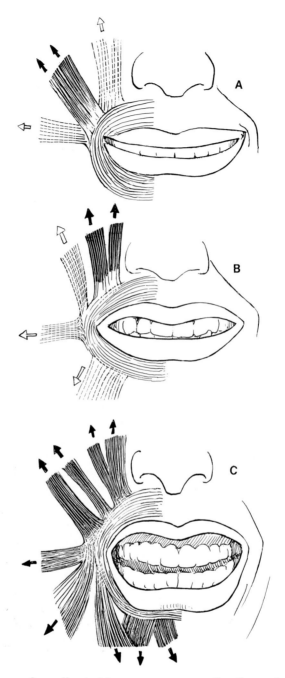

Fig. 18-7. Anatomy of a smile. **A,** Most common type of smile results from dominant pull by zygomaticus major lifting angle of mouth. There is minimal or no counteraction from depressors. **B,** More action and dominance from levator labii superioris produces "canine" smile. There is usually some counteraction from depressors, but none from platysma. **C,** "Full-denture" smile is least common (only 2% according to Rubin) and results from all elevators and depressors of lips and angles contracting. Platysma muscle action is usually significant. (After Rubin.[28] From Baker, D.C., and Conley, J.: Avoiding facial nerve injuries in rhytidectomy, Plast. Reconstr. Surg. **64:**781, 1979.)

It has already been stressed that patients with atrophy or hypoplasia of the platysma muscle may have very little protection of the marginal mandibular branch of the facial nerve at the level of the lower border of the mandible. Also, in patients with atrophic skin and subcutaneous tissue, its vulnerability is obviously increased. Any dissection beneath the platysma muscle at this level may cause injury. Only about 15% of the nerve filaments of the marginal mandibular branch communicate with the major buccal system in the middle third of the face, making spontaneous, complete return of movement unlikely in most of these cases. Fortunately, however, the marginal mandibular nerve normally consists of two or three branches, so that injury to only one branch may cause no more than a slight weakness, which may eventually improve spontaneously.

INCIDENCE OF FACIAL NERVE INJURY IN RHYTIDECTOMY

The incidence of injury to the facial nerve during a standard rhytidectomy has been reported as being between 0.4% and 2.6%.[21] A review of the larger reported series of face-lifts and the accompanying complications (Table 18-1) shows 50 cases of paralysis in about 6500 face-lifts, for an average of 0.7%.[1] Of these 50 paralyses, only 7 were reported as being permanent (0.1%). The most frequently injured branches were the temporal and the marginal mandibular. Most patients had recovered from these injuries within 6 months. There were no reports of complete facial paralysis except for two cases mentioned by Castañares.[3]

Nearly all of the published reports that evaluate complications concern the standard face-lift with subcutaneous undermining. However, a recent oral report by Peterson (at the 1977 meeting of the American Society for Aesthetic Plastic Surgery) and a published report by Connell,[5] in which the platysma muscle was transected, listed no cases of facial paralysis. Owsley[25] also reported the use of a platysma-SMAS technique on 145 patients, with no facial nerve injuries. Lemmon and Hamra[18] reported 10 cases of facial nerve palsy in 577 face-lifts in which they used the Skoog technique; there was complete recovery of function in all 10 cases within 6 months. All of these newer, deeper face-lifts obviously require more time with more precautions taken in doing the dissection under direct vision, often with the use of fiberoptic lights under the skin flaps. This undoubtedly helps to prevent facial nerve injuries while these more risky procedures are being done.

MANAGEMENT OF NERVE INJURIES

Partial facial paralysis after a rhytidectomy may come as an unexpected surprise to the surgeon and the patient postoperatively, or the surgeon may have become aware of it during the operative procedure.

When the transection of a facial nerve branch is recognized during the operation, the surgeon should attempt to repair it by microsurgical techniques. Most often, however, such injuries are not

Table 18-1. Facial nerve injuries in rhytidectomy

Year	Author	Face-lifts	Paralyses	%	Temporal	Buccal	Mandibular	Recovered	Time
1970	Conway[7]	325	2	0.6	2			0	
1971	McGregor[21]	524	14	2.6				All	6 months
1972	Greenberg McDowell[20]	105	2	1.9			2	1	
1972	Pitanguy[27]	1600	3	0.2	3			?	
1974	Castañares[3]	?	(12)	?	3	5	4	All	5 months
1977	Baker Gordon Mosienko[2]	1500	8	0.5	5	1	2	7	6 months
1977	Stark[30]	500	2	0.4	2			All	6 months
1977	Leist Masson Erich[17]	324	3	0.9	3			0	
1977	Peterson	174	0						
1977	Owsley[25]	145	0						
1978	Thompson Ashley[31]	922	6	0.7				5	1 year
1978	Lemmon Hamra[18]	577	10	1.7		1	9	All	6 months
TOTAL		6551	50	0.7	18	7	17	43	

From Baker, D.C., and Conley, J.: Avoiding facial nerve injuries in rhytidectomy, Past. Reconstr. Surg. **64:**781, 1979.

recognized during the surgery, and testing with a nerve stimulator may be ineffective because the nerve is anesthetized. Most of these injuries are first noted in the postoperative period, and the choice in management is between immediately reopening the wound and exploring nerve branches, or waiting 3 to 6 months before making a decision. Clinical experience tells us that more than 80% of facial nerve injuries following a rhytidectomy will have a spontaneous return of function within 6 months, so waiting is usually the more prudent choice.

However, the surgeon should carefully reevaluate the operative technique used in search of some technical error made that could be corrected (such as a deep suture plication). It is important to evaluate the number of muscles affected and then to decide whether to reopen the wound and attempt a reapproximation or to wait for some spontaneous improvement. Usually it is best that any decision be made in accordance with the patient's complete understanding and wishes. If a high suspicion of specific nerve injury exists, reexploration may be warranted to identify the suspected branch of the facial nerve and to reestablish its integrity if it has been cut. An immediate approximation of the cut ends will then offer the best chance for some return of movement, even though there may be some residual weakness.

If one decides to wait and observe, then serial testing by electromyography and electroneurography may help in determining whether the affected muscles have the capability of rehabilitating themselves spontaneously. The limitations of these tests must be recognized, however, since they cannot definitely prognosticate either the degree or the quality of recovery. Their results can only suggest a trend.

Conservative management may include exercises, physiotherapy, or other noninvasive methods to keep patients actively involved in their own recovery. More important, as emphasized by Castañares,[3] is a close rapport between patient, surgeon, and office staff, with constant and gentle reassurance and sympathetic understanding and attention given during frequent office visits.

Upper facial paralysis

The degree and the permanency of the paralysis may be established by electrical testing of the facial nerve and recording the chronaxial levels. If these levels remain high for more than 3 months, most likely there will be no return of movement to the brow.

If the paralysis persists, the frontalis muscles will atrophy, with resulting ptosis of the brow. Any improvements at this stage will involve an equalization of the movement of the forehead by a selective cutting of the corresponding nerve on the opposite side.[4] This may be carried out through the temporal incision used in the facelift, with identification of the responsible nerve by electrical testing. At this anatomical level there are frequently two or three filaments requiring lysis (this is determined by electrical stimulation). They should be sectioned step by step until the brow is paretic. Even with this approach to nerve lysis, equalization of movement of the brow does not result in every case. Occasionally, after the operation the paralysis of the normal side may not be as much as desired, and a "second look" may be necessary. In equalizing the brow, one should always attempt to save the filament that goes to the corrugator muscle, to the eyebrow, and to the orbicularis muscle, since this retains an active and lively expression about the eyebrows. Not uncommonly, however, patients with a paralysis of the frontal branch prefer to have a smooth, immobile forehead on the other side with minimal frown lines.

Middle facial paralysis

If the paresis is recognized postoperatively, it is reasonable to wait, because almost all of these nerves will recover considerably during a period of months because of collateral budding from the network that these nerves have with each other. The result may be complicated, however, by a slight motor tic. If a persistent or troublesome tic or spasm of the face should develop, then consideration may be given to a selective lysis of the particular nerve filament causing it.[4] This is accomplished by exposing the branch, doing electrical testing, and then performing a neurotomy. The weakness that develops in the muscle systems supplied by this nerve will be marked in the beginning, but over a period of 6 months there will be considerable return of movement via the network pathways. Unfortunately, in some instances when the balance becomes restored, there may be a reappearance of the tic, but this is usually not as marked as it was originally.

A persistent paralysis of the marginal mandibular branch may be handled by lysis of the opposite mandibular branch after an interval of 1 year. A neurotomy at this level will place the lower lip in relative balance. Again, this may be difficult to accomplish permanently because of variations in the network connections of the distal branches of the facial nerve. A combination of this procedure with a selected myectomy, accomplished through a mucosal incision (as described by Rubin[28]) gives more assurance of permanent symmetry.

The need to repair the defect depends on its significance to the patient and the effect on the overall appearance. For a very mild, partial weakness, one may elect to do nothing.

SUMMARY

Injury to the facial nerve in rhytidectomy has been occurring in less than 1 percent of cases, and spontaneous return of function has taken place within 6 months in more than 80% of these injuries. With the introduction of newer and more aggressive techniques of platysma muscle and subplatysmal flaps and SMAS dissections, the risk of injury to facial nerve branches is obviously increased. Although there has not yet been an increase in the facial nerve injuries reported, these techniques are still relatively recent additions to the face-lift operation—and usually they have been done by more experienced surgeons, taking more time and working under direct vision with more careful dissection. Obviously, more care is needed to prevent injuries in these extensive dissections.

REFERENCES

1. Baker, D.C., and Conley, J.: Avoiding facial nerve injuries in rhytidectomy: Anatomical variations and pitfalls, Plast. Reconstr. Surg. **64**:781, 1979.
2. Baker, T.J., Gordon, H.L., and Mosienko, P.: Rhytidectomy, statistical analysis, Plast. Reconstr. Surg. **59**:24, 1977.
3. Castañares, S.: Facial nerve paralysis coincident with, or subsequent to, rhytidectomy, Plast. Reconstr. Surg. **54**:637, 1974.
4. Clodius, L.: Selective neurectomies to achieve symmetry in partial and complete facial paralysis, Br. J. Plast. Surg. **29**:43, 1976.
5. Connell, B.F.: Contouring the neck in rhytidectomy by lipectomy and a muscle sling, Plast. Reconstr. Surg. **61**:376, 1978.
6. Converse, J.M., and Coburn, R.J.: The twitching scar, Br. J. Plast. Surg. **24**:272, 1971.
7. Conway, H.: The surgical face lift—rhytidectomy, Plast. Reconstr. Surg. **45**:124, 1970.
8. Correia, P., and Zani, R.: Surgical anatomy of the facial nerve as related to ancillary operations in rhytidectoplasty, Plast. Reconstr. Surg. **52**:549, 1973.
9. Davis, R.A., et al.: Surgical anatomy of the facial nerve and parotid gland based upon a study of 350 cervico-facial halves, Surg. Gynecol. Obstet. **102**:385, 1956.
10. Dingman, R.O., and Grabb, W.C.: Surgical anatomy of the mandibular ramus of the facial nerve based on the dissection of 100 facial halves, Plast. Reconstr. Surg. **29**:266, 1962.
11. Ellenbogen, R.: Pseudo-paralysis of the mandibular branch of the facial nerve after platysmal face-lift operation, Plast. Reconstr. Surg. **63**:364, 1979.
12. Guerrerosantos, J.: The role of the platysma muscle in rhytidoplasty, Clin. Plast. Surg. **5**:29, 1978.
13. Habal, M.B.: Parotid retention cysts as a complication of rhytidectomy, Plast. Reconstr. Surg. **61**:920, 1978.
14. Huber, E.: Evolution of facial musculature and facial expression, Baltimore, 1931, The Johns Hopkins University Press.
15. Hueston, J.T., and Cuthbertson, R.A.: Duchenne de Boulogne and facial expression, Ann. Plast. Surg. **1**:411, 1978.
16. Kaye, B.L.: The extended face lift with ancillary procedures, Ann. Plast. Surg. **6**:335, 1981.
17. Leist, F., Masson J., and Erich, J.B.: A review of 324 rhytidectomies, emphasizing complications and patient dissatisfaction, Plast. Reconstr. Surg. **59**:525, 1977.
18. Lemmon, M.L., and Hamra, S.T.: Skoog rhytidectomy: a five-year experience with 577 patients, Plast. Reconstr. Surg. **65**:283, 1980.
19. Loeb, R.: Technique for preservation of the temporal branches of the facial nerve during face-lift operations, Br. J. Plast. Surg. **23**:390, 1970.
20. McDowell, A.J.: Effective practical steps to avoid complications in face lifting, Plast. Reconstr. Surg. **50**:563, 1972.
21. McGregor, M.W., and Greenberg, R.L.: Rhytidectomy. In Goldwyn, R.M., editor: The unfavorable result in plastic surgery, Boston, 1972, Little, Brown & Co.
22. Mitz, V., and Peyronie, M.: The superficial musculoaponeurotic system (SMAS) in the parotid and cheek area, Plast. Reconstr. Surg. **58**:80, 1976.
23. Moffat, D.A., and Ramsden, R.T.: The deformity produced by a palsy of the marginal mandibular branch of the facial nerve, J. Laryngol. Otol. **91**:401, 1977.
24. Nelson, D.W., and Gingrass, R.P.: Anatomy of the mandibular branches of the facial nerve, Plast. Reconstr. Surg. **64**:479, 1979.
25. Owsley, J.Q., Jr.: Platysma-facial rhytidectomy: a preliminary report, Plast. Reconstr. Surg. **59**:843, 1977.
26. Pitanguy, I., and Ramos, A.S.: The frontal branch of the facial nerve: the importance of its variations in face lifting, Plast. Reconstr. Surg. **38**:352, 1966.
27. Pitanguy, I., Ramos, H., and Garcia, L.C.: Filosofia, tecnica e complicacoes das ritidectomias atraves de observaçao e analise de 2600 casos pessoais consecutivos, Rev. Bras. Cir. **62**:277, 1972.
28. Rubin, L.: The anatomy of a smile: its importance in the treatment of facial paralysis, Plast. Reconstr. Surg. **53**:384, 1974.
29. Skoog, T.: Plastic surgery: new methods and refinements, Philadelphia, 1974, W.B. Saunders Co.
30. Stark, R.B.: A rhytidectomy series, Plast. Reconstr. Surg. **59**:373, 1977.
31. Thompson, D.P., and Ashley, F.L.: Face-lift complications: a study of 922 cases performed in a 6-year period, Plast. Reconstr. Surg. **61**:40, 1978.

Chapter 19

Secondary rhytidectomy: basic considerations

Bernard L. Kaye

Consideration of a secondary rhytidectomy raises four basic questions:

1. *When?* How much time should elapse after a primary rhytidectomy before a secondary operation is considered?
2. *Why?* What are the indications for a secondary procedure?
3. *How often* can it (or should it) be performed?
4. *How many* times can it be done?

WHEN
Patient's goals

If a patient's goal is to turn back the aging clock so as to continue the aging process from a younger baseline, the patient's own individual rate of aging must determine the interval between primary and secondary rhytidectomies (e.g., 2 to 3 years or 5 to 7 years).[11]

Some patients want to delay the aging clock as much as they can in order to "fix" their apparent age for as long as possible. Such individuals would benefit from an early secondary rhytidectomy, as early as 1 or 2 years following the initial procedure. Some degree of recurrent skin sag must be expected after any face-lift operation, because facial skin is a material that stretches. A patient who wishes to look about as good 2 years after the primary operation should be informed that an early secondary face-lift will be indicated. This secondary procedure can be expected to last longer, however, since the primary operation removes some of the "stretch" in the skin, making the effects of the secondary operation last longer. Thus subsequent renewal procedures can be done at increasingly longer intervals. Individuals who wish

to try to "fix" their apparent age should plan on a second face-lift 1, 2, or 3 years after the initial procedure, and even a third procedure 5 to 7 years after the second one.

Physical findings

Neck. Usually the earliest recurrence of the aging appearance is in the neck, especially if the first operative procedure was a conventional skin-redraping rhytidectomy. Patients often experience dissatisfaction and disappointment with the reappearance of looseness of neck skin and prominence of the medial platysma bands. These manifestations may stimulate the surgeon to consider neck procedures at the time of the secondary rhytidectomy (see subsequent discussion).

Jowls. Recurrent fullness of the jowls is an indication for a secondary rhytidectomy. Individuals experiencing this problem can benefit from an additional skin rhytidectomy, often supplemented by repositioning or plication of the underlying superficial musculoaponeurotic system (SMAS).*[11,13,15]

Nasolabial folds. Nasolabial folds are normal expression lines, and their complete elimination is practically impossible. Patients should be informed that these folds will probably recur early after the initial edema subsides and the skin restretches. Improvement of nasolabial folds can be obtained by a secondary rhytidectomy, either with wide undermining or with support of the underlying fascial tissue.[12,19] Direct external excision

---

*Provided it was not done at the time of the primary procedure.

might be required to deal with very severe naso-labial folds.[2,3]

Descent of the upper third of the face. The ordinary primary rhytidectomy, dealing with the lower two thirds of the face, is usually sufficient to treat the majority of aging deformities.[7] However, the upper third of the face (forehead, eyebrows, lateral upper eyelids, root of the nose) is not immune to the effects of time and gravity, and these effects may become more obvious, either in contrast with the already-lifted lower two thirds of the face or with the continued passage of time, or both.

Ancillary procedures such as a forehead lift should be considered in a secondary rhytidectomy[10] if they were not done during the primary operation.

WHY
Surgeon's outlook

Advantages and disadvantages. Whether a secondary rhytidectomy is more or less difficult than the primary procedure depends on several factors:

1. The delayed flaps can be dissected more easily in a previously established and less bloody plane than in the primary rhytidectomy. On the other hand, any previous hematoma with its resultant scarring could make the dissection more difficult, and the delay phenomenon could produce more bleeding from the undersurface of the flap.

2. Favorably placed previous scars can serve as guides to secondary incisions (Fig. 19-1, *A*). Unfavorably placed scars can increase the risk of skin slough after a secondary operation. This additional risk should be explained to the patient before surgery.

3. More realistic expectations and attitudes may be expected from the experienced patient undergoing a secondary procedure, although it would be unwise to carry this presumption too far, since many patients forget much of their earlier postoperative experience. It is prudent to repeat the thorough patient education process prior to a secondary rhytidectomy, to remind the patient of what might be expected in the postoperative period.

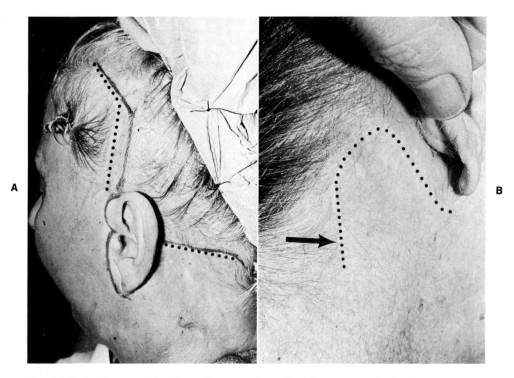

Fig. 19-1. A. Proposed incisions for secondary rhytidectomy marked adjacent to previous, favorably placed scars. **B,** Unfavorably placed vertical neck scar from previous rhytidectomy.

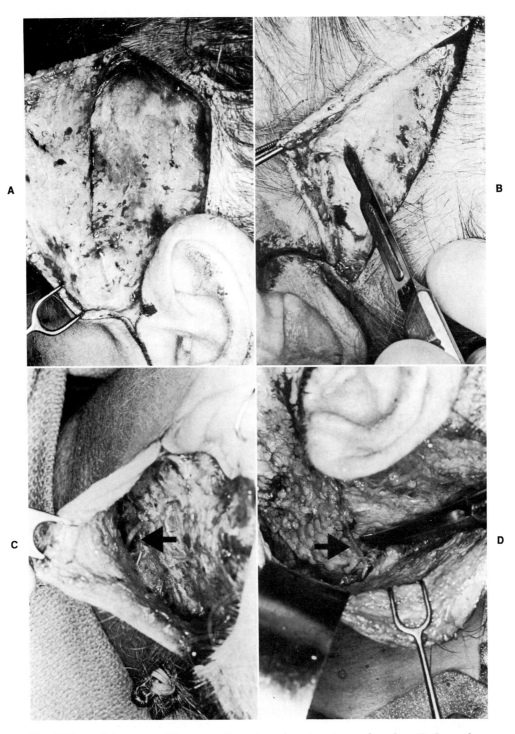

Fig. 19-2. A, Primary rhytidectomy, dissection plane in temporal region. **B,** Secondary rhytidectomy, dissection plane in temporal region. Considerable scarring requires sharp dissection. **C,** Primary rhytidectomy, lateral cervical region; greater auricular nerve is readily apparent. **D,** Secondary rhytidectomy, lateral cervical region; greater auricular nerve is bound down in scar tissue.

Specific problems. Some problems should be anticipated in the performance of a secondary rhytidectomy:

1. *Scarring.* Previous hematoma and scarring can render the dissection plane more difficult, but, more important, scarring can cause distortion of anatomy. Such distortion may be particularly pronounced around the marginal mandibular nerve or greater auricular nerve if a previous dissection involved these structures (Fig. 19-2).

2. *Undermining.* A secondary rhytidectomy usually requires as much undermining as a primary rhytidectomy if it is a straightforward skin redraping (Fig. 19-3). As an alternative, or in addition, underlying fascial tissues (SMAS)[11,12] may be repositioned if previous scarring has not rendered this procedure hazardous. If a SMAS procedure was done in the primary operation, it would be best to avoid it in a secondary procedure because of distortion due to scarring and increased risk of motor nerve injury.

3. *Skin excision.* Perhaps the greatest difference between the primary and the secondary rhytidectomy is that there is *much less skin to be removed* in the secondary procedure, whether one adopts wide undermining and redraping of the skin, repositioning of underlying tissues, or both (Figs. 19-4 and 19-5). Those surgeons who are accustomed to preexcising their skin strips prior to undermining might find it safer to do their undermining before excision, to avoid removing too much skin.

Patient's outlook

Advantages

1. The results of a secondary procedure often last longer than those of a primary rhytidectomy. This is because the skin, having been made less elastic by the primary procedure, holds better and stretches less after secondary procedures. However, the longer the time interval between operations, the more this advantage diminishes.

2. The lessened tissue trauma and usually easier dissection of the secondary procedure may produce easier postoperative recovery, as may the experienced patient's better idea of what to expect postoperatively.

Disadvantages

1. A secondary rhytidectomy produces a less dramatic change than that of a primary procedure. Although a primary face-lift may result in a patient's looking significantly younger, the secondary rhytidectomy is more of a maintenance than a rejuvenative procedure and, at best, can be expected to keep the patient looking approximately the same age (Figs. 19-6 and 19-7). The patient should be thoroughly informed about how much to expect from a secondary procedure.

2. Hair management is made more difficult if the incisions of the secondary rhytidectomy

Text continued on p. 170.

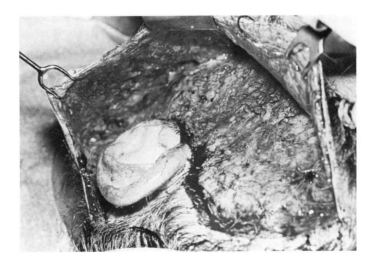

Fig. 19-3. Extent of undermining in secondary rhytidectomy. Alternatively, or in addition, underlying SMAS may be taken up if not done previously.

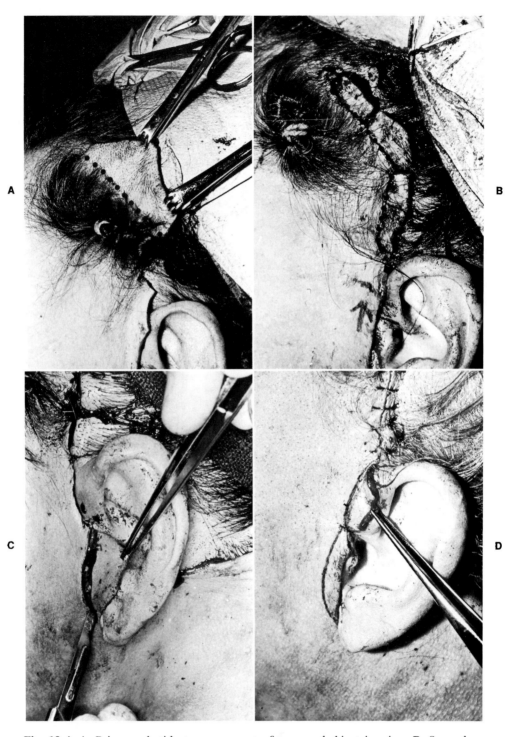

Fig. 19-4. A, Primary rhytidectomy, amount of temporal skin trimming. **B,** Secondary rhytidectomy, much less temporal skin trimming. **C,** Primary rhytidectomy, generous preauricular skin trimming. **D,** Secondary rhytidectomy, conservative preauricular skin trimming.

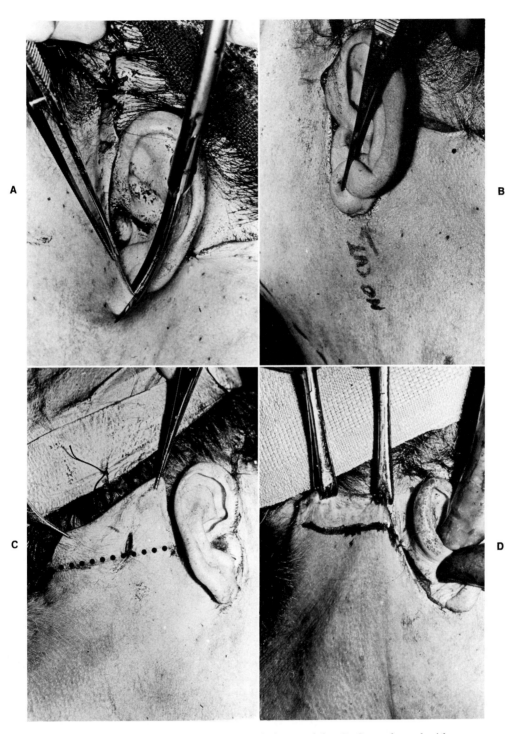

Fig. 19-5. A, Primary rhytidectomy, cutting below earlobe. **B,** Secondary rhytidectomy, "no cut" below earlobe. **C,** Primary rhytidectomy, more postauricular and occipital skin trimming. **D,** Secondary rhytidectomy, minimal postauricular and occipital trim.

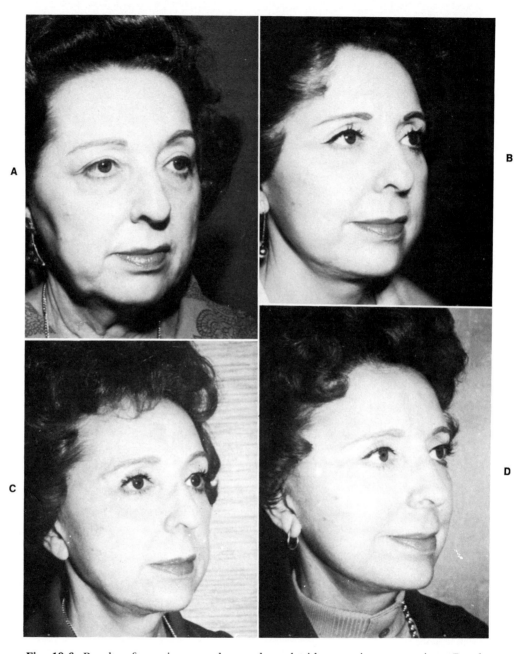

Fig. 19-6. Results after primary and secondary rhytidectomy in same patient. Result from secondary operation was less dramatic. **A,** Preoperative photograph. **B,** Patient 14 months postoperatively. **C,** Patient 5½ years postoperatively. **D,** Patient 6 months after secondary rhytidectomy.

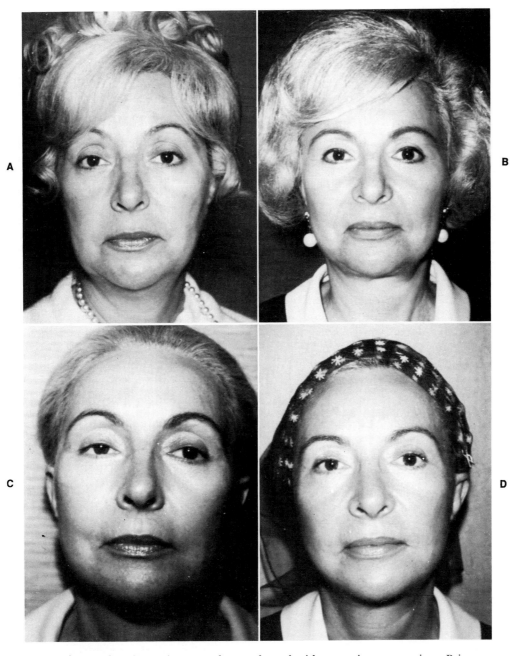

Fig. 19-7. Results after primary and secondary rhytidectomy in same patient. Primary operation was more rejuvenative, whereas secondary procedure was more maintenance. **A,** Preoperative photograph. **B,** Patient 13 months postoperatively. **C,** Patient 2½ years postoperatively. **D,** Patient 2 years after secondary rhytidectomy.

are made within the hairline, thus raising the temporal and occipital hairlines higher (see subsequent discussion).

3. A pulled look can result from a secondary rhytidectomy if the skin is tightened too much or if the flap is stretched too much in a posterior direction rather than in the more favorable superior direction.

HOW OFTEN
Factors causing early recurrence of the aging deformity

Age at the time of the primary rhytidectomy. Early recurrence of the aging deformity is more likely when the primary rhytidectomy is done at an older age than when the initial procedure is undertaken relatively early (e.g., in the third or fourth decade). Patients who elect to have a primary rhytidectomy in their sixties or seventies should be advised to expect early recurrence of the deformity, which may necessitate a secondary rhytidectomy as early as 1 or 2 years after the primary procedure.

Extent of the initial deformity. Patients who suffer from severe sagging and wrinkling and an extensive initial deformity are more likely to require an early secondary rhytidectomy than are patients who have a less severe initial deformity.

Old acne. Skin that has been scarred by severe acne in the past has a tendency to restretch more quickly after the primary rhytidectomy than does normal skin.

Weight loss. Recurrence of facial skin laxity is accelerated by significant weight loss. Therefore it is very important that any planned weight loss be accomplished *before* the primary rhytidectomy.

Poor physical or emotional health. Biological aging can be hastened by both physical and mental illness. Following a rhytidectomy the existence of significant physical illness or emotional problems such as anxiety or depression may necessitate an early secondary procedure to restore the younger appearance.

Poor personal care. Personal habits can play a significant role in accelerating the aging process after a rhytidectomy. Overexposure to the elements, especially the sun, and the excessive use of alcohol and tobacco may age the skin prematurely.

Heredity. The individual's genetic makeup, which determines the rate of biological aging, is the single most important factor in recurrence of aging following the primary rhytidectomy. A pa-

tient whose parents were relatively youthful looking into their seventies may reasonably expect to retain the beneficial effects of a primary rhytidectomy for a longer period of time than may a patient whose parents had aged rapidly and who might therefore require an early secondary operation.

Racial characteristics of the skin may also play a part in the way facial tissues resist aging. Individuals with fair, thin skin seem to age more rapidly than those with darker, thicker skin.

HOW MANY TIMES

If the following precautions are observed, additional rhytidectomies can be performed as long as there is loose skin to be excised:

1. Be careful not to excise too much skin; in secondary operations, there is always less excess skin than one expects.
2. Be careful not to pull the skin too tightly. Skin loses much of its elasticity after several rhytidectomies and can be easily overpulled. In cases where the patient has also previously undergone a chemical skin peel, elasticity may be virtually nil, and the skin might take on the nonelastic characteristics of silk or linen. Most of the traction should be exerted in an upward rather than a posterior direction, since recurrence is linked with the effects of gravity. The "fish-face" look can be avoided by pulling drooping corners of the mouth upward rather than posteriorly.

ANCILLARY PROCEDURES
Forehead lift

As previously stated, the primary rhytidectomy often involves only the lower two thirds of the face, but the upper third (forehead, eyebrows, lateral upper eyelids, root of the nose) does not escape the ravages of time and gravity. When a secondary rhytidectomy is being planned, it is often wise to consider a forehead lift as well, if it is indicated and was not performed during the original operation.

Sagging of the forehead and eyebrows with ptosis of the lateral portions of the upper eyelids are primary indications for a forehead lift. Transverse wrinkling of the forehead, glabellar frown, transverse wrinkling at the root of the nose, and drooping of the nose are all secondary indications for a forehead lift (Fig. 19-8). A partial resectioning of the frontalis muscle prolongs the result of the forehead lift.[10,20]

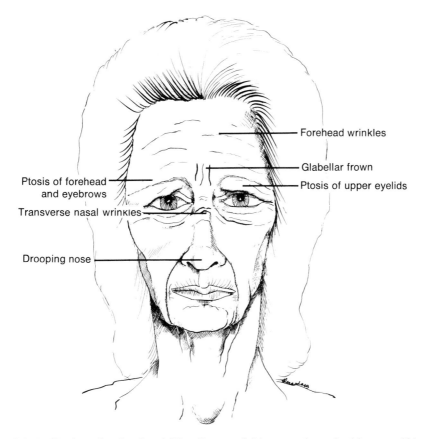

Forehead wrinkles

Glabellar frown

Ptosis of forehead
and eyebrows

Ptosis of upper eyelids

Transverse nasal wrinkles

Drooping nose

Fig. 19-8. Indications for forehead lift, often useful in secondary rhytidectomy if it was not done previously. (From Kaye, B.L.: The forehead lift: a useful adjunct to face lift and blepharoplasty, Plast. Reconstr. Surg. **60:**161, 1977.)

Special neck procedures

The neck is one of the first areas to exhibit recurrence of the aging deformity following a primary rhytidectomy. Recurrent looseness of skin appears, as well as recurrence of one or both medial borders of the platysma muscle, webbing in prominent bands across the hollow of the neck.

Numerous surgical procedures have been devised to deal with this problem, including medial incision of the platysma bands, creation of a superiorly based medial muscle flap that is retracted laterally,[5] excision of the medial borders of the platysma,[14] partial transection of the medial border of the platysma in its center to create superiorly and inferiorly based muscle flaps that are pulled laterally,[8] partial lateral and/or medial transection of the platysma,[12] complete transection and lateral rotation of a superiorly based platysma flap,[4,5] and lateral traction on the lateral border of the platysma, which is raised as a flap without transection of muscle fibers.[19] (Results of

unilateral trials have cast doubts on the effectiveness of this last maneuver.[16]) Other medial border procedures include imbrication of the medial borders of the platysma,[18] Z-plasty of the medial borders of the platysma,[21] and various external incisions[1,2,6] that result in external scarring of the skin.

Temporal hairline procedures

One effect of the secondary rhytidectomy is to raise the temporal hairline and sideburns. This rarely presents difficulties for men, since they can simply begin shaving lower on the preauricular skin, thus allowing the sideburns to start growing at a lower point. However, it can cause problems in hair management for women. There are several ways of dealing with this problem. Sheehan's maneuver can be performed, in which a posteriorly based triangle of skin just below the inferior border of the sideburn is excised and the defect closed,[17,18] which lifts the posterior cheek skin

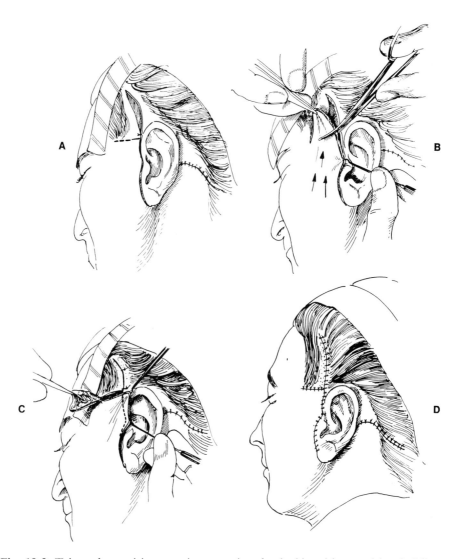

Fig. 19-9. Triangular excision to raise posterior cheek skin without raising hairline excessively. (From Rees, T.D., and Guy, C.L.: Patient selection and techniques in blepharoplasty and rhytidectomy, Surg. Clin. North Am. **51:**364, 1971.)

without raising the sideburn excessively (Fig. 19-9). An alternative procedure is to make the temporal incisions below and anterior to the hairline, although this tends to leave obvious scars, especially in patients with darker complexions.

My preferred method involves placing the upper anterior incisions within the hairline for the first two operations. When the lower border of the temporal hairline has finally been elevated above the level of the upper border of the ear concha (usually after a second operation), I then make the temporal incision just below the border of the temporal hairline (Fig. 19-10). This rarely presents difficulties for my patients, since most have already become accustomed to wearing their temporal hair lower over the preauricular area to disguise the elevation of the temporal hairline from previous surgery. Most patients usually prefer to continue doing so, rather than to have the temporal hairlines elevated even further. Therefore they usually select a pre-hairline incision when the alternatives are explained to them. In cases where the patients' temporal hairline has been raised very high, a multistaged rotation of hair-bearing scalp flaps to the temporal and preauricular regions may be indicated.[9]

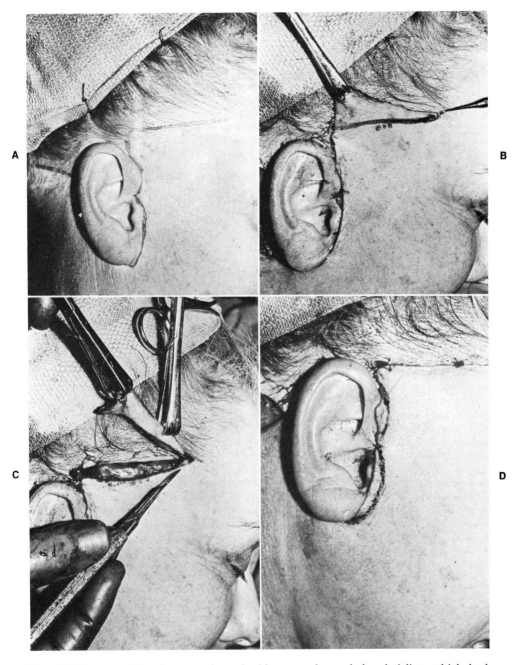

Fig. 19-10. A, Incision for secondary rhytidectomy drawn below hairline, which had been raised in previous operation. **B,** Amount of skin to be resected. **C,** Resection of skin. **D,** Closure of horizontal incision. Also note minimal preauricular skin excision in repeat rhytidectomy (tertiary in this patient).

SUMMARY

If the secondary rhytidectomy is viewed as a maintenance rather than a rejuvenating procedure, it can provide significant benefits to the patient. The disadvantages for the patient, including elevation of the temporal and occipital hairlines and the risk of a pulled look if too much skin is excised or if traction is exerted in an unfavorable (posterior) direction, should be weighed against the advantages of longer-lasting operative results and relative maintenance of the appearance at a "fixed" apparent age. The surgeon's experience with secondary procedures may vary for the reasons discussed in this chapter.

The most important point to keep in mind regarding the secondary rhytidectomy is that there is far less skin to be excised than in a primary rhytidectomy. The surgeon performing a secondary rhytidectomy for the first time should be prepared to modify his surgical methods if necessary to take account of this major difference.

REFERENCES

1. Cannon, B., and Pantazelos, H.H.: W-plasty approach to submandibular lipectomy. In Hueston, J.T., editor: Transactions of the Fifth International Congress of Plastic and Reconstructive Surgeons, Melbourne, 1971, Butterworths, Ltd.
2. Carlin, G.A., and Gurdin, M.M.: Ancillary procedures for the aging face and neck, Surg. Clin. North Am. **51:**371, 1971.
3. Castañares, S.: Two ancillary procedures for face lifting operation. In Hueston, J.T., editor: Transactions of the Fifth International Congress of Plastic and Reconstructive Surgeons, Melbourne, 1971, Butterworths, Ltd.
4. Connell, B.F.: Contouring the neck in rhytidectomy by lipectomy and a muscle sling, Plast. Reconstr. Surg. **61:**376, 1978.
5. Connell, B.F.: Cervical lifts: the value of platysma muscle flaps, Ann. Plast. Surg. **1:**32, 1978.
6. Cronin, T.D., and Biggs, T.M.: The Z-plasty for male "turkey gobbler" neck, Plast. Reconstr. Surg. **47:**534, 1971.
7. Fredricks, S.: The lower rhytidectomy, Plast. Reconstr. Surg. **54:**537, 1974.
8. Guerrerosantos, J.: The role of the platysma muscle in rhytidoplasty, Clin. Plast. Surg **5:**29, 1978.
9. Juri, J., Juri, C., and Antueno, J.: Reconstruction of the sideburn for alopecia after rhytidectomy, Plast. Reconstr. Surg. **57:**304, 1976.
10. Kaye, B.L.: The forehead lift: a useful adjunct to face lift and blepharoplasty, Plast. Reconstr. Surg. **60:**161, 1977.
11. Kaye, B.L.: The secondary rhytidectomy. In Goulian, D., and Courtiss, E.H., editors: Symposium on surgery of the aging face, St. Louis, 1978, The C.V. Mosby Co.
12. Kaye, B.L.: The extended face lift with ancillary procedures, Ann. Plast. Surg. **6:**335, 1981.
13. Mitz, V., and Peyronie, M.: The superficial musculo-aponeurotic system (SMAS) in the parotid and cheek area, Plast. Reconstr. Surg. **58:**80, 1976.
14. Millard, D.R.: Submental and submandibular lipectomy in conjunction with a face lift, in the male or female, Plast. Reconstr. Surg. **49:**385, 1972.
15. Owsley, J.Q., Jr.: Platysma-fascial rhytidectomy: a preliminary report, Plast. Reconstr. Surg. **60:**843, 1977.
16. Rees, T.D., and Aston, S.J.: A clinical evaluation of the results of submusculo-aponeurotic dissection and fixation in face lifts, Plast. Reconstr. Surg. **60:**851, 1977.
17. Rees, T.D., and Guy, C.L.: Patient selection and techniques in blepharoplasty and rhytidectomy, Surg. Clin. North Am. **51:**364, 1971.
18. Rees, T.D., and Wood-Smith, D.: Cosmetic facial surgery, Philadelphia, 1973, W.B. Saunders Co.
19. Skoog, T.: Plastic surgery: new methods and refinements, Philadelphia, 1974, W.B. Saunders Co.
20. Viñas, J.C., Caviglia, C., and Cortinas, J.L.: Forehead rhytidoplasty and brow lifting, Plast. Reconstr. Surg. **57:**445, 1976.
21. Weisman, P.A.: Simplified technique in submental lipectomy, Plast. Reconstr. Surg. **48:**463, 1971.

Chapter 20

Secondary face-lift procedures

John R. Lewis, Jr.

Secondary face-lifts are carried out for three chief reasons: (1) to improve the appearance of the patient who has gradually had a recurrence of relaxation of facial tissues with aging or weight loss, (2) to improve areas of the face that were not adequately improved by the primary lift, and (3) to correct complications occurring with the primary lift. Obviously, the extent of the secondary lift may vary from that of the primary lift according to the indications and the areas to be given primary consideration. Secondary procedures and primary procedures should both be problem oriented, both as to planning and execution, with the idea of avoiding problems and complications.

LONG-TERM OR SUBSEQUENT FACE-LIFT (RENOVATIVE LIFT)
Incisions

The secondary face-lift has much in common with the primary lift, in that the incision lines are made in essentially the same locations, the undermining and support of the deep tissues is repeated, and the careful layer closure and management of the superficial musculoaponeurotic system (SMAS) in the cheeks and the platysma in the neck is essentially the same as in the primary lift (Fig. 20-1). Even the management of the upper and lower lids may be essentially the same. However, one may need to vary the incision lines, depending on the location of the incisions for the primary lift. If the surgeon is the same one who performed the primary lift, it is likely that the incision lines will be in locations suitable for simple excision of the scar line and a repeat of the lift. If the incision lines vary, they may be modified in the secondary lift to improve them. The scar in the temporal scalp may be wide with some alopecia around it. In this case the incision should be

beveled to preserve the hair roots. For many years I have recommended this procedure and emphasized it at the very first meeting of the American Society for Aesthetic Plastic Surgery. The beveling of the incision to preserve the hair roots usually will permit adequate healing with a minimal scar in hair-bearing areas, such as the temporal and occipital scalp areas, and helps to avoid alopecia about the incision line. If the incision was managed in this way in the primary lift, simple excision of the scar line in the secondary lift procedure with the beveled incision line is all that is necessary. If there is alopecia with widening of the scar line, this is managed in a similar fashion in the secondary lift. Sometimes a wide area of alopecia does not allow for full resection of the bald area.

In instances in which this cannot be fully accomplished, management of the alopecia by any number of hair graft techniques can be carried out at the same procedure, and sometimes in subsequent procedures.

The incision in front of the ear may have been made straight or away from the ear in the primary procedure (Fig. 20-2) and may have elevated the hairline (Fig. 20-3). The new incision is brought closer against the ear with a curve into the supratragal notch and out again to break up the line of the scar and to make it less noticeable. If the previous incision was made inside the tragus, one may need to modify the secondary incision line to improve the scar line, or to follow the same scar line, as the case may be. I personally prefer an incision in front of the tragus, which leaves only a fine-line scar when a layer closure is carried out.

Management of the scar at the earlobe can be most important. In many secondary lifts one must

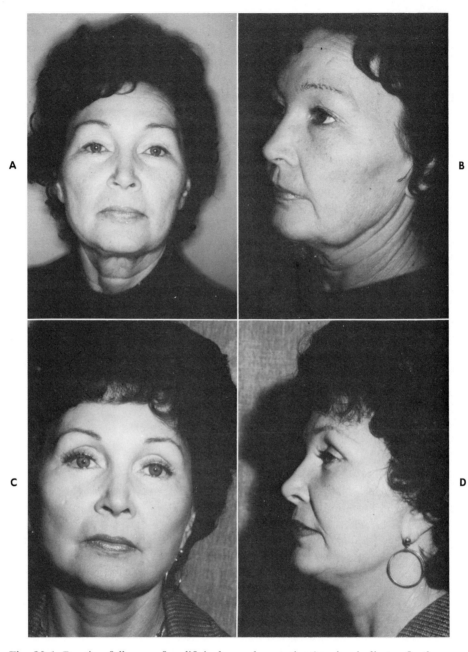

Fig. 20-1. Routine follow-up face-lift is done when patient's aging indicates further surgery because of sags, droops, or wrinkles, usually 7 to 10 years after first procedure, or earlier for smaller partial procedures. **A** and **B,** Patient's appearance before 9-year follow-up meloplasty, **C** and **D,** Appearance following secondary meloplasty.

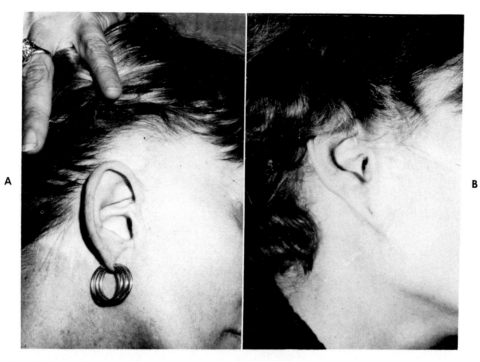

Fig. 20-2. A, Scar about ear is resected and brought closer to ear for closure in layers, breaking up line of scar by small triangle of skin shaped into supratragal notch. **B,** Contracted earlobe, which pulls down into cheek, is corrected by small fold-under flap, which allows roundness of lobe and avoids pull on lobe by advancing cheek skin upward in front of and behind ear as in original meloplasty procedure.

correct a contracture of the earlobe (Fig. 20-2). In some instances the earlobe may have been pulled down into the cheek or jawline, eradicating the normal rounded lobe. This is usually corrected simply by making a little wedge resection and rounding the lobe by folding the skin onto the lobe and against the cheek. There are other ways of managing this, as I have described in the past, but this is the simplest and does suffice in most instances. Displacement of the lobe anteriorly is often seen and is corrected by placing the lobe more posteriorly in the secondary procedure. Obviously, there should be no pull on the lobe itself in the repair.

Management of the incision line on the back of the ear should be the same as in the primary procedure, in that the incision should be made slightly up on to the back of the concha so that, with time and the normal tension of the tissues, it will pull downward into the postauricular sulcus. If the incision is made in, or lateral to the sulcus, the subsequent scar will pull down and backward from the ear. The incision line in the occipital scalp should be made a little higher than the original incision line in order to excise the previous

scar. When the original incision line was made along the hairline, the surgeon may wish to follow this same incision line in the subsequent procedure. However, the desirable location is usually higher in the occipital scalp, so that a good part of the original scar is excised and the lower hairline is brought somewhat forward toward the back of the ear in the process. This leaves some of the original scar only along the hairline inferiorly. If this scar is wide, hypertrophic, or very obvious, then one may modify the incision line posteriorly and resect the previous scar as part of the repeat face-lift.

Management of the eyelid incisions is usually simple in that any secondary blepharoplasty follows the same incision lines unless the previous surgeon has made the upper lid incision line too close to the cilia or in the lower lids, too far from the cilia. Sometimes the incision line may be followed across the lid but tapered more upward laterally and away from the original incision line in order to achieve the best result. Likewise, the lower lid incision line may follow a part of the previous incision line and then taper upward and laterally in the lateral portion in an attempt to

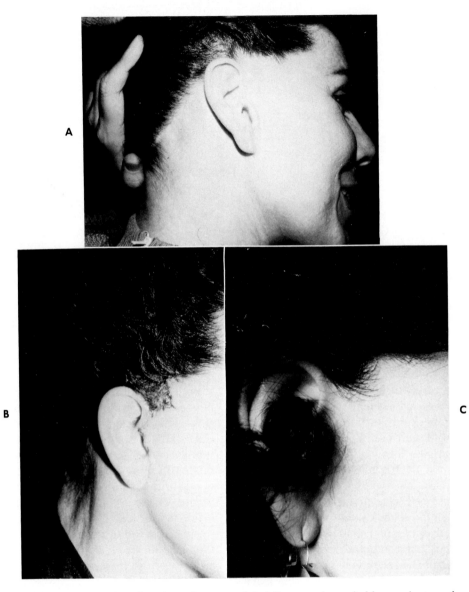

Fig. 20-3. A, Excessive elevation of temporal hairline can leave bald area in temple. Hairline may be so high that no sideburn remains. Reconstruction of sideburn and of temporal hairline may be accomplished as isolated procedure or as part of secondary face-lift procedure. **B,** Rotation flap from above and behind ear is brought forward in front of ear to create sideburn. **C,** Long-term result at 2 years. This problem can also be corrected by plug grafts or strip grafts of scalp from occipital area and improved by stippling with brown pigment between grafts to give impression of thicker hair growth.

move the incision line further superiorly to hide it better. One can see that the secondary face-lift may be easier or harder, depending on the initial surgeon's choice of incision lines and method of repair.

Undermining

Undermining for the primary and the secondary face-lifts probably should be about the same. One undermines relatively widely in the cheek and in the neck, but I avoid undermining widely in a narrow area along the lateral aspect of the jawline itself. This avoids the flattening that may occur across the angle of the jaw in front of the earlobe and leaves better venous return and lymphatic exchange in the area. It does not limit one in snugging and shaping the cheek and neck. If one prefers wide undermining of the SMAS in front of the ear, and elevation of the platysma and SMAS in continuity, one may need to do some further undermining in this area, but I prefer another method of deep support: the double-tiered overlap support of the facial fascia.*

Undermining in the temple, as in other areas, may be more difficult in the secondary lift. Even if the original undermining was in the relatively avascular plane superficial to the temporal fascia, often there are some fibrous adhesions, which make the dissection a little more difficult as one elevates the flap again in this same plane. If there was an unusually tight closure, hematoma, and/or infection (which should be rare), the dissection may pose more difficulty, of course. If the original undermining was more superficial, one has the choice of undermining again in a more superficial plane, which may be made considerably more tedious by the scar tissue left from the original surgery, or one may undermine in the deeper plane, superficial to the temporal fascia, which is usually better. The support of the skin in the temple may not be quite as effective as with more superficial undermining, but it is a safer procedure, with less likelihood of a spreading scar and/or alopecia. Usually, hemostasis is no more difficult in the secondary lift than in the primary lift in the temporal area or, for that matter, in the cheek and neck.

However, undermining in the cheek must be done even more carefully than in the primary face-lift, since the more superficial branches of the facial nerve have been pulled somewhat upward and backward in the primary lift. This makes them more accessible to the dissecting instrument and thus more easily injured during the secondary procedure. It is important to proceed cautiously not only with the dissection, but with electrocoagulation of bleeding vessels in the mid and anterior cheek. Undermining in the neck should probably proceed as indicated for a primary lift; one should judge this on the basis of the need and on what deep procedures are required.

Deep support

Deep support in the cheek and in the neck may be of equal or more importance in the secondary procedure, since presumably the patient is older and the tissue more relaxed (Figs. 20-4 to 20-7). Much has been written about the support of the SMAS in the posterior cheek and the support of the platysma by simple pull-back, partial division, or complete division and rotation-advancement. I still prefer the use of multiple-tiered support of the facial fascia (SMAS), the first tier supporting the fascia upward to the zygomatic fascia in front of the ear, and the second tier lower in the cheek to support the nasolabial area, corner of the mouth, and the jowl. This jowl area support also starts the tightening in the submental area, even before support in the neck. In some instances, the multiple-tiered support includes even a third tier, which may be required for optimum support (Fig. 20-4).

Deep support in the neck depends on the need. If the relaxation is primarily of skin and subcutaneous tissue, the platysma need not be divided. However, if the platysma is relaxed, conservative undermining and support (Skoog procedure) are carried out or else a division of the posterior portion of the platysma is made to create a sling beneath the jawline (Rees procedure) (Figs. 20-1, 20-6, and 20-7).

As far back as my training period 30 years ago (with Dr. Claire Straith), we were supporting the platysma backward to the fascia overlying the sternomastoid or the mastoid fascia. This was improved and popularized by Skoog, and even more extensive division and support of the platysma have been popularized in more recent years by a number of excellent surgeons, including Connell, Peterson, Guerrerosantos, Rees, and others. My preference still is a partial posterior division of the platysma, a safe, middle-of-the-road proce-

---

*EDITOR'S NOTE: I believe that platysma-SMAS procedures may be performed during a secondary rhytidectomy provided that they were not done in the primary operation. I would hesitate to attempt to repeat such platysma-SMAS operations for fear of scarring, anatomical distortion, and changes to facial nerve branches. (B.L.K.)

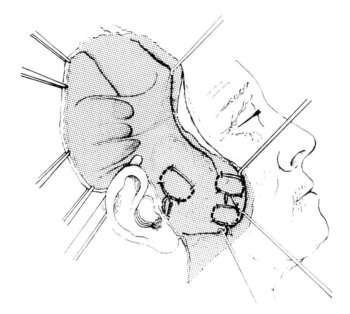

Fig. 20-4. Multiple-tiered deep cheek support. Deeper sutures support fat and fascia of cheek to zygomatic fascia, and two or three or more sutures imbricate fat pad and fascia (SMAS) of cheek, supporting it upward, once superior support has been secured. (From Lewis, J.R.: Atlas of aesthetic plastic surgery, Boston, 1973, Little, Brown & Co.)

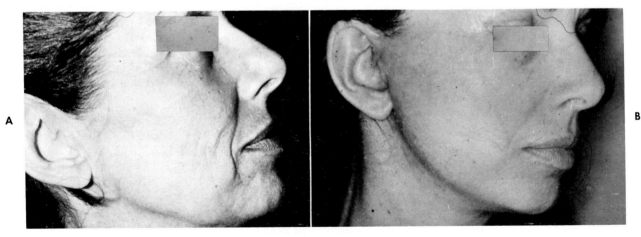

Fig. 20-5. A, Patient with recurrent changes of aging primarily involving upper lid and nasolabial fold area. Partial lift in combination with upper blepharoplasty and minor lower blepharoplasty, was considered adequate. **B,** Appearance following cheek lift from behind earlobe up into midtemple, which did adequate smoothing of nasolabial area.

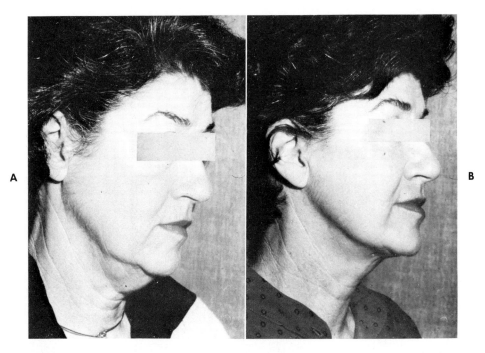

Fig. 20-6. A, Patient with lasting result from blepharoplasty and reasonably lasting result from cheek lift. With weight gain and loss and with continued aging, patients neck is area requiring surgery the most. **B,** Appearance following secondary temple, cheek, and neck lift with submental lipectomy and with rotation-advancement of platysma for support laterally. Considering extent of patient's neck problems, result is considered acceptable.

dure with few postoperative complications and little morbidity as compared with complete division of the platysma. However, all rules are made to be broken, and, at times, particularly in the heavy, thick neck, complete division of the platysma may be indicated.

In the secondary meloplasty, the submental and submandibular resection of fat must be considered, and anterior resection or plication of the platysma may also be indicated (Figs. 20-6 and 20-7). In some instances I still use a Z-plasty of the platysma as originally recommended by Weiseman.

Deep support in the secondary face-lift is of equal importance to that in the primary face-lift, and may in some instances be even more important. The original lift may not have accomplished all that might have been desired, and the original procedure may have been carried out even before such great importance was placed on this deep support.

SECONDARY FOREHEAD LIFT

The coronal lift is usually a more lasting part of the complete meloplasty when it is performed,

and rarely is an early repeat lift required. However, aging is not consistent in different races, families, or even individuals; as some people age, they sag in the forehead and brows, whereas others sag more in the cheeks, and still others in the neck. It is quite common to see people of advanced age who need only a minor blepharoplasty, whereas younger patients may need an extensive blepharoplasty. As with secondary cheek and neck lifts, when a repeat coronal lift is required, one seldom excises as much skin as in the original lift. However, this does vary. It is important, in my opinion, to bevel the incision in the frontal scalp just as one does in the temporal scalp to avoid a bald area along the incision line. Just as in the primary lift, there may be more ptosis on one side of the forehead as characterized by more wrinkling of that side, and/or by more drooping of one eyebrow. Obviously, more support is given to the side needing it.

LIPECTOMY

Resection of the excess fat of the neck may be required in the secondary face-lift because of variation in weight and changes occurring during

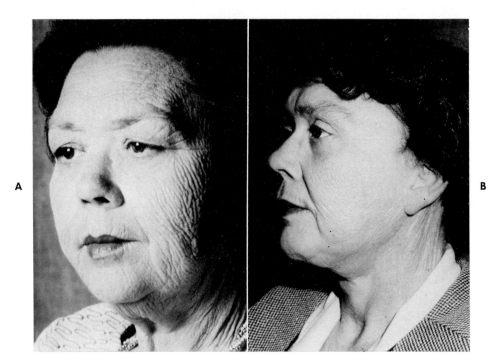

Fig. 20-7. A, Patient with long history of obesity and with marked weight loss over past 2 years with resultant wrinkles of facial and neck skin. Patient has submental fat hypertrophy, submandibular fat hypertrophy, prominent platysma bands, and marked blepharoptosis of upper lids posing a functional problem. **B,** Patient was managed by snug temple, cheek, and neck lift; submandibular and submental fat resection; rotation-advancement of platysma laterally with partial lateral division of muscle; chemical peel of upper and lower lips and chin extending slightly lateral to nasolabial sulcus; and upper blepharoplasty. One year following surgery, patient obviously needs secondary procedure to include additional submental fat resection and possibly more tightening of platysma laterally, as well as chemical peel of remainder of face, particularly cheeks and overlapping lower portion and vermilion of upper lip and corners of mouth. It is quite possible that patient would benefit a great deal from repeat full face-lift at this point in time. Patient continued to lose weight after her meloplasty, although she was certain she had reached her bottom point at time surgery was scheduled. Compromise procedure would be small trim of fat in submental area and full face peel.

the time span between the procedures. Even if a submental lipectomy was performed at the primary lift, a submandibular resection of fat may now be indicated (Figs. 20-6 and 20-7). This may be combined with platysma muscle and skin support to give the best neck contour (Figs. 20-1 and 20-6).

CHEMICAL PEEL

The chemical peel may be needed only for upper lip and/or glabellar wrinkles; alternatively, it may benefit the whole face (Fig. 20-7). A secondary peel may even be required for areas previously peeled, most commonly for the skin at the vermilion border. A peel of the undermined cheek skin or eyelid skin has obvious dangers; so a delay of 3 months following meloplasty is advised for the full face peel.

SECONDARY BLEPHAROPLASTY

Secondary procedures for the eyelids are often less necessary than are procedures on the cheeks and neck. However, there are variations in this, and usually some degree of further support of the lids is necessary when secondary face-lifts are carried out. It may be that resection of the fat pads and of the deep hernias may not be required. However, skin resection may be indicated, particularly in the lateral portion of the upper lid and to some degree in the lateral portion of the lower lid. Obviously, if there have been recurrent hernias, these should be corrected.

MENTOPEXY

Continued aging may cause changes in the chin itself, indicating a mentopexy for correction of the progressive sagging, particularly in the edentulous patient. This "witch's chin" is rather simply corrected by the procedure of Gonzalez-Ulloa,[2] by my procedure,[3] or by a combination of the two procedures. Sometimes, for the mild ptosis, a small augmentation at the point of the chin may be all that is required.

SECONDARY MELOPLASTY

In secondary meloplasty, it is presumed that the patient is several years older than at the time of the primary meloplasty, at least for the routine secondary procedures. Because of this, one would expect to find more wrinkling of the skin in connection with atrophy and aging, as well as more skin blemishes and lesions such as seborrheic keratoses, actinic keratosis, and papillomas. It is usually desirable to remove these skin lesions and

blemishes at the same time as the meloplasty. It is common practice to carry out a chemical peel to the midface area, including the upper lip, lower lip, chin, glabella, and forehead; one may safely peel out into the temple if one has undermined in the deep fascial plane.

SECONDARY FACE-LIFT FOR FURTHER CORRECTION (CORRECTIVE LIFT) AND SECONDARY PROCEDURES FOR COMPLICATIONS (PROBLEM LIFT)

The secondary face-lift performed because of an inadequate or excessive resection and repair, or because of complications that occurred during the surgery or following it, may take a variety of forms. Although complications and/or an incomplete or inadequate result may be due in part to a lack of confidence or a lack of proper caution, patients heal so differently that it is impossible to get the near-perfect result in every case. Do not be unjustly critical of the surgeon who did the first surgery, as you would hope a later surgeon would not be unjustly critical of you.*

How does one properly correct problems either initially or in the secondary face-lift or blepharoplasty? The most important two factors are (1) the proper analysis of the problem, and (2) the proper correction of the problem. It is important first to realize exactly what the problem is and what is causing it in order to correct it properly. This usually requires experience with some of the subtle problems and variations that occur in aesthetic plastic surgery in general and especially about the eyelids and cheeks.

Surgical repair and secondary meloplasty may involve the coronal lift or various types of forehead and brow lifts. However, the most common reasons for secondary lifts within a few months of the original surgery are poorly healed wounds with hypertrophic or wide scars, uneven support with more relaxation of one nasolabial or jowl area than the other, ptosis of one eyebrow and/or oversupport upward of the opposite eyebrow, relaxation of the submental area, and possibly alopecia. Surgery for these problems should be deferred until tissue is well healed, so that the secondary revision has an excellent chance of success. Often, small discrepancies and asymmetries will correct themselves in the course of the healing, and with physiotherapy and reassurance, the

---

*EDITOR'S NOTE: Sound and ancient advice (Matthew 7:12). (B.L.K.)

patient will usually manage to get through this waiting period and be happy with the ultimate result.

If secondary procedures are required, they should be planned carefully to correct the defect and/or deformity that is present. Secondary resections of the scars of the scalp should be made in a beveled fashion to preserve the hair roots and minimize alopecia about the resulting incision line. Wider areas of alopecia should certainly be treated by the use of hormone lotions (or the injection of dilute corticosteroid) and expectant waiting. Consultation with a dermatologist with a special interest in hair problems can be worthwhile. Wider areas of alopecia may even require punch grafts, a strip graft, or a small rotation flap.

Recession of the hairline

Elevation of the hairline in the temple, more likely to follow multiple face-lifts, can be an annoying problem (Fig. 20-3, *A*). Some elevation of the hairline must be expected in an extensive lift of the cheeks and temples, but some degree of compromise is also indicated. When it is necessary to raise the hairline markedly, one may use a marginal hairline incision with careful closure to minimize the resulting scar. If the hairline of the frontal and temple scalp has been raised considerably, it may be that a subsequent lift of the forehead should be carried out at the frontal hairline, particularly when the forehead extends upward and then backward before the hair growth starts. Subsequent lifts back in the hair of the frontal scalp will only widen the forehead and increase the need for the patient to use a hairstyle that hides the receding hairline. Most patients would prefer to hide the resulting fine-line scar rather than have frontal recession of the hairline, but it should be discussed before surgery.

Correction of recession of the temporal hairline with a relative loss of the sideburns can be corrected by a forward rotation flap of scalp from above and behind the ear (Fig. 20-3, *B* and *C*). This may take the form of a modified S-plasty or Z-plasty. Stippling of points of pigment with a needle to simulate hairs may give the appearance of thicker hair growth. The same type of tattoo stippling may be used in small bald areas such as result above the ear following double rotation flaps for reconstruction of the sideburn. Similarly, one may use plug grafts to plug into this area so that there will be no bald area behind the resulting sideburn.

Incisions about the ear

If the original incision in front of the ear was made straight, it is best to curve the secondary incision line into the supratragal notch to make it less obvious.

Correction of contractures of the earlobes and other deformities is often called for in the secondary meloplasty. The tightly pulled earlobe can be corrected by a small wedge resection, rolling the skin up between the lobe and cheek to round it off as a fold-under flap (Fig. 20-2). More severe contractures may also require a little rotation-advancement from the back of the ear forward to close the defect, but this is rarely necessary. Large redundant lobes may be shortened in a somewhat similar fashion, resecting tissue as a single wedge or as multiple conjoined wedges to give a nicely rounded and pleasant-appearing lobe. If openings for earrings are present (perforated ear lobes), these may usually be salvaged, unless there is a very large redundant lobe needing marked reduction. In that case the openings must be replaced at the time of surgery or later.

Scars that are on the back of the ear are simply excised in the process of the secondary lift. When these scars have drifted backward and downward to become more obvious, then the incision line is placed on the back of the concha so that, with tension and time, the resulting scar will fall in the postauricular crease. From the sulcus this incision extends upward and around into the occipital scalp, preferably not along the hairline. The original scars are resected, and again an attempt is made, as with primary meloplasty, to even up the hairline. This is more important in the male patient, but it should be done in the female patient also, unless it decreases the efficiency and effectiveness of the neck lift, which usually is not the case. If the original scar was made along the posterior hairline downward on the neck, this same incision line may be used if it is necessary to resect a wide or hypertrophic scar. If it is desirable to use a higher incision, as usually is the case, one simply uses the incision straight back into the occipital scalp, resecting the topmost portion of the original scar and pulling the inferior hairline forward to eradicate or improve the offset. If a wide offset is required in the hairline, it is best to make it high behind the ear rather than low, where it is more obvious.

Fat hypertrophy

Persistent fullness in the submandibular and submental areas may require a secondary lipectomy in these areas, and it may be desirable to do a rotation-advancement of the platysma in the secondary procedure if it was not carried out adequately in the primary one (Fig. 20-7). A submental lipectomy and/or approximation or resection of submental platysma bands may be required. When needed, this may be carried out relatively early at 3 or 4 months after surgery. Secondary procedures are usually delayed longer to allow for better tissue healing and softening of scar tissue.

Sloughs and scarring

More severe complications, such as sloughs and wide scars, are managed by resecting the scar tissue in an attempt to simulate the lift procedure without making additional scars in other directions. The tissue of the neck may often be advanced further upward and backward behind the ears to resect scars and make them less obvious. Scars in the cheek are managed in a similar fashion, as are those in the temple and scalp.

Prominent bands of the neck may not be platysma bands, but sternomastoid bands. A resection or section of the sternal heads of the sternocleidomastoid through a small transverse incision just above the clavicle will manage to soften these lines and make them less prominent.[1]

Prominence of nasolabial folds

Severe secondary nasolabial relaxation and folds may require direct resection (Fig. 20-8), the need for which is usually obvious before the primary operation. However, at the primary procedure one wishes to do a snug lift upward and posteriorly, which pulls on the nasolabial area, and the patient should be warned that a later, secondary nasolabial resection may be required. When the nasolabial resection is performed, a layer closure with a final running intracuticular skin suture is used, perhaps to be followed by a surgical abrasion later to blend the scar line further. This usually gives a good result with a minimal scar that simulates the nasolabial fold. Obviously, care should be taken not to overresect in the subcutaneous tissue for fear of cutting the terminal branches of the facial nerve to the lips. Usually, no resection of subcutaneous tissue is needed; rather, repair by plication, which aids in filling the nasolabial depression, should be done.

Ptosis of the brows

There are certain procedures that may be required in the secondary face-lift, either at the subsequent routine face-lift procedure (when the additional procedure may not have been indicated earlier) or as a relatively early secondary procedure when the face-lift did not fully accomplish adequate support. One must, of course, be sure that a brow lift is needed, rather than an upper blepharoplasty.

The brow lift may be carried out as a resection along the line of a prominent forehead crease. This would usually be done only with a markedly wrinkled forehead in the male patient. The most common brow lift is carried out as a resection of skin at the top of the eyebrow, in which case the incision is made obliquely through the skin to protect the hair roots and to mask the incision line as well as possible. A careful repair must of necessity be carried out, and the highest part of the eyebrow is usually in the mid or lateral portion, rather than in the medial portion, which tends to give the patient a startled look rather than a more youthful and happy one.

For a number of years I have used a modified brow lift, employing an incision in the eyebrow itself and undermining through this incision above the eyebrow. Support of the orbicularis at the incision line upward to a higher point on the occipitofrontalis has given good, subtle elevation of the eyebrow. This may be an isolated brow lift on an outpatient basis, or it may be used in conjunction with a total face-lift or upper and lower blepharoplasty. The technique is simple, has been relatively problem free, and has given good long-term results. The elevation is usually less marked than with the direct excision above the eyebrow or along a forehead scar or crease, but it does compare favorably with a moderate coronal lift.

Skin wrinkles

The chemical peel procedure may be planned as a procedure subsequent to the healing of the meloplasty incisions, since one would hesitate to do a peel over undermined skin without waiting at least 3 or 4 months for adequate healing and regrowth of the circulation into the skin from the base. However, one may carry out a central face peel at the same time as a meloplasty procedure, and it is usually safe to peel the entire forehead and temples when a routine meloplasty (even with a high temporal lift) has been carried out. One would obviously hesitate to peel the forehead along with a coronal lift.

A peel around the mouth, to the lips, chin, and nasolabial areas of the cheeks, may be safely carried out along with the meloplasty, since the peel does not involve undermined skin (Figs. 20-

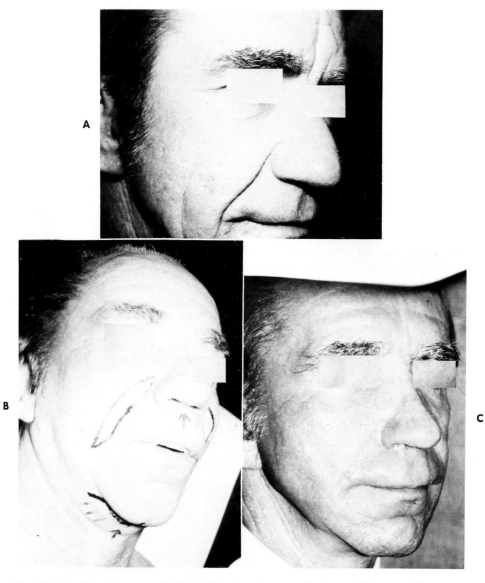

Fig. 20-8. A, Prominent nasolabial fold and sulcus may be impossible to eradicate completely by meloplasty laterally. **B,** Patient should be forewarned that secondary procedure may be required with later direct excision of nasolabial fold as outlined. **C,** Appearance following secondary direct excision of nasolabial folds and sulci.

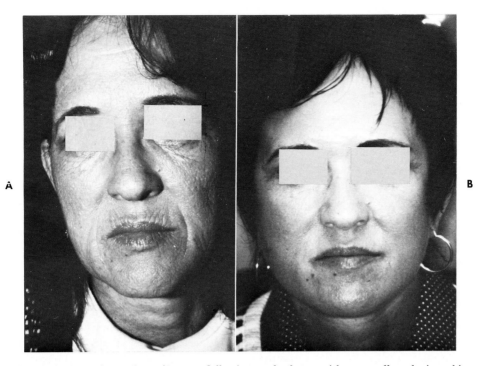

Fig. 20-9. A, Patient, about 7 years following meloplasty, with generally relaxing skin with coarse texture and with wrinkles of whole face, particularly around eyes and mouth, with worst ones being in upper lip. **B,** Appearance 1 year following surgery. Despite patient's rather dark pigmentation, forehead and glabellar peel and peel of full circle about mouth, including nasolabial areas, lips, and chin, was carried out, along with conservative secondary meloplasty and conservative upper and lower blepharoplasty.

6, 20-7, and 20-9). However, it is wise to use measures to minimize edema from the peel in order to keep it from lessening the effect of the meloplasty itself by swelling and stretching.

A secondary procedure (peel or dermabrasion) for wrinkles may be required when the initial peel did not completely eradicate them. However, one should never promise the patient that the peel will eradicate the wrinkles, but only that they will be improved. A secondary peel may be carried out after several months to improve the wrinkles further, but the secondary peel must be carried out a little more carefully because of the previous peel, especially in patients with a thin dermis.

Pigment problems

A secondary peel or surgical abrasion may be required because of sharp demarcation of pigmentation following a chemical peel. This is often seen at the jawline or slightly above the jawline when the peel is not blended into the adjacent skin, but it may occur in any area of the face. Occasionally, healing will result in splotchy areas of pigmentation and depigmentation. In such cases,

surgical abrasion of the area, blending it out to a natural crease or junction line where possible, has given better results than secondary peels, which tend to leave yet another demarcation line. Obviously, after a peel, the patient should avoid the sun for several weeks and use a sun screen for several months to minimize the effects of the actinic and ultraviolet rays.

Submental depression

The depressed submental area with fullness on either side is the result of either overly zealous central fat resection or inadequate lateral fat resection. It may also be due in part to prominent lateral platysma bands (Fig. 20-7). Obviously, a resection of the lateral fat of the submental area, with or without excision or repair of the platysma bands, is indicated. Sometimes a turnover flap of fat from the lateral area to the central area may be required, but usually simply approximating the platysma in the submental area will aid in satisfactorily filling the central depression. A Z-plasty of the platysma often gives an excellent result also.

Mask-face

Last, perhaps the most difficult problem presented to the surgeon for a possible secondary face-lift, other than large areas of slough, is the masklike appearance of the face. This may result following repeated face-lifts with excessive tightening of the skin, or with dermal scarring. It may result from an overzealous peel or from repeated peels. It may also result to a degree from overtightening in certain areas of the face, such as across the jawline or below the cheek bones, and not tightening the remainder of the face to the same degree. The patient with a thin dermis is more likely to have this type of result, but no face can be considered completely exempt. Often, no further surgery is indicated; time, gentle massage, and reassurance may be all that is needed. Even with scarring of the skin itself by overzealous or repeated peels combined with surgical stretching of the skin, moderate improvement would occur with time. The best treatment is the avoidance of overstretching the skin and a more conservative peel routine.

Direction of support in the cheeks

A similar type of mask-face with tightening in some areas may occur when the facial skin is pulled straight posteriorly, rather than upward and backward.* This tends also to pull the earlobe forward, which is a less natural position and tends to pull the corner of the mouth downward, which

---

*EDITOR'S NOTE: "Fish-face" deformity. (See Chapter 19.) (B.L.K.)

produces a tight, flat contour across the jawline below and in front of the earlobe. A secondary procedure may be carried out only after a long period of massage and should involve elevation of the cheek skin, rather than posterior support, and repositioning of the earlobe more posteriorly. One often cannot excise additional skin except for the scar line itself, since the skin has already been pulled too tightly.

SUMMARY

In summary, the best treatment of problems resulting from face-lift procedures, whether early or late, is the proper evaluation of the patients' problems and the proper execution of the surgical procedures. Then one is less likely to have anything but routine long-term followup face-lifts to perform except for a minimum of early corrections due to variations in patient healing. It must be remembered that there is great variation in healing in different patients and in different races, and indeed even in the same patient at different times, depending on the patient's general health and physical and emotional state at the time.

REFERENCES

1. Beers, M.D.: Surgical sectioning of the sternal origins of the sternocleidomastoid muscles as an adjunctive aid to rhytidoplasty: a new procedure. In Lewis, J.R., editor: Textbook of plastic surgery, Boston, Little, Brown & Co. (In press.)
2. Gonzalez-Ulloa, M., and Stevens, E.: Ptosis of the chin: the witch's chin, Plast. Reconstr. Surg. **50:**54, 1972.
3. Lewis, J.R.: Atlas of aesthetic plastic surgery, Boston, 1973, Little, Brown, & Co.

Editorial comments
Part II

A previous shortcoming in rejuvenative facial surgery was failure to recognize the importance of the upper third of the face: the forehead–eyebrow–upper eyelid complex. This area is no less immune to the ravages of time and gravity than is the lower two thirds of the face. Forehead-brow lifts were unpopular in the past because the results were thought not to last very long. In my opinion, the concept of reducing the pull of the frontalis muscle by either incising, striating, or removing a strip of muscle has contributed significantly to the lasting qualities of the operation. The forehead lift usually outlasts a face-lift, and we find that we need to do far fewer secondary forehead lifts than secondary face-lifts.

In recent years we have come to understand the limitations of upper lid blepharoplasty, particularly when there is redundant eyelid skin laterally. Lateral upper lid blepharochalsis (as well as central and medial excess upper lid skin) can be compared to an excessively long pair of pants or skirt: it is obvious that one must pull the garment up to the proper waist level before judging how much to shorten the bottom. Likewise, one must raise the forehead and brows to the proper level before resecting excess upper lid skin. This can be done by a conventional coronal forehead lift, by a partial lateral (temple lift) procedure, or even by a direct lateral excision (provided one is prepared to deal with the lateral scar).

Obviously, if one is going to raise the forehead and brows, this procedure should be done before the upper lid blepharoplasty, in order to gauge how much "material" one has left to resect in the upper lids. Even more caution is needed in performing a forehead-brow lift in a patient who has had a previous upper lid blepharoplasty.

Fortunately, the forehead lift is an operation that is relatively free of problems. Massive hematoma and necrosis are the only serious complications, and these are rare. The massive hematoma is easy to diagnose because of the severe pain that accompanies it.

The middle third of the face may present special problems, such as excessive cheek fullness, correctible by cheek fat pad excision, or inadequate cheek prominence, which may be improved by malar augmentation with alloplastic materials.

Male face-lifts present special problems because of the beard, thicker skin, and male scalp hair distribution, as well as certain "extras" such as heavy nasolabial folds and severe "turkey gobbler" neck deformities. The advent of longer hairstyles in men has made the incisions for the male face-lift much easier to place, and, except in men with severe baldness, the incisions can be the same as in the female face-lift. Platysma-SMAS procedures have improved the results and duration of male face-lifts significantly and, in my experience, have almost eliminated the need for special external incision procedures, such as those for turkey gobbler deformities.

I believe that there is a place for coronal forehead lifts in selected male patients. These are men with low, drooping brows, severe lateral upper eyelid overhang, and redundancy and wrinkling at the root of the nose, who still have enough hair to hide the coronal incision. Unless there is some peculiar hair loss timing in their family history, one can assume that most men who have reached face-lift age will probably keep most of the hair that they have left by that time. When doing a forehead lift in a male patient, one must be careful to be more conservative in the amount of lift and in the amount of skin excision than in the female patient. Men look odd with high, arched eyebrows, whereas conservative elevation of the brows can relieve them of a tired, bloodhound look.

I believe that the playtsma-SMAS procedures that I have been doing for the past 7 years have improved my face-lift results and their duration significantly. Initially I thought it would be easy to prove that they produce a better, longer-lasting face-lift. Proof has been more elusive than I had imagined. Comparison of patients done with as opposed to without platysma-SMAS procedures is invalid, because we are comparing different people with different intrinsic rates of aging, different skin structure, and so on. Doing platysma-SMAS procedures on one side of the face only would not yield valid results for comparison, even if we could get volunteers to submit to such operations, because of the "hammock effect" from the pull of the platysma-SMAS elevation on one side. There is at least one valid method for proof of the efficacy of this double-layered technique. That would be to operate on a series of identical twins, doing the platysma-SMAS lift on one of each pair of twins, and then have a group of impartial observers evaluate them a year later and try to tell "which twin had the Toni." Unfortunately, as of this writing, I have yet to encounter a set of identical twin volunteers.

In my own practice I have abandoned complete transection of the platysma and now do only a partial lateral and partial medial platysma transection low in the neck. Following complete transection, I used to see occasional patients with unsightly fullness in each lateral submental region, which I postulate was caused by (1) loss of platysma support for ptotic submaxillary glands and (2) bunching of the transected upper half of the platysma as it rolled up like a window shade. I have not seen this deformity as frequently or to the same degree since I began leaving an intact central strip of platysma.*

One certain result of my platysma-SMAS procedure has been a significant increase in the operating time required for face-lifts. Because of this, I no longer do multiple rejuvenative procedures at one operation. Instead, I stage them on 2 successive days if they are done with the patient under local anesthesia, or on 2 alternate days with 1 day in between if they are done with the patient

under general anesthesia. My usual order of procedures is to do the forehead, eyelids, and nose at the first stage and then do the face, neck, and perioral peel-abrasion at the second stage. Dividing these multiple procedures into two stages has proved to be very satisfactory for both patient and surgeon.

There are three circumstances in which I will not do platysma-SMAS procedures:

1. In a younger patient with slight deformity, a skin lift is usually sufficient.
2. If a patient has had a previous platysma-SMAS procedure and is to have a secondary rhytidectmy, I omit procedures on the underlying tissues for fear of producing motor nerve injury in tissues that are distorted from previous surgery and scarring in the underlying layers.
3. I would not do a platysma-SMAS procedure in a professional wind instrument musician for fear of possibly disturbing the *embouchure* (the adjustment of the lips to the mouthpiece of the instrument, which is the sum total of strength, sensitivity, flexibility, and agility in the lip musculature produced by years of training and practice). For several years I have inquired at every meeting I have attended as to whether anyone had any experience with platysma-SMAS procedures in professional wind instrument players. So far, no one has come forth with any report.* I would welcome correspondence from any surgeons who have had such experience with this type of patient.

Although Davis of Argentina had been doing facial fat sculpturing for many years, it has become popular in this country relatively recently. One potential problem related to defatting of underlying tissues is the production of contour deformities. Another is possible injury to branches of the facial nerve, particularly the marginal mandibular branches, which may be inadequately protected by a thin layer of overlying platysma muscle. I have two suggestions for avoiding these problems:

1. Defat only after the underlying platysma-SMAS layers have been transposed to their new positions. By this means, the surgeon

---

*Kaye, B.L.: The extended face-lift with ancillary procedures, Ann. Plast. Surg. **6**:335, 1981.

*Subsequent to this writing, one of my face-lift patients, who is also a plastic surgeon, told me that he had difficulty pronouncing certain words for nearly 1 year after his platysma-SMAS procedure.

can see exactly how and to what degree the defatting is affecting the overlying facial contour (instead of defatting a given area and then finding, to one's consternation, when that area is transposed to its new position, that one has defatted too much). Moreover, it is easier to defat the platysma-SMAS after it is put on a stretch by having been transposed and sutured to its new position; one is far less likely to inadvertently pick up underlying muscle and nerve under these circumstances.

2. Defat conservatively. Even thin faces have some underlying fat, which is necessary for normal gliding and mobility of the skin.

Finally, I agree with Dr. Owsley that the platysma-SMAS operation is a safe procedure when done by qualified, experienced surgeons. In his chapter, Dr. Owsley cites 273 patients done without permanent nerve injury. In a subsequent paper (1983)* his series has increased to 435 patients done without permanent nerve injury.

B.L.K.

___

*Owsley, J.Q., Jr.: SMAS-platysma face lift (update), Plast. Reconstr. Surg. **71:**573, 1983.

Part III

Blepharoplasty

Chapter 21

Preoperative considerations in blepharoplasty

Gilbert P. Gradinger

In all elective surgery procedures, the surgeon needs enough preoperative information to accurately evaluate the patient for surgery. The acquisition of general health information should precede the acquisition of specific information. In a first office visit, the patient is given the responsibility of initiating this process by filling in a form (Fig. 21-1) supplying a medical history.

A nurse, in the privacy of an examination room, can then assist the patient in completing the form, at the same time obtaining additional history and obtaining and recording the patient's vital signs. The nurse's assistance helps assure a good start in gathering this information because it prevents the patient from feeling isolated while waiting for the physician, it establishes professional contact with the patient, it assures the patient that primary consideration is being given to his or her general health, it helps to calm an understandably anxious patient, and it provides the physician with valuable information at the onset of the consultation.

The discussion is an important part of the preoperative evaluation. The word *discussion* has been substituted for *consultation* to emphasize bilaterality for communication between patient and surgeon. In this discussion the surgeon should assume nothing about what the patient desires. The discussion should be directed so that important information is not omitted or fragmented. The surgeon needs to learn what the patient wishes to discuss (e.g., eyelid, face, or nose) and what the patient's concerns are (e.g., bags, loose skin, dark circles, tired look, crow's-feet, wrinkles, or swelling). The surgeon also needs to know if the patient feels that there is a physical impairment resulting from the eyelid problem (e.g., interference with vision, heaviness, or drooping), if the patient has an eye problem (e.g., irritation, dryness, visual loss, need for glasses, or glaucoma), if the patient has seen an ophthalmologist (for glasses or other problems), and whether it is the upper or the lower lids (or both) that are causing the patient concern. (It can be embarrassing to assume or suggest.)

EXAMINATION
Observation

During the initial discussion, good eye contact with the patient is essential. Contact (1) shows interest and attentiveness, (2) initiates the examination, and (3) allows observation of expression and animation habits (information that can subsequently be fed back when expectations are discussed).

The periorbital area is evaluated in relation to the entire face. The different components of the periorbital area are then evaluated separately.

Bony orbit

Configuration of the bony orbit—is it satisfactory, or is it encroaching on the globe and lids in such a way as to give the eye and lids a constricted appearance?

Eyebrows

The relationship of the brow to the bony orbit is critical in achieving a good blepharoplasty result. Is the brow situated either at the level of the supraorbital rim or above it, or is it ptotic and descending toward the free lash margin? Are the brows symmetrical in their position?

Account # _____

PATIENT INFORMATION FOR MEDICAL RECORDS

Date _____

Patient _____

       (last name)   *(first)*   *(middle)*

Age _____   Sex F _____ M _____

Date of Birth _____

Address _____

          (street/box number)

Telephone _____

Social Security _____

_____

  (city)   *(state)*   *(zip code)*

Single   Widowed   Divorced

Married   Name of Spouse _____

Name of Person Responsible for Bill _____

Patient employed by _____ Business Phone _____

Business Address _____ Occupation _____

Spouse or parent employed by _____ Business Phone _____

Business Address _____ Occupation _____

Patient referred by _____

Have you consulted or been treated by another plastic surgeon for this condition? _____

HEALTH INSURANCE INFORMATION

Name of Insurance Co. _____ Policy Number(s) _____ Policy Holder

Name of Insurance Co. _____ Policy Number(s) _____ Policy Holder

Is this a work related injury? Yes _____ No _____ Industrial Insurance Carrier _____

MEDICAL HISTORY

Family Physician _____

Patient's Height _____ Weight _____

	Yes	No		Yes	No
Drug sensitivities or allergies, If yes			Heart disease		
which drugs?			High blood pressure		
			Diabetes		
Problems with local anesthetic?			Epilepsy		
Do you bruise easily?			Glaucoma or cataracts		
Bleeding tendency			Psychiatric counseling		
Breathing or lung problems					

Present Medications	Past Illnesses & Surgeries	For Office Use
		P. *B.P.*

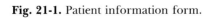

Fig. 21-1. Patient information form.

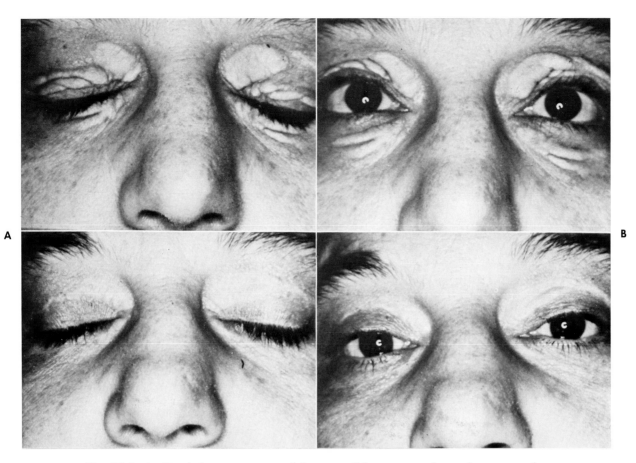

Fig. 21-2. A, Xanthelasma, upper and lower eyelids, preoperative and postoperative views, eyes closed. **B,** Xanthelasma, upper and lower eyelids, preoperative and postoperative views, eyes open.

Skin

The skin must be evaluated for its general quality, texture, tone, wrinkling, laxity, pigmentation, and presence of surface blemishes, such as scars, lesions, or xanthelasma plaques (Fig. 21-2). It is extremely important to note evidence of edema.

Subcutaneous tissue

Particularly in the upper lid, it is important to determine if there appears to be excess subcutaneous tissue, which one would expect to encounter superficial to the orbital septum. This is most likely to be present toward the brow and laterally.[1] It must be excised at the time of surgery to prevent an otherwise well-performed blepharoplasty from having a disappointing result.

Muscle

Particularly on the lower lid, clinical evaluation of the status of the orbicularis oculi muscle is crit-

ical. One can readily determine whether there is hypertrophy or atrophy. A lid that shows bulging muscle in the pretarsal region and below will require partial resection of that muscle. On the other hand, a lid that shows very little evidence of muscle and is concave in the pretarsal area is apt to be flaccid and will require additional muscle support in the blepharoplasty procedure. It is at this point in the examination that the "snap test" can be conducted on the lower lid to determine whether the lid has good tone—after the lid is gently pulled away from the globe, releasing it should result in its immediate reapproximation to the globe in normal position.

Submuscular fat and lacrimal gland

There are three potential spaces in the upper and lower lid. These spaces are created by the emergence of ligamentous and tendinous structures attaching to the globe. The medial and central spaces of the upper lid and the medial, cen-

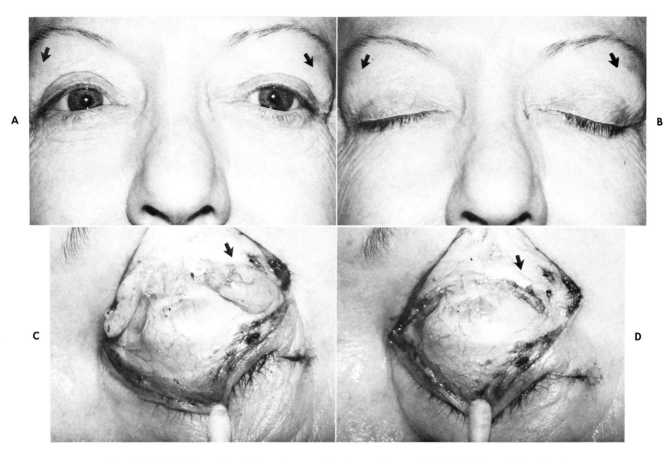

Fig. 21-3. A, Patient who had undergone blepharoplasty and had visibly ptotic lacrimal glands; eyes open. **B,** Patient who had undergone blepharoplasty and had visibly ptotic lacrimal glands; eyes closed. **C,** Operative identification of lacrimal glands and medial fat pocket. Central fat pocket had apparently been resected at original surgery. **D,** Following resection of ptotic portion of lacrimal gland and medial fat pocket.

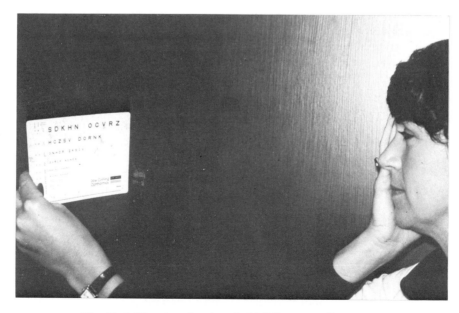

Fig. 21-4. Visual acuity chart held 2 feet away from eyes.

tral, and lateral spaces of the lower lid are potential areas of fat protrusion. The lateral space of the upper lid is a potential space for the protrusion of the lacrimal gland and/or fat. Protrusion in these spaces should be evaluated with the patient's eyes open and closed, as well as with gentle pressure applied to the globe with the lids closed, to better define protrusion of tissue in these areas.

Fig. 21-3 illustrates a patient who was seen 1 year after she had undergone a bilateral upper lid blepharoplasty. The surgeon had apparently overlooked ptotic lacrimal glands. Operative photographs show that the central fat pad was excised, but the medial fat pocket and lacrimal gland were not corrected. Heeding the advice given by Owsley[7] and others to open the orbital septum all the way across the lid lessens the likelihood of overlooking these structures.

Ptosis

The upper lids should be evaluated for ptosis. With normal frontal gaze, the lid margins should rest above the pupil, but there should be no scleral show above the limbus. (The normal covering of the upper cornea is about 1 mm with the eyes in the primary position.[2]) Ptosis must be recognized, classified, and corrected. It may be an initial complaint of the patient, or it may have been unrecognized. It definitely will be recognized postoperatively. If there is unilateral or bilateral ptosis, the degree of asymmetry and the lid apertures must be measured. Levator function must be evaluated with the brow stabilized to eliminate frontalis action. A standard blepharoplasty will not correct true ptosis. It may seem to improve it for a brief postoperative period, but invariably the ptosis reappears.

Either transcutaneous levator resection or the Fasanella-Servat[4] transconjunctival approach can be performed independently or in combination with a blepharoplasty. The Fasanella-Servat operation, involving a levator resection, is a conjunctival tarsal resection that incorporates resection of a portion of Müller's muscle. If there is not fair (5 to 7 mm) or good (8 mm or more) levator function, correction of severe ptosis usually requires one of the sling procedures.

Lower lid position

It is very important to evaluate the level of the lower lid in forward gaze. If scleral show or lateral sagging of the lid is not recognized preoperatively, one will most assuredly end up with in-

creased scleral show or an ectropion postoperatively. (See Chapter 27.)

Visual acuity

Gross visual acuity in each eye should be tested and recorded using either a wall-mounted or hand-held chart (Fig. 21-4). (See Chapter 26 in which Dr. Weis discusses the 2% incidence of amblyopia in the general population.) Preexisting visual loss undiagnosed preoperatively may later be claimed to have been caused by surgery. Many surgeons will not do a lower lid blepharoplasty in a patient who is blind in one eye.

Tear production

Any patient with symptoms of chronic eye irritation or dryness is tested for tear production. The Schirmer test is easily performed and should be readily available in all offices (Fig. 21-5). In the presence of diminished tear production, an ophthalmological consultation can be very helpful therapeutically and in determining the advisibility of surgery. Postoperatively patients should have artificial tear drops (e.g., Lacril) instilled in each eye. These drops are then sent home with the patient with instructions for their continued use. Nighttime ointments (e.g., Lacri-Lube), placement of soft lenses (e.g., Silfot, High Water Soft Lens), and pellets (e.g., Lacrisert) that, when inserted, release artificial tears over a 24-hour period are all useful adjuncts in the prevention of exposure keratitis and keratoconjunctivitis sicca.

Conjunctival integrity

Fluorescein and a blue Concept flashlight,* or rose bengal establishes the *diagnosis of* conjunctival or corneal irregularities or abrasions. These tools are invaluable aids preoperatively and postoperatively if there is concern (Fig. 21-6).

Visual fields

It is a simple matter to check monocular and binocular *gross* visual fields, as well as extraocular muscle function, by asking the patient to follow a moving finger with the head stabilized in the forward position. Many patients seeking blepharoplasty have laxity of skin of the upper lids to the degree that it drapes over the free margins of their lids and interferes with peripheral or in some instances even frontal vision. This may

---

*Concept Blu-Spot cobalt blue diffuse light, Concept, Inc., Clearwater, Fla.

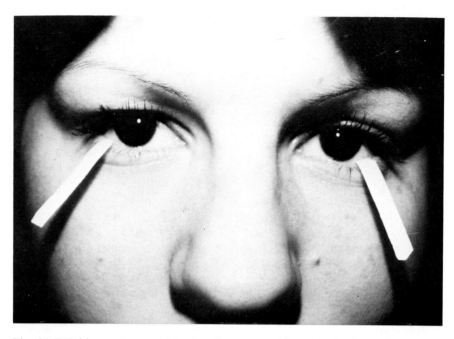

Fig. 21-5. Schirmer tear test. Wetting filter paper 15 mm in 5 minutes is normal.

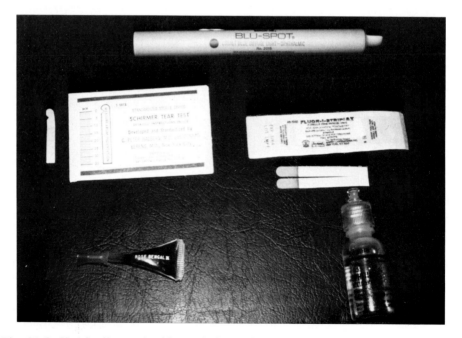

Fig. 21-6. Simple diagnostic aids: topical anesthetic (Ophthaine); fluorescein (Fluor-I-Strip); blue light (Concept Blu-Spot); Schirmer tear test.

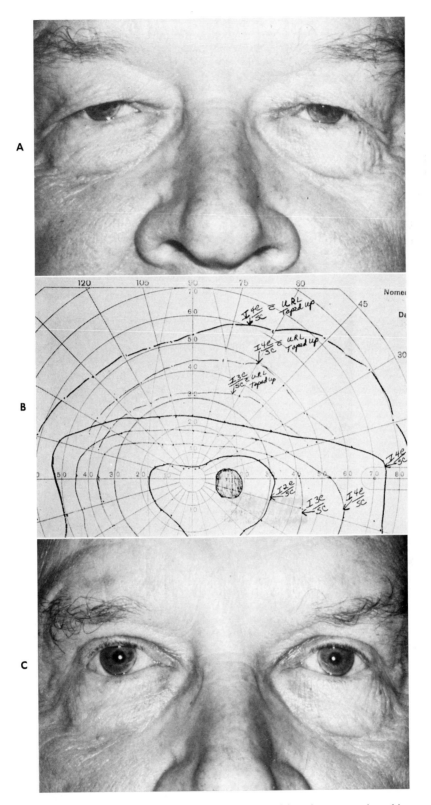

Fig. 21-7. A, Preoperative forward gaze in neutral position demonstrating skin crossing visual axis. **B,** Preoperative visual field examination demonstrating extent of improvement when lid is taped up (eliminating excess skin). **C,** Postoperative forward gaze in neutral position.

cause a medical disability. Such patients can be referred to an ophthalmologist, who performs and records on a chart the patient's *exact* visual fields. This test is performed first with the patient's lid and skin in the normal position and then with the eyebrow and upper lid skin taped up so as to eliminate this skin as a visual obstacle (Fig. 21-7). (Submitting a patient's preoperative photographs along wth the ophthalmologist's visual field charts will substantiate to an insurance company that surgery was indeed performed to improve vision.)

Ophthalmoscopic examination

The ophthalmoscope can be used to determine the clarity of the anterior and posterior chambers and the lens, as well as to examine the retina. Obviously, if there is any question about the ophthalmoscopic findings, the patient should be referred to an ophthalmologist.

Bells' phenomenon

It is worthwhile to check each patient for adequacy of Bell's phenomenon. With normal function, the globe rotates superiorly when the eyelids are closed. This protects against accidental corneal injury or exposure keratitis. This test is easily performed by the examiner stabilizing the patient's eyebrow in a cephalic direction with the eyes open and then asking the patient to close his or her eyes. If the patient's Bell's phenomenon is

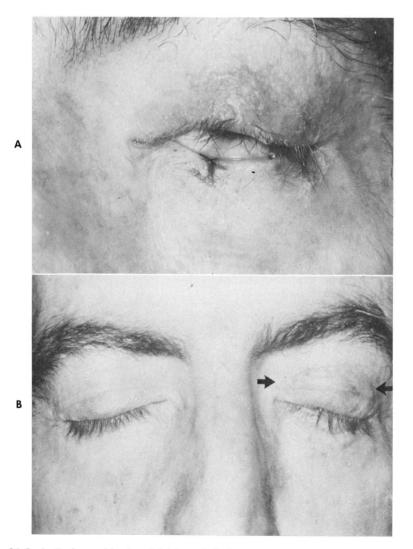

Fig. 21-8. A, Patient with cicatricial lagophthalmos. Good Bell's phenomenon has protected eye from serious exposure problems. **B,** Upper lid after release of contracture and full-thickness skin graft.

normal, no pupil and little cornea will be visible in the eye in which the lid has been held open. Because a temporary lagophthalmos usually occurs at the time of upper lid blepharoplasty, this mechanism is a great protection for the patient (Fig. 21-8).

Special examination

Whenever the patient's symptoms, physical findings, or simple diagnostic procedures indicate the need for further testing, the patient should be referred to an ophthalmologist for additional studies. In addition to the visual field test mentioned above, these tests may include slit-lamp examination, pressure readings for suspected glaucoma, and tonometry for exophthalamos or enophthalamos.

PHYSICIAN-TO-PATIENT PRESENTATION

Having completed the history and physical evaluation, the surgeon is now ready to make a recommendation to the patient. It may be helpful for the surgeon to start with a simple statement such as, "I believe that the things that concern you about your upper and lower eyelids can be improved with surgery," or "I have real concern that surgery will not lead to the kind of improvement that you expect, and therefore I recommend that you not have surgery." Such statements immediately let the patient know where the surgeon stands.

The patient can now be advised that if a decision is made to go ahead with surgery, he or she will receive a detailed explanation of preoperative plans (including lab work, shampooing, diet, and medications), general events surrounding the surgery, and the anticipated postoperative recovery. The surgeon should also accept the responsibility for giving the patient a general description of what to expect. This description might be as follows:

Surgery is done as an outpatient at the hospital (or office surgery suite) with sedation and local anesthesia. A day or two before surgery, routine laboratory tests are performed. You will receive typewritten instructions on your preparation for surgery and advising you to arrive 1 hour before the scheduled surgery. The nurse will check you in and prepare you for surgery by administering medication that will have a calming effect and remove tension, which almost all patients experience preoperatively. The nurse will also check your temperature, pulse, and blood pressure and start an intravenous infusion, which is used to administer addi-

tional medication during surgery. Your blood pressure and heart rate are monitored throughout surgery. The surgery begins with my measuring and diagramming on your eyelid skin. Then a local anesthetic is injected in the skin to numb the area for surgery. The surgery will take approximately 1 to 1½ hours. The time will pass quickly for you, and we will see to it that you are kept in a calm state throughout the operation. Although you may doze off, there will be times when I may ask you to open and close your eyes.

The patient is now assured that the surgeon personally will be doing the surgery. This is a secret concern of many patients. The most important elements of postoperative care are then outlined for the patient. These include eyedrops, cold compresses, and elevation of the head and bed.

A simple diagram is done in front of the patient on his or her chart, indicating the location of incisions and resultant scars. It also shows the anticipated removal of skin, fat pockets, and muscle. This gives the patient a better understanding of how the surgery is done without being unnecessarily technical. It also substantiates in the patient's chart that the surgeon has indeed presented this material to the patient. It is a good time for the surgeon to point out that wherever there is an incision, there is a scar and that although scars are permanent, the incisions are placed in such a manner as to make them as inconspicuous as possible.

HEALTH PROBLEMS

In patients with health problems, other preoperative considerations must be made.

Hypertension

Patients whose hypertension is well controlled with medication should continue taking that medication up to and including the morning of surgery and postoperatively. β-Blockers (such as propranolol) protect the cardiovascular system against the deleterious effects of epinephrine (Adrenaline).[3] Propranolol and epinephrine compete for β-receptor sites. Patients taking propranolol preoperatively may respond to epinephrine by developing hypertension and bradycardia.[1] The chronotropic and inotropic effects of epinephrine are negated.

Dilute (1:800,000) concentrations of epinephrine provide adequate cutaneous hemostasis.[8] It has been my experience that drug reactions and interactions related to epinephrine can be virtually eliminated by using 0.5% lidocaine hydrochloride (Xylocaine) and adding epinephrine to a concentration of 1:500,000. Skin blanching, indistinguishable from that achieved with stronger concentrations, is achieved. Most studies would indicate that no arrhythmias occur with epinephrine doses of 5 μg/kg.[8] A concentration of 1:200,000 epinephrine equals 5 μg/ml. If 1:600,000 epinephrine is used, one should be able to use a volume three times the patient's weight in kilograms with almost complete freedom from arrhythmias. Patients in whom hypertension is first diagnosed at the time of the initial consultation should be evaluated and treated before surgery.

Edema

Many patients use diuretics. In such individuals the serum potassium level should be measured and an ECG obtained. An altered ECG (depressed ST segments, lengthened QT interval, and depression or inversion of T waves) is an indication for postponing surgery until potassium depletion is effectively corrected. Rapid intravenous administration, which corrects the serum level without restoring the intracellular component, is of little or no value.[3]

Diabetes

The brittle ketone-prone diabetic patient is probably not a good candidate for blepharoplasty. Any surgery should be in consultation with the patient's internist. It is better to allow patients with ketone-resistant, maturity-onset diabetes to become mildly hyperglycemic during surgery rather than risk hypoglycemia.[3]

Hyperthyroidism and hypothyroidism

Hyperthroidism and hypothyroidism need medical control, and each has aesthetic considerations (exophthalmos and edema, respectively). Certainly, these conditions should be well controlled medically before the patient can be considered for elective surgery, such as blepharoplasty.

Aspirin and aspirin-containing compounds

Aspirin and aspirin-containing compounds interfere with normal blood clotting. The deleterious effects of one aspirin can last as long as 10 days. (The average life of a platelet is 10 days.) Patients should be advised to discontinue the use of aspirin 2 weeks before surgery and for 10 days after surgery. Patients should check all medications with their pharmacist to find out if they contain aspirin or other drugs that may cause abnormal bleeding. (The surgeon should check also.)

Bleeding time may be prolonged secondary to aspirin injestion.

Smoking

Patients are encouraged to stop smoking before and after surgery. Local edema is increased by smoking. The blood pressure and pulse rate are increased.

LABORATORY TESTS

Laboratory tests to be considered for each patient include:
1. CBC
2. Urinalysis
3. Preoperative coagulation panel (PTT, PT, bleeding time, platelet count, thrombin time)
4. Serum potassium
5. ECG

USUAL POSTOPERATIVE PROBLEMS

The usual postoperative problems should also be outlined for the patient, with suggested therapy and explanations as to why they occur and how long they will last.

Pain

The need for pain medication usually lasts only 2 to 3 days. Severe pain should be investigated.

Swelling and bruising

Ice compresses, elevation, and rest help to minimize swelling and bruising. Patients should be advised that within 2 weeks they will be able to use makeup and disguise most of the bruising. They should also know that it may be 3 to 4 weeks before they are completely comfortable with their appearance in a social setting.

Lagophthalmos

Patients undergoing upper lid blepharoplasty need to be advised that when they close their eyes, they may not shut completely. They will not be aware of this, but whoever is with them will. They should be told not to be concerned about it, since it is a temporary condition that may last for several days to a few weeks.

Increased scleral show

Patients need to know that when they look in the mirror, they may see more of the "white of the eye" showing above the lower lid margin than was present preoperatively. This may last from several weeks to several months.

Tightness

Postoperatively patients will become aware of the simple act of blinking and a feeling of rightness associated with it. This also may last for a period of several weeks to several months. If patients know this ahead of time, they will not be concerned about it.

Asymmetry

Dr. Gorney has shown us that all faces are asymmetrical. Patients become acutely aware of this postoperatively. The use of the reversal mirror* (patients see themselves reversed from what they usually see when they look in the mirror) is a valuable preoperative aid in establishing patient awareness of asymmetry. If patients are told preoperatively that they should expect some slight differences in the appearance of their eyes, depending on the location of incisions and other postoperative factors, they will accept it more willingly postoperatively.

*Meddev Corp., Los Altos, Calif.

Blurred vision and tearing

It is common, in the early postoperative period, for patients to experience some blurring of vision, some matting of material in the eye, and increased tearing. Again, if they know to expect this, they will handle it much better.

POSSIBLE COMPLICATIONS

The detail with which possible postoperative complications is discussed varies greatly among different surgeons and also depends on how much a patient wishes to hear. The patient is considering volunteering for surgery and is entitled to know the risks.

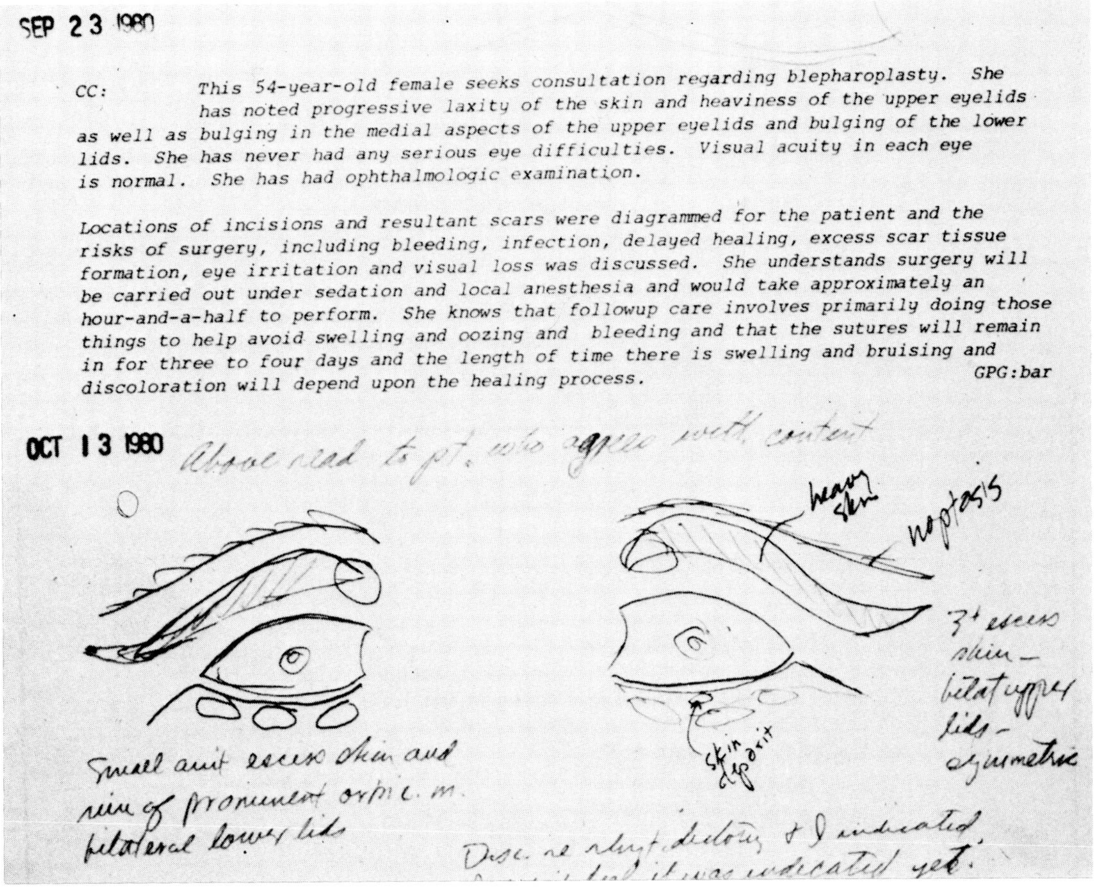

SEP 23 1980

CC: This 54-year-old female seeks consultation regarding blepharoplasty. She has noted progressive laxity of the skin and heaviness of the upper eyelids as well as bulging in the medial aspects of the upper eyelids and bulging of the lower lids. She has never had any serious eye difficulties. Visual acuity in each eye is normal. She has had ophthalmologic examination.

Locations of incisions and resultant scars were diagrammed for the patient and the risks of surgery, including bleeding, infection, delayed healing, excess scar tissue formation, eye irritation and visual loss was discussed. She understands surgery will be carried out under sedation and local anesthesia and would take approximately an hour-and-a-half to perform. She knows that followup care involves primarily doing those things to help avoid swelling and oozing and bleeding and that the sutures will remain in for three to four days and the length of time there is swelling and bruising and discoloration will depend upon the healing process.

GPG:bar

OCT 13 1980

Fig. 21-9. Patient's record, including typewritten consultation that was read to patient at second office visit. Diagram of surgery plan is also drawn for patient and serves as preoperative review for surgeon.

SURGERY SCHEDULING

K   PT. W/C _____

G

         _____
          (sched. by/date)

Name: _Jane Doe_____ age: _____

phone: _____ #2 phone: _____

    Surg/date/time: _____ hours: 1½

local ____✓____   general _____

out pt. ___✓____   in pt. _____

   Surg. room/hosp: Hosp. O.P. or Office Surgery Suite

Procedure: Bilat. U+L bleph_____

_____

_____

Diagnosis: _____

Assist: _____ confirmed: _____

Ref. Dr. _____ phone: _____ advised: _____

Pt. advised: _____ Info. sheet: _____

Photos taken: _____ photo. consent: _____
          surg. consent: _____
Prosthesis/other needs: _____

_____

       Fee quote: **2,000 IA** by: _____
            ✓
IA date noted: _____
IA billed: _____
IA received: _____

other: CBC, U.A._____
  ____ Pre surg. hemorrhagic panel

_____

Fig. 21-10. Surgery scheduling slip that I fill out for secretary's use in giving information to patient and making surgical arrangements. Checkmark under *2000* indicates that I have quoted fee to patient. Absence of a checkmark under *IA* indicates that I have not told patient that it is payable "in advance" of surgery. A checkmark under *NIA* would have meant "not in advance."

These possible complications include:

A. General
   1. Bleeding
   2. Infection
   3. Delayed healing
   4. Excessive scar tissue formation
B. Lid complications
   1. Ectropion
   2. Ptosis
   3. Lagophthalmos
   4. Asymmetry
   5. Vascular changes in skin
   6. Hypesthesia
   7. Overresection of fat
   8. Underresection of fat
   9. Persistent lacrimal gland ptosis
C. Ocular complications
   1. Corneal abrasion
   2. Keratoconjunctivitis sicca
   3. Diplopia
   4. Loss of vision

These complications are well covered in the various chapters on blepharoplasty within this text, and it is not within the scope of this chapter on preoperative considerations to go into detail regarding them.

CONCLUSION OF THE CONSULTATION

It is important that the patient not feel pressured to make a decision regarding surgery at the conclusion of the initial consultation. I do not believe, however, that it is necessary to see every prospective surgical patient more than once. If I feel that the patient's expectations are realistic in terms of what I think can be accomplished, I am satisfied to arrange for surgery at that time.

Patients are advised that they, in turn, should feel comfortable with what I have told them and understand that we are talking in terms of improvement—not perfection. Whether or not a decision is made regarding surgery at the time of the first consultation, the patient is encouraged to return to ask additional questions or obtain further information. At the time of a second office visit, the typewritten consultation from the first visit is read to the patient (Fig. 21-9). This reassures the patient that individualized, personal attention and concern is being given to the patient's problems. It also allows an opportunity to correct any omissions and to reaffirm our goals.

Fees, photos, scheduling, and arrangements

Each of us has our own comfort zone and our own time constraints. I do not bring up the subject of fees unless patients ask. If they ask, then I tell them what the surgery fee will be. If they have not asked, at the conclusion of the consultation, I say to them, "It is necessary to take photographs of you for our record. After I do this, I will introduce you to our secretary, who will discuss other information that is going to be important to you in your decision." After taking the photographs, I take the patients to our secretary's office and introduce them. Our secretary is given the surgery scheduling slip that I have filled out at the conclusion of the consultation (Fig. 21-10). This is all the information the secretary needs in order to assist patients in making their decision:

1. What the procedure is
2. Where it will be performed
3. How long it will take
4. Whether the patient is to be under local or general anesthesia
5. Whether the patient is to be an inpatient or an outpatient
6. The fee and whether it is *IA* (in advance or *NIA* (not in advance)

REFERENCES

1. Aston, S.J., and Foster, C.A.: Propranolol-epinephrine interaction: a potential disaster, Plast. Reconstr. Surg. **72:**74, 1983.
2. Beard, C.: Ptosis, St. Louis, 1976, The C.V. Mosby Co., pp. 80-84.
3. Etherington, L.: Symposium of problems and complications in aesthetic plastic surgery of the face, Monterey, Calif., January 28, 1980.
4. Fasanella R.M., and Servat, J.: Levator resection for minimal ptosis: another simplified operation, Arch. Ophthalmol. **65:**4, 1980.
5. Mathews, W.A.: Symposium on disasters in plastic surgery, II, Newport Beach, Calif., March 31, 1982.
6. Mustarde, J.C.: Problems and possibilities in ptosis surgery, Plast. Reconstr. Surg. **56:**381, 1975.
7. Owsley, J.Q., Jr.: Resection of the prominent lateral fat pad during upper lid blepharoplasty, Plast. Reconstr. Surg. **65:**4, 1980.
8. Siegel, R.J., Vistnes, L.M., and Iverson, R.E.: Effective hemostasis with less epinephrine, Plast. Reconstr. Surg. **51:**129, 1973.
9. Souther, S.G., Corboy, J.M., and Thompson, J.B.: Fasanella-Servat operation for ptosis of upper eyelid, Plast. Reconstr. Surg. **53:**123, 1974.

Chapter 22

Applied anatomy in upper lid blepharoplasty

John Q. Owsley, Jr.

An exact understanding of functional anatomy is a necessary foundation for successful eyelid surgery. In this chapter it is my intent to review some current studies of the anatomy of the upper eyelid in order to recommend several useful techniques for upper lid blepharoplasty. For a more detailed description of the anatomy of the orbital-eyelid region, I recommend Beard and Quickert's text,[2] *Anatomy of the Orbit.* This dissection manual, now in its second edition, is an invaluable source of text and illustrations. In the present discussion I would like to emphasize several points that are described in greater detail in that source.

The orbicularis oculi muscle in the upper lid is divided into three parts: the pretarsal, preseptal, and orbital portions. The pretarsal portion is the most active during involuntary reflex blinking, and the preseptal and orbital portions are called into use for tight squinting. It is the preseptal portion of the orbicularis muscle that is exposed by the initial removal of the redundant skin strip during upper lid blepharoplasty. Removal of a portion of the preseptal orbicularis muscle has been a standard technique in Oriental blepharoplasty for many years.[3,5,13] More recently, it has been included as a routine part of upper lid blepharoplasty in white patients.[1] Removal of a strip of preseptal orbicularis muscle across the entire width of the upper eyelid does not cause any functional deficit in either the blinking or squinting function of the muscle.

The muscle strip resection greatly enhances exposure of the orbital septum and the area of its fusion with the levator expansion where it inserts at the superior border of the tarsus. It is this fusion of the levator expansion and the orbital sep-

tum that defines the inferior margin of the preaponeurotic space containing the medial and central preaponeurotic fat pads and laterally the lacrimal gland. The gland is normally maintained in a small fossa behind the lateral superior border of the bony orbit. In certain patients with a bulky lateral hooding condition of the upper lid, a lateral fat pad is encountered overlying the orbital septum in the region of its attachment to the superior lateral orbital rim. This fat pad extends over the lateral portion of the orbital rim toward the outer extreme of the eyebrow. The lateral fat pad is easily dissected away from the underlying orbital septum and periosteum of the bony rim but is quite adherent to the undersurface of the overlying orbicularis muscle. Resection of the lateral fat pad in conjunction with removal of the strip of orbicularis muscle is necessary for adequate correction of the lateral hooding deformity.[12]

Splitting the entire orbital septum transversely to the lateral bony rim opens the preaponeurotic space widely to reveal the extent of the fat pads. I favor this exposure rather than teasing the redundant fatty tissue through small stab incisions for several reasons:

1. I frequently encounter large vessels coursing through the fat pads that could be injured either by blind injection of a local anesthetic or by excessive traction during dissection without adequate visualization. In either case the result can be brisk bleeding with the possible development of a retrobulbar hematoma.

2. A ptotic lacrimal gland is encountered with more frequency than was previously recog-

nized. The contribution of the gland to the lateral fullness of the upper lid is to be recognized and should be corrected by suture replacement of the gland into its normal fossa.[7] (See Editorial Comments following this chapter.)

3. The prominent central fat pad is fusiform and extends laterally to the area of attachment of the orbital septum to the bony rim. It contributes to fullness all across the upper lid and must be adequately delivered for appropriate resection. Frequently, sharp dissection is necessary for complete delivery of the fat in the lateral part of the lid. I prefer cross-clamping of the dissected fat pad and electrocoagulation of the cut edge for secure hemostasis. Electrocautery is also useful for additional obliteration of residual prominent fat, particularly in the area of the medial fat pad following initial cross-clamping and resection.[11]

4. Removal of the muscle strip, opening the orbital septum widely, and resection of the fat pads expose the levator expansion where it inserts at the superior edge of the tarsus. Closure of the skin incision along this level results in adherence of the scar line to the underlying levator, where it fuses with the orbital septum. This scar adherence deepens the palpebral sulcus while minimizing the fold and enhances the exposure of the pretarsal portion of the lid in a pleasing manner.

Some controversy exists regarding the anatomical basis for the upper eyelid sulcus and fold. The fold is commonly obscure or absent in Oriental patients, and numerous techniques have been published for the creation of a well-defined sulcus and fold in Oriental upper lid blepharoplasty.[10,14] Variations or elaborations of such techniques have been adopted by some surgeons for routine use in white patients in any effort to create a controlled level or definition of the upper lid sulcus.[6,15]

In his 1932 text entitled *Anatomy of the Human Orbit*, Whitnall[16] states that the superior eyelid fold is created by the insertion of the levator aponeurosis into the skin at the level of the fold and that it is the contraction of the levator that causes the fold to become deeply recessed. According to Whitnall, the cutaneous insertion of the levator expansion is into the skin of the fold of the preseptal portion of the lid by means of vertically radiating fibers of delicate connective tissue. This classical description of the levator insertion and its role in the creation of the superior eyelid fold has been widely accepted.

In 1962 Isaksson[8] reviewed the literature regarding the anatomy of the insertion of the levator aponeurosis. He concluded that the connective tissue lamellae that stretch forward from the fused junction of the levator and the orbital septum blend with the other loose connective tissue of the upper lid in the supratarsal region. According to his observations, the so-called cutaneous insertion is not a well-defined structure that deserves to be looked on as part of the levator aponeurosis.

According to Isaksson, the idea of a distinct cutaneous aponeurotic insertion does not conform with two readily observable facts. First, the eyelid skin is freely movable over the underlying orbicularis muscle in the area of the lid fold. Second, the fold is obliterated by the injection of anesthetic fluids or the development of edema, which could not be the case of the skin were firmly attached to the levator expansion. Of course, when fluid is absorbed, the fold immediately reappears at its preexisting position when the lid is elevated.

Isaksson's views have since been supported by the electron microscopy studies published by Kuwabara, Cogan, and Johnson[9] in 1974. These authors found that the levator aponeurosis blends with the orbital septum where it attaches to the superior edge of the tarsus and then passes in front of the tarsus to insert chiefly into the fiberous septa that extends from the tarsus, separating the bundles of the orbicularis muscle, to insert into and firmly attach the pretarsal skin to the tarsus.

Studies by Collins and Beard[4] published in 1978 have confirmed Isaksson's study. Their anatomical experiments have provided strong supporting evidence that there is no direct insertion of the levator expansion into the skin. According to them, the loose connective tissue of the eyelid does not appear to have any organized direction and appears equally haphazard in orientation in the pretarsal, preseptal, and skin fold regions. However, as Isaksson significantly pointed out, the thickness of the subcutaneous tissue increases markedly above the level of the palpebral fold. Below the lid fold the subcutaneous tissue is thin in association with snug adhesion between the skin and the underlying orbicularis and the tarsus, which is responsible for the typically smooth unwrinkled appearance of the pretarsal skin.

When the levator contracts and elevates the tarsus, the overlying snugly attached orbicularis muscle and pretarsal skin move up as a unit. The normal supratarsal fold is thereby created as the unattached and therefore mobile skin above the tarsus, with its thicker subcutaneous layer, folds over the adherent pretarsal skin. In effect, the lid sulcus is secondarily created by the folding of the supratarsal portion of the lid.

This description of the anatomy of the palpebral fold is typical in whites with rare exception and is also the case in Orientals in whom the lid fold is present. In certain individuals the upper lid fold is obscure and the pretarsal skin exhibits loose adherence with one or several fine wrinkles near the palpebral margin. This appearance is probably associated with a thicker layer of subcutaneous tissue in the pretarsal region and less-firm adhesion between the skin and the underlying pretarsal orbicularis and tarsus. This situation occurs commonly in Oriental individuals but is rare in whites. It is in such patients that supratarsal fixation by suture attachment between the skin to the levator expansion at the level of the superior border of the tarsus is necessary to eliminate the loose folding quality of the pretarsal skin and create a sharply defined palpebral cleft and fold.

In those patients undergoing blepharoplasty in whom the palpebral sulcus and fold exist in a normal location, removal of excess skin, muscle, and fatty tissue as previously described will deepen the sulcus, minimizing the fold, and improve exposure of the pretarsal skin. Routine deep suture fixation is unnecessary in those patients in whom the fold preexists at a normal level.

REFERENCES

1. Baker, T.J., Gordon, H.L., and Mosienko, P.: Upper lid blepharoplasty, Plast. Reconstr. Surg. **60:**692, 1977.
2. Beard, C., and Quickert, M.H.: Anatomy of the orbit, New York, Aesculapius Publishers, Inc.
3. Boo-Chai, K.: Plastic construction of the superior palpebral fold, Plast. Reconstr. Surg. **31:**556, 1964.
4. Collins, R., Beard, C., and Wood, I.: Experimental and clinical data on the insertion of the levator palpebrae superioris muscle, Am. J. Ophthalmol. **85:**792, 1978.
5. Fernandez, L.R.: Double eyelid operation in the Oriental in Hawaii, Plast. Reconstr. Surg. **25:**257, 1960.
6. Flowers, R.S.: Bicentennial blepharoplasty, Motion picture presented at the annual meeting of the American Society of Plastic and Reconstructive Surgeons, September 1976.
7. Horton, C.E., Carraway, J.H., and Potenza, A.D.: Treatment of a lacrimal bulge in blepharoplasty by repositioning the gland, Plast. Reconstr. Surg. **61:**701, 1978.
8. Isaksson, I.: Studies on congenital genuine blepharoptosis, Copenhagen, 1962, Munksgaard.
9. Kuwabara, T., Cogan, D., and Johnson, C.: Structure of the muscles of the upper eyelid, Arch. Ophthalmol. **93:**1189, 1975.
10. Millard, D.R., Jr.: Oriental peregrinations, Plast. Reconstr. Surg. **16:**319, 1955.
11. Owsley, J.Q., Jr.: Blepharoplasty variations. In Goulian, D., and Courtiss, E.H., editors: Symposium on surgery of the aging face, St. Louis, 1978, The C.V. Mosby Co.
12. Owsley, J.Q., Jr.: Resection of the prominent lateral fat pad during upper lid blepharoplasty, Plast. Reconstr. Surg. **65:**4, 1980.
13. Sayoc, B.T.: Plastic construction of the superior palpebral fold, Am. J. Ophthalmol **38:**556, 1954.
14. Sayoc, B.T.: Surgery of the Oriental eyelid, Clin. Plast. Surg. **1:**157, 1974.
15. Sheen, J.H.: Supratarsal fixation in upper blepharoplasty, Plast. Reconstr. Surg. **54:**424, 1974.
16. Whitnall, E.: The structure and muscle of the eyelids. In Anatomy of the human orbit, London, 1932.

Editorial comments
Chapter 22

A word of caution regarding suture fixation of the lacrimal gland to the posterior aspect of the orbital rim is that personal experience has shown that this can cause ptosis postoperatively (Fig. 1). Frequently the ptosis, or bulging, of the lacrimal gland can only be seen when the patient's eyes are closed (Fig. 2). With elevation of the lid, the gland disappears behind the orbital rim. If the gland is fixed to the periosteum at a level lower than it normally achieves with opening, limitation of lid elevation can ensue. I have experienced this, and secondary surgery was necessary to release the gland. This resulted in complete correction of the ptosis. Since I presented this problem at a sym-

posium on postoperative complications of blepharoplasty, another plastic surgeon reported on the same complication corrected by secondary surgery.

The portion of the gland that is ptotic does not contain the lacrimal duct. There is no clear-cut evidence that excising this portion of the gland has long-term deleterious effects. If the gland-periosteum suture technique is performed, one should be absolutely certain that no orbital septum or fibers of the lateral expansion of the levator muscle are used to support the gland in its fossa.

G.P.G.

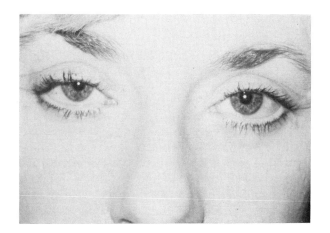

Fig. 1. Ptosis of right upper lid 3 months postoperatively.

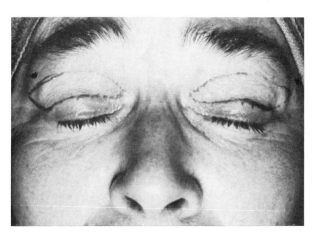

Fig. 2. Bilateral lacrimal gland ptosis that had not been detected with patient's eyes open.

Chapter 23

Correction of crow's-feet with orbicularis oculi muscle flaps: a technique to improve crow's-feet and lateral canthal skin folds

Sherrell J. Aston

Skin folds and wrinkles in the lateral canthal area and lateral brow ptosis are improved little by standard blepharoplasty and facioplasty techniques. The difficulty in improving lateral canthal skin folds and lateral brow ptosis is suggested by the different operative procedures reported.

Rees[9] noted that lateral and wide extensions of upper and lower lid blepharoplasty incisions help correct lateral canthal skin folds and wrinkles, but when the maximum amount of skin has been removed, persistent skin folds may remain in the lateral canthal area. A brow lift or temporal lift with undermining of the temporal skin medially as far as the brow and lateral canthus may subsequently improve the skin folds and wrinkles.[8] Viñas, Caviglia, and Cortinas[11] and Kaye[5] recommended a bicoronal flap forehead rhytidectomy and brow lift, with wide undermining beyond the lateral canthus to the zygomatic arches, to improve crow's-feet lines and lateral brow ptosis. González-Ulloa and Stevens[3,4] reported a racquet incision to join upper and lower lid blepharoplasty incisions and to create a triangular flap of skin lateral to the canthus, which is then raised toward the upper lid as the wounds are sutured. Lewis[6,7] advised Z-plasties at the lateral extension of upper and/or lower lid blepharoplasty incisions to help correct ptosis in the lateral canthal area. Courtiss, Webster, and White[2] described a double W-plasty to allow maximum excision of skin in the lateral portion of the upper eyelids.

Lateral orbital skin folds and wrinkles and lateral brow ptosis are primarily due to three fac-

tors: (1) senile degeneration of the skin, (2) laxity and ptosis of the orbicularis oculi muscle and lateral brow ptosis as part of the aging process, and (3) the accordian-like activity of the orbicularis oculi muscle during movements of facial expression, which accentuates folds and wrinkles as the muscle shortens and the overlying skin does not. It is this third factor that contributes significantly to crow's-feet in the younger patient who has lines and wrinkles in excess of those anticipated for the younger age. Very often, patients with this problem demonstrate greater and more frequent expressive facial animation.

Skoog[10] suggested that the lateral orbital portion of the orbicularis oculi muscle could be splayed out and sutured in the splayed position to help smooth overlying skin and prevent excessive wrinkling at the lateral canthus. Skoog also noted that the orbicularis oculi muscle could be split laterally and the cut ends separated without disturbing eyelid function. I devised the technique of orbicularis oculi muscle flaps described here following the suggestions of Skoog noted above.[1]

TECHNIQUE

The lateral orbital portion of the orbicularis oculi muscle is exposed through the temporal and preauricular face-lift incision. Dissection from lateral to medial over the course of the temporal branch of the seventh cranial nerve is performed by rotating a fingertip into the skin flap and downward to separate the skin flap from underlying fascia (Fig. 23-1). The orbicularis oculi mus-

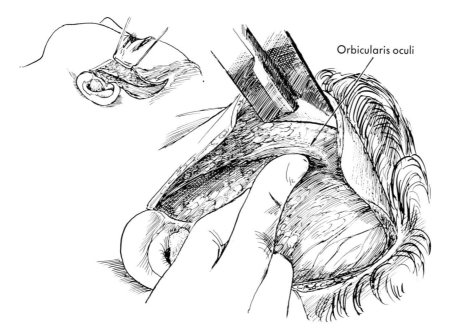

Fig. 23-1. Temporal portion of face-lift skin flap is elevated with care to avoid frontal branch of facial nerve and to expose orbicularis oculi muscle. (From Aston, S.J.: Orbicularis oculi muscle flaps: a technique to reduce crows feet and lateral canthal skin folds, Plast. Reconstr. Surg. **65:**206, 1980.)

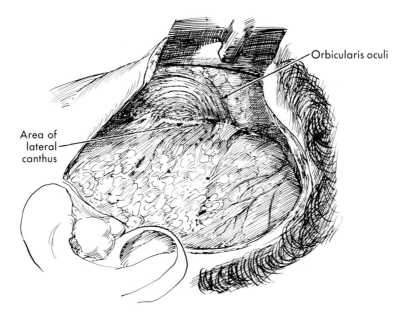

Fig. 23-2. Orbicularis oculi muscle attached to skin flap. (From Aston, S.J.: Orbicularis oculi muscle flaps: a technique to reduce crows feet and lateral canthal skin folds, Plast. Reconstr. Surg. **65:**206, 1980.)

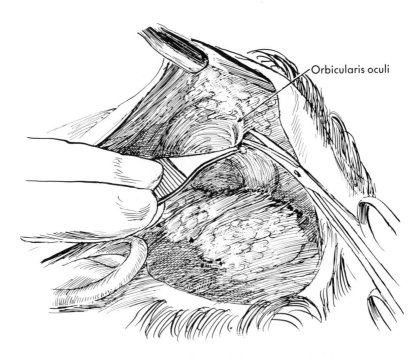

Fig. 23-3. Orbicularis oculi muscle is dissected from temporal skin flap. (From Aston, S.J.: Orbicularis oculi muscle flaps: a technique to reduce crows feet and lateral canthal skin folds, Plast. Reconstr. Surg. **65:**206, 1980.)

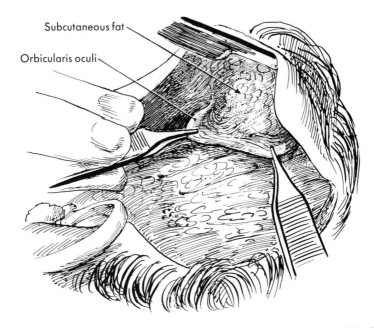

Fig. 23-4. Orbicularis oculi muscle is splayed out. (From Aston, S.J.: Orbicularis oculi muscle flaps: a technique to reduce crows feet and lateral canthal skin folds, Plast. Reconstr. Surg. **65:**206, 1980.)

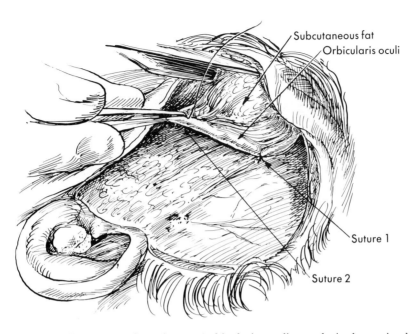

Fig. 23-5. Desired amount of tension on orbicularis oculi muscle is determined, and splayed-out orbicularis oculi muscle is sutured into position. (From Aston, S.J.: Orbicularis oculi muscle flaps: a technique to reduce crows feet and lateral canthal skin folds, Plast. Reconstr. Surg. **65:**206, 1980.)

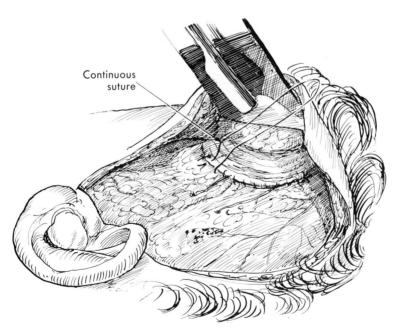

Fig. 23-6. Completion of muscle suturing. (From Aston, S.J.: Orbicularis oculi muscle flaps: a technique to reduce crows feet and lateral canthal skin folds, Plast. Reconstr. Surg. **65:**206, 1980.)

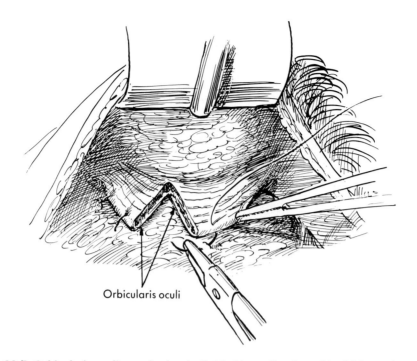

Orbicularis oculi

Fig. 23-7. Orbicularis oculi muscle ring is divided laterally when skin folds are large and orbicularis oculi muscle is thick. Separated muscle ends are sutured under tension. (From Aston, S.J.: Orbicularis oculi muscle flaps: a technique to reduce crows feet and lateral canthal skin folds, Plast. Reconstr. Surg. **65:**206, 1980.)

cle is present 3 to 5 cm lateral to the orbital rim and is closely adherent to the undersurface of the skin flap (Fig. 23-2). The muscle is thicker and more clearly defined in some patients than in others. Dissection in the correct plane frees the muscle from the temporal fascia and leaves the muscle attached to the skin flap. Dissection is then continued medially to the orbital rim.

The lateral border of the orbicularis oculi muscle is held with tissue forceps, and small, blunt scissors are used to separate the muscle from the thin layer of subcutaneous fat between the muscle and overlying skin (Fig. 23-3). The muscle is dissected from the skin flap as far medially as the lateral orbital rim; it is splayed out with two pairs of forceps; the skin flap is draped over the muscle flap held by the forceps, and traction is placed on the muscle (Fig. 23-4). The cephaloposterior pull on the muscle transmitted to the skin of the lateral canthal area and eyelids is observed, and the desired tension is determined. The splayed-out muscle is sutured into position with two stitches of chromic catgut at the cephalad and caudad limits of the expanded muscle (Fig. 23-5). A running catgut stitch is placed along the lateral border of the muscle between the two positioning sutures (Fig. 23-6).

When skin folds at the lateral canthal area are large and the orbicularis oculi muscle is thick, the muscle ring is divided in a lateral-to-medial direction at a point lateral to the lateral canthus (Fig. 23-7). The divided ends of the muscle are separated, splayed out in a cephaloposterior direction, and sutured to the temporal fascia under the desired amount of tension. Excessive tension on the divided muscle will cause an undesired "pull" at the lateral canthus that may persist for several months postoperatively. When muscle flap suturing is done, the overlying skin flap is redraped and the surgical procedure is completed.

Frequently during upper lid blepharoplasty I excise a strip of preseptal orbicularis oculi muscle beginning at the lateral limit of the upper lid skin excision. Therefore the excision includes a portion of the lateral orbital orbicularis oculi muscle. This does not interfere with the lateral-to-medial approach to the orbicularis oculi muscle for developing a muscle flap.

DISCUSSION

Patients selected for the technique described in this chapter have all had lateral canthal skin folds and wrinkles (crow's-feet lines) that were not anticipated to be eliminated by routine blepharo-

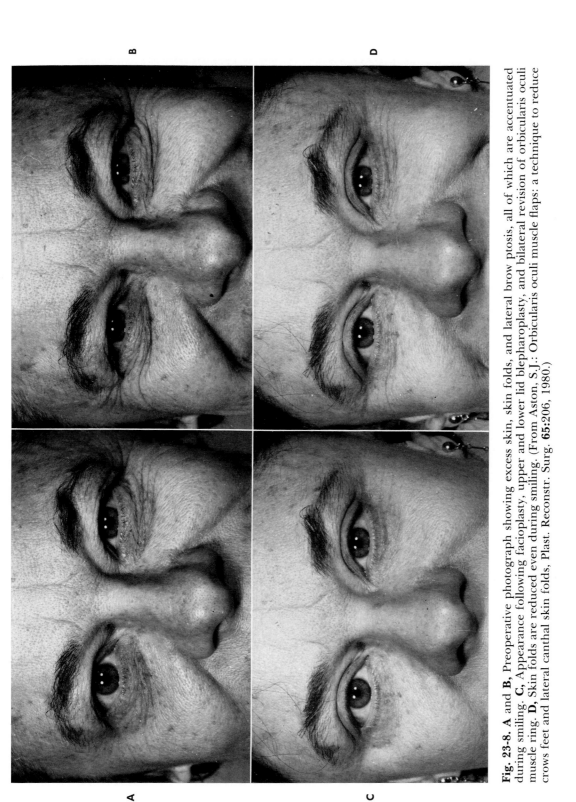

Fig. 23-8. A and **B,** Preoperative photograph showing excess skin, skin folds, and lateral brow ptosis, all of which are accentuated during smiling. **C,** Appearance following facioplasty, upper and lower lid blepharoplasty, and bilateral revision of orbicularis oculi muscle ring. **D,** Skin folds are reduced even during smiling. (From Aston, S.J.: Orbicularis oculi muscle flaps: a technique to reduce crows feet and lateral canthal skin folds, Plast. Reconstr. Surg. **65:**206, 1980.)

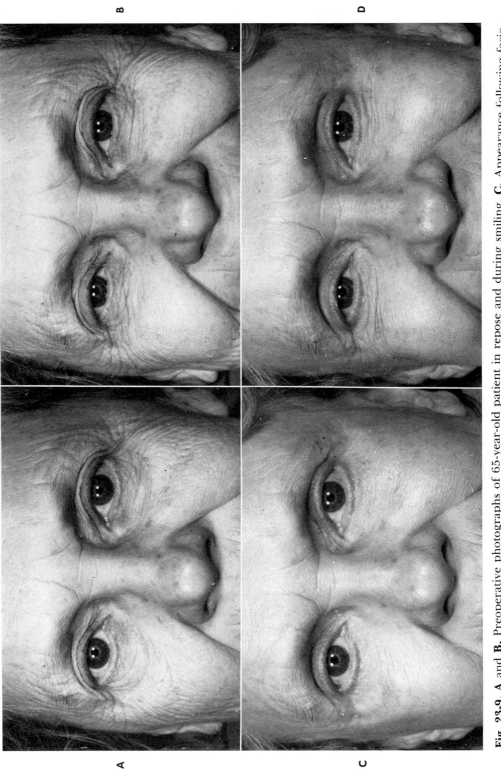

Fig. 23-9. A and **B,** Preoperative photographs of 65-year-old patient in repose and during smiling. **C,** Appearance following facioplasty, upper and lower lid blepharoplasty and orbicularis oculi muscle flaps with splaying out of muscle on right side and muscle ring division on left side. **D,** During smiling, orbicularis oculi muscle activity at lateral canthus is greater on undivided side (*right*) as compared with divided side (*left*), where folds and wrinkles are absent. (From Aston, S.J.: Orbicularis oculi muscle flaps: a technique to reduce crows feet and lateral canthal skin folds, Plast. Reconstr. Surg. **65:**206, 1980.)

plasty and/or facioplasty. All patients have undergone orbicularis oculi flaps at the time of facioplasty alone, facioplasty and upper lid blepharoplasty, lower lid blepharoplasty, or both upper and lower lid blepharoplasty.

In order to study the effects of the orbicularis oculi flaps, the technique has been varied in different patients as follows.

1. The orbicularis oculi muscles were dissected bilaterally from the overlying skin flaps, splayed out, and sutured to the temporal fascia.
2. The orbicularis oculi muscle ring was divided bilaterally and the cut ends of the muscle separated and sutured to the temporal fascia.
3. As an attempt to evaluate the effects of dividing the muscle ring, the orbicularis oculi muscle was divided and sutured unilaterally and the contralateral muscle was splayed out and sutured to the temporal fascia.

Skin folds and wrinkles in the lateral canthal area are reduced by orbicularis oculi muscle flaps more than would be anticipated following facioplasty or facioplasty and blepharoplasty (Fig. 23-8). Laxity, ptosis, and the accordian-like activity of the orbicularis oculi muscle are reduced by dissecting the lateral orbital portion of the muscle from the overlying skin and splaying it out in the cephaloposterior direction. In addition, some elevation of lateral brow ptosis has occurred in most patients who have undergone this technique.

Unilateral division of the orbicularis oculi muscle has caused a greater reduction of folds and wrinkles during movements of facial expression on the side of muscle division as compared with contralateral splaying out of the orbicularis oculi muscle (Fig. 23-9). Muscle ring division is most useful for correction of very large skin folds, deep wrinkles, and heavy ptotic lateral brows.

There have been some complications with the orbicularis oculi muscle flap technique. One patient who had bilateral muscle ring division showed unilateral pull on the lateral upper lid, caused by greater posterior traction placed on the upper limb of the separated muscle flap, as compared with more cephaloposterior traction on the contralateral side. Two patients have had complete unilateral temporal nerve paralysis in the early postoperative period. In the first patient in which this occurred, I was confident that the nerve was not traumatized during surgical dissection, and nerve injury by nylon sutures affixing the orbicularis oculi muscle to the temporal fascia

was postulated. The preauricular and temporal skin incision was opened, the temporal skin flap elevated, and the nylon sutures removed. The patient had complete return of frontalis motor function between the second and third postoperative months. Chromic catgut sutures are now used for muscle flap suturing. The second patient with transient temporal nerve paralysis had a great deal of scarring in the temporal area as a result of a childhood injury. There was some difficulty in dissecting the orbicularis oculi muscle at the time of the surgical procedure. Complete return of frontalis muscle function occurred within 6 weeks following surgery.

Eyelid function has not been disturbed in any patient in this series—even in those patients with orbicularis oculi muscle ring division. Innervation of the orbicularis oculi muscle occurs from the temporal trunk of the seventh cranial nerve with numerous small branches coming into the lateral portion of the orbicularis muscle. It is no doubt the numerous branches innervating the muscle that are not disrupted during the surgical procedure that maintain motor function postoperatively.

REFERENCES

1. Aston, S.J.: Orbicularis oculi muscle flaps: a technique to reduce crows feet and lateral canthal skin folds, Plast. Reconstr. Surg. **65:**206, 1980.
2. Courtiss, E.H., Webster, R.C., and White, M.F.: Use of double W-plasty in upper blepharoplasty, Plast. Reconstr. Surg. **53:**25, 1974.
3. Gonzalez-Ulloa, M., and Stevens, E.F.: The treatment of palpable bags, Plast. Reconstr. Surg. **27:**381, 1961.
4. Gonzalez-Ulloa, M., and Stevens, E.F.: Senile eyelid: esthetic correction. In Smith, J.W., and Converse, J.M., editors: Proceedings of the second international symposium on plastic and reconstructive surgery of the eye and adnexa, St. Louis, 1967, The C.V. Mosby Co.
5. Kaye, B.L.: The forehead lift, Plast. Reconstr. Surg. **60:**161, 1977.
6. Lewis, J.R.: Atlas of aesthetic plastic surgery, Boston, 1973, Little, Brown & Co.
7. Lewis, J.R.: The Z-blepharoplasty, Plast. Reconstr. Surg. **60:**161, 1977.
8. Rees, T.D., and Guy, C.L.: Patient selection and techniques in blepharoplasty and rhytidoplasty, Surg. Clin. North Am. **51:**353, 1971.
9. Rees, T.D.: Blepharoplasty. In Rees, T.D., and Wood-Smith, D., editors: Cosmetic facial surgery, Philadelphia, 1973, W.B. Saunders Co.
10. Skoog, T.: Plastic surgery, Philadelphia, 1974, W.B. Saunders Co.
11. Viñas, J.C., Caviglia, C., and Cortinas, J.L.: Forehead rhytidoplasty and brow lifting, Plast. Reconstr. Surg. **57:**445, 1976.

Editorial comments
Chapter 23

The problem of the elimination of crow's-feet, or periorbital wrinkling, remains a vexing one. Dr. Aston has shown that significant improvement is possible. The prospective patient must be advised that complete elimination of these wrinkles is not possible. Removal of excess skin, muscle, and protruding fat effects the tried-and-true benefits one can anticipate following blepharoplasty.

G.P.G.

Chapter 24

Variations in blepharoplasty technique

John R. Lewis, Jr.

The fact that there are a number of blepharoplasty techniques and variations should indicate that a single technique is not the ideal answer in every case. The earlier corrections of the drooping soft tissue of the lids and/or the removal of bags had to do with simple skin resection. This resection was carried out wherever the droop occurred. As refinements in technique developed, the incisions were made in unobstrusive locations, such as in the upper lid fold and just below the cilia of the lower lid. Later techniques used the creases ("smile lines") in the external canthal area to extend the eyelid incisions.

Further progress in the development of blepharoplasty techniques recognized the need also to eradicate the hypertrophic fat pads in the medial and intermediate compartments of the upper lids and in the medial, intermediate, and lateral compartments of the lower lids when these were bulging. The actual herniation of intraorbital fat against or through weakened orbital septa was later recognized. This necessitated teasing these hernias out and resecting them. For many years the actual skin resections remained the same except for the gradual elongation of the upper lid skin resection laterally and upward and of the lower lid skin resection laterally and downward.

The simplest and most straightforward technique should be the best for the average case and indeed for most cases so long as scars are minimized. This is the crescent-shaped resection of excess skin from the upper lid from the area of the major crease of the upper lid and an excision of the excess skin from just below the cilia of the lower lid. In each instance some lateral extension of the incision beyond the external canthus is required to excise the excess laterally to avoid a straight-up-and-down pull. No matter what the

technique, the principle of resection of the excess fat pads and/or hernias of the upper and lower lids is necessary in many instances to achieve a good result.

This straightforward upper and lower lid blepharoplasty (Fig. 24-1) has been described by a number of surgeons and has been popularized in recent years by Castañares, Morel Fatio, Rees, and others. A similar technique has been followed by many of the American pioneers in aesthetic surgery, including Aufricht, Straith, and others. There are instances when a variation in the technique for blepharoplasty may be indicated to

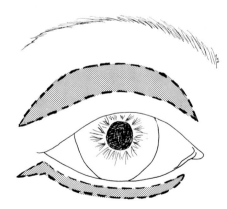

Fig. 24-1. Original basic crescent-shaped resection of excess skin from upper lid followed curve of major crease at supratarsal fold and tapered downward toward internal canthus and laterally downward toward external canthus. Resection of skin from lower lid was narrow strip below cilia with abrupt incision inferiorly or inferolaterally from a point short of lateral canthus. Usually resection was simple skin excision without resection of hernias and without muscle resection.

achieve a superior result. Some of these variations have been described by Castañares, Gonzalez-Ulloa, Lewis, Demere, Beare, Sheen, Flowers, and others.

INDICATIONS FOR BLEPHAROPLASTY

The purpose of the upper and lower lid blepharoplasty is the reduction of the redundant soft tissue of the upper and lower lids. This additional unwanted tissue may be in the form of wrinkled or relaxed skin, which is primarily a reflection of the aging of the skin, or simply an inherited tendency. It may be seen as a bulge beneath the skin, denoting a hypertrophy of the underlying fat pad, a weakness of the orbital septum, or both. Frequently the two problems are concurrent, the skin being excessive and relaxed and the underlying fat pads hypertrophic and prominent because of a weakened septum; in addition, there may be true herniations of intraorbital fat into the lid, bulging against the weakened orbital septum.

The ptosis of the soft tissues of the lids and the hernias may vary considerably from slight wrinkling of the lid skin with the face at rest to frank bagginess of the lids, and from slight puffiness just below the central portion of the eyes to obvious bulges across the upper and lower lids. There may be changes that only hint at fatigue, dissipation, unhappiness, or aging, or there may be marked changes that cause a visual problem, with the upper lid tissues dropping down against the upper lashes and even over the pupil itself. These patients usually have deep forehead wrinkles from keeping the eyebrows elevated in order to see properly.

The patient usually comes for treatment with complaints such as "I look so old"; "People say I look unhappy"; "I look tired to myself and to everyone else"; "Everyone thinks I am older than I am"; "My father had eyes like these"; or simply, "Look at these eyelids!" The psychological aspects of blepharoplasty are profound and beyond the scope of this chapter, but one who looks tired and unhappy is likely to be so.

In the usual case where there is a need for aesthetic blepharoplasty, the patient's eyelids may be handled very satisfactorily by the relatively standard technique of separate upper and lower lid blepharoplasty. The incisions usually follow easily concealed lines, running along the major crease of the upper lid and falling just below the cilia of the lower lid, where there is a natural shadow line. Lateral to the external canthus a natural wrinkle

or smile line is followed. It is best that the inexperienced surgeon master the standard techniques before attempting the variations of these techniques. However, as with other procedures, there are a number of variations of the blepharoplasty techniques that may often be of aid. Often the indication is not a clear-cut and definite one, and the surgeon's judgment, which must of necessity be based on experience, dictates the procedure to be followed. Obviously, the degree of the deformity indicates the extent of the surgery, and the type of deformity and the result desired dictate the surgical technique.

OTHER TECHNIQUES
Low resection

Always the patient should understand that no incision is made through the skin without leaving a scar, but also that an attempt is made to make the necessary scar as fine line and in as inconspicuous a location as possible. However, in the very markedly redundant lower lid with a pouch at the junction of the lower lid and cheek (secondary bags), there may be a rare indication for a direct excision of the tissue rather than an excision just below the cilia. The indication should be rather strong, since the scar will be in a much more noticeable location, and one must prepare the patient for the fact that the scar will be present (Fig. 24-2). Although the low resection may be carried out at the primary procedure, in other instances the low resection may be a secondary procedure when the primary lower lid blepharoplasty has not accomplished adequate improvement of the low-lying bag. Usually a much more conservative resection is carried out in these cases, since the relaxed skin superior to this area has already been tightened. One may cause an ectropion by an excessive lower resection as well as by overdoing the higher one.

Lateral resection

Early in my practice, I found that by varying the lower lid incision from the usual line following downward and laterally from the external canthus to an incision that curved upward above the lateral canthus and then around to the end point almost straight laterally, a better result was obtained. This supports the lower lid better opposite the external canthus, and when healing has occurred, the natural tension will cause the incision to lie along the crease almost straight laterally from the external canthus. It makes an incision

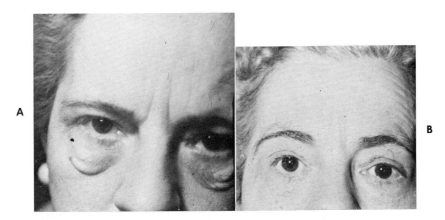

Fig. 24-2. A, Patient with low-lying bags at base of eyelids at their junction with cheeks. Besides bags there are large xanthelasmas of both lower lids involving lower portion of lids. In cases of this sort direct excision of bags and/or tumors may be indicated, rather than blepharoplasty with incision just below cilia. **B,** Appearance following resection of bags and tumors directly, leaving incisions at junction of eyelids and cheeks bilaterally. Note that there is still some widening of orbital commissure of patient's right eye. This cleared with time and gentle massage upward and laterally on right lower lid.

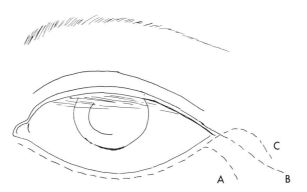

Fig. 24-3. Incision for lower lid blepharoplasty should usually follow just below cilia of lower lid. Most common incision line followed is line *A*, which goes downward and laterally along crease below external canthus. A better result can often be obtained by carrying lower lid incision further laterally and extending laterally and only slightly downward, as in line *B*. I feel that an even superior method is curve of line *C*, which goes up to a point superior to external canthus and then curves laterally and slightly downward. With time, pull of tissues of lid and cheek straighten out line *C* so that it lies almost straight laterally along natural crease opposite external canthus. It not only leaves incision line that is not usually noticed, but also gives good support to lower lid without pull of cheek and lid on lateral portion of lower lid or external canthus.

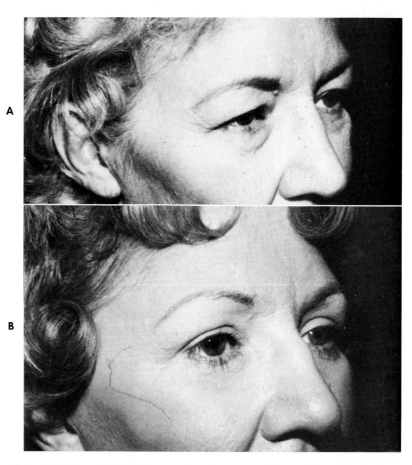

Fig. 24-4. A, Patient with blepharoptosis of upper and lower lids with considerable sag of soft tissues of upper lids down against upper lid lashes and over external canthi. There is a marked bagginess of lower lids, particularly at junction of lower lids and cheeks. **B,** Appearance following upper and lower lid blepharoplasty with resection of wide ellipse of skin from upper lid and with incisions made according to line *C* in Fig. 24-3 for lower lid repair. Note that curved incision has been straightened out and falls along natural crease opposite external canthus.

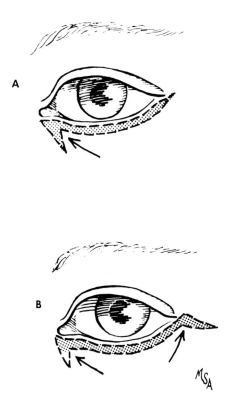

Fig. 24-5. A, Resection of skin from lower lid obliquely below internal canthus may occasionally be used instead of lateral resection. Tension of skin of lid is then pulled upward, then medially, for tension carried medial to internal canthus. When there is rather definite line at junction of nose and lower lid, this incision line is usually hidden. Repair of eyelid is done when medial resection has been carried out. For mildly ptotic skin (blepharochalasis) or hernias with minimal skin resection, this technique may serve quite well. **B,** I resect skin medially and laterally more often than from medial aspect alone. This technique limits length of lateral skin incision by taking part of excess skin out medially. Tension is carried lateral to external canthus and medial to internal canthus. Care must be taken to avoid tension in vertical direction, which might cause ectropion. Combination of resections medially and laterally may limit width of resection on either side and make lateral extension quite short. This may be brought about by extensive blepharochalasis where great deal of skin resection is required or may be chosen as method of choice in fairly youthful face where lateral resection is to be minimized.

that is seldom noticed and, in addition, avoids the pull of an oblique incision downward and laterally from the external canthus (Figs. 24-3 and 24-4). It is important not to crowd the external canthus too closely with the incision as it passes along the infraciliary line just at the external canthus. It is also important not to carry the incision abruptly superiorly at this point, because it creates a fold. However, a gentle curve, convexly upward, allows the end of the incision to return to the horizontal line opposite the external canthus or below the level of the horizontal crease. Obviously, variations in the height of this incision are made depending on the appearance of the eyelids and of the external canthus, as well as on the nature of the tissues itself. Rarely do I make an incision downward and laterally from the external canthus, because this incision is likely to pull even more medially and downward with the ravages of time and the relaxation of the tissues.

Medial resection

Although the excess skin of the lower lid is ordinarily pulled laterally and upward, in order to take the tension lateral to the external canthus, a part of the excess skin may be resected medially. This variation is as a rule a wise one only if a large amount of skin must be resected, for it can be helpful in limiting the extent of the lateral incision line (Fig. 24-5, *A*).

More often than not, when a medial resection is carried out, one compromises and resects a part of the tissue medially and part laterally, minimizing the resection just below the cilia to avoid vertical tightness, which could lead to an ectropion (Fig. 24-5, *B*).

Muscle resection (lower lid)

When the orbicularis oculi muscle is hypertrophic, resulting in a fullness just below the cilia of the lower lid, a deeper resection is frequently indicated. These patients may require only a minor resection of skin but also require a trim of the orbicularis just below the cilia to smooth out this limited area of fullness. This strip of musculature is often excised with the skin in the "muscle flap" technique.

Muscle flap technique

The superficial undermining of the skin of the lower lid allows for tightening of the skin in an upward and lateral direction, creating tension lateral to the external canthus to avoid any pull on the lower lid margin. The reduction of the hernias is then carried out by spreading the muscle fibers and by dividing the orbital septum to expose the hypertrophic fat pads and/or fatty hernias.

The muscle flap technique and variations of it allow for a thicker flap of lower lid skin and musculature, which directly exposes the fatty hernias. There are instances when this technique would seem to have advantages, such as for the markedly relaxed flaccid lid or for the younger patient with fatty hernias but little skin relaxation. I have used more often a separate muscle flap support in the lower lid, undermining between the skin and the underlying musculature and then supporting these two layers separately to achieve the best result. This technique, or the routine blepharoplasty with superficial undermining, is best for the lid with considerable skin relaxation and wrinkling and for the lid with marked relaxation in the lower portion (toward the cheek). A more superficial undermining allows for better smoothing and tightening of the relaxed lid skin, even if a separate muscle flap support is needed deeply.

However, this deeper incision through skin, subcutaneous tissue, and muscle brings one directly over the hernias and hypertrophic fat pads. For the lid that is relatively normal in skin area and without folds of skin at the base of the lid, and that has large hernias bulging against the lower lid skin, this technique is good. It allows one to trim the fat pads and hernias directly and to excise the excess of soft tissue from the lid. When there is fullness of the soft tissue just below the cilia of the lower lid, this allows for trimming of the muscle to the desired degree to smooth out this portion of the lid. It allows for a moderate snugging of the skin of the lid but does not allow an extensive skin excision or extensive skin tightening, because the skin is left attached to the muscle.

Whenever the lower lid has excessively large hernias, there may be a need to expose more thoroughly the underlying hernias and/or hypertrophic fat pads. This may be done through the superficial undermining and an additional elevation of soft tissue to expose these hernias. This amounts to a variation of the muscle flap technique. However, usually the simple separation of the muscle fibers over the hernias (a "buttonhole" opening) adequately allows for the teasing out of these fatty tumors and their resection. For the most part, this latter technique is the simplest, the most conservative, and the safest, and it serves quite satisfactorily.

Separate skin and muscle flaps

As mentioned in the previous section, I frequently use separate skin and muscle flaps for support of the lower lid in lower lid blepharoplasty (Fig. 24-6). By undermining in a superficial plane and separating the skin from the underlying orbicularis, the skin may be tightened adequately in an upward and lateral direction, avoiding any undue pull on the lower lid margin. Support is carried upward and lateral to the external canthus. However, the deep support in the lid may be inadequate because of a flaccid, senile lid with soft tarsal support and redundant musculature. There may be a tendency toward ectropion or entropion. Support to this type of lid is best achieved by a separate muscle flap support to the lateral orbital periosteum. The muscle along the infraciliary area may be pulled upward and laterally to secure it to the lateral orbital periosteum for correction of incipient ectropion of the flaccid lid, or the muscle just below the ciliary line may be pulled laterally and slightly downward when there is a tendency toward entropion. In that case the muscle inferior to the first muscle support may be brought upward and laterally to tighten it firmly, crisscrossing the first muscle flap to achieve some upward pull and tightening of the base of the lid while everting the margin of the lid. This is, of course, the opposite of the pull one would wish to achieve when correcting an ectropion. In that case one would snug the lid in both areas, but particularly support the upper portion of the lid to bring it close to the globe.

Once the muscle flap or flaps have been brought upward and secured to the lateral orbital periosteum, the skin is brought upward and laterally and the excess excised. *It is important that the upper lid skin resection and closure of the wound in the upper lid be carried out before determining the amount of skin to be resected from the lower lid.* It is also important to accomplish the muscle flap support of the lower lid before determining the amount of skin to be resected from the lower lid, since both the muscle flap support of the lower lid and the upper lid blepharoplasty have a tendency to elevate the external canthal area and the lateral part of the lower lid. It is easy to excise skin from the lower lid excessively if this rule is not followed.

Upper lid skin resection laterally

Variations in upper lid repair are dictated by the degree of the blepharoptosis and blepharochalasis. When there is no particular ptosis of the

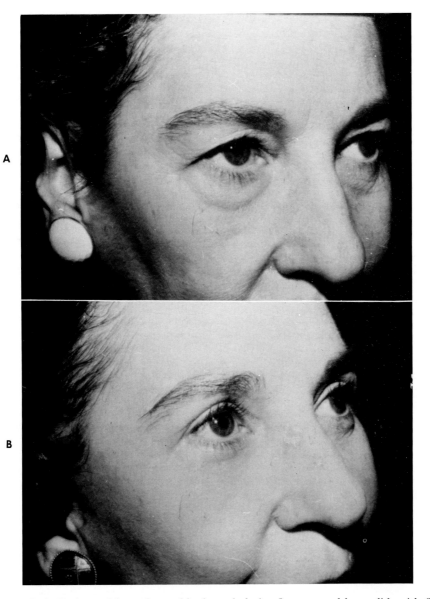

Fig. 24-6. A, Patient with moderate blepharochalasis of upper and lower lids with fatty hernias of upper and lower lids as well. Aside from skin to be resected from upper lids and minimal skin resection from lower lids, primary problem is one of flaccidity of lower lids with lack of lower lid support. **B,** Following upper and lower lid blepharoplasty with resection of skin and hernias from upper lids and fatty hernias from lower lids, minimal skin resection was carried out from lower lids, but separate muscle flap support was carried to lateral orbital periosteum. Skin was supported upward and laterally as separate layer.

soft tissues lateral to the external canthus, the resection of skin may be limited simply to the upper lid. Cases of this sort are infrequent but may be helped considerably by the very conservative resection of the relaxed skin. This is particularly applicable to those patients who do not have hypertrophic fat pads or hernias and who have relatively high eyebrows.

The upper lid, which is markedly ptotic, with excess skin extending far medially and far laterally, may require a long lateral extension of the resection. This should be carried upward and laterally, following the natural expression lines, but should not extend farther than the line of the eyebrow. If it seems to extend beyond the line of the curve of the eyebrow downward and laterally, a small V resection downward in the line of the eyebrow will take care of the residual dog-ear.

Upper lid skin resection medially

When the redundancy and relaxation extend far medially, one is tempted to extend the incision up onto the nose to achieve an adequate resection of skin, or even to extend the incision onto the nose and actually cross the nasal bridge (as has been described). This can be hazardous insofar as

the residual scar is concerned and may result in tightness above the internal canthus. An alternate procedure is the Y-V resection, in which a part of the resection is taken downward and medially and a part upward and medially to achieve a resection of skin without extending the incision further medially. Another type of resection that may keep the incision shorter is resection of the dog-ear upward and laterally following the shadow curve of the upper lid above the internal canthus. This still amounts to a modified Y-V procedure (Fig. 24-7).

Upper lid muscle resection and tarsal fixation

Resection of a strip of the orbicularis muscle of the upper lid is indicated by a full heavy upper lid with redundant skin. The resection of the excess skin from the upper lid along with the underlying fatty hernias may still leave a full upper lid because of the heaviness of the orbicularis. This in itself indicates some resection of orbicularis across the upper lid, or at least in the lateral half of the upper lid and somewhat lateral to the external canthus. The closure of the upper lid skin incision after removal of the excess skin tends to

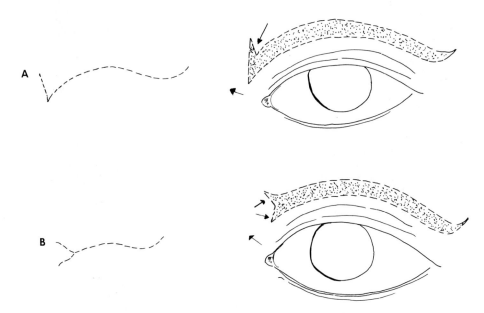

Fig. 24-7. A, Resection of small dog-ear of skin *(arrows)* above medial end of upper lid resection may help to shorten medial extension of incision line. Dog-ear should curve upward along natural shadow line of upper lid, and its closure should cause no additional noticeable scar. **B,** V-Y closure *(arrows)* is also useful in shortening medial extension of upper resection. One must also avoid extending resection line downward too close to internal canthus because of tight band that may occur.

crowd the soft tissue together in the upper lid. This is usually taken care of by the resection of the lateral and intermediate fat pads and the medial fatty hernia if present. If there is still some fullness in the upper lid, particularly in the lateral portion of the upper lid and the external canthal area, this is a strong indication to resect a strip of the orbicularis.

Usually the excision of an upper lid muscle strip is accompanied by a tarsal fixation procedure. One may depend on enough adherence of the overlying skin to the underlying tarsus following resection of the orbicularis to create a reasonable upper lid fold. This is all that is required for the average eyelid, which has a reasonable height of insertion of the levator and Müller's muscle. When there is an abnormal level of insertion of the levator and Müller's muscle and there is a very low supraorbital fold, then it is usually advisable to do a tarsal fixation. This may be done simply by using interrupted silk sutures that catch a deep bite of the tarsus with skin closure, or more satisfactorily by using buried sutures to accomplish this support of the skin to the tarsus. I use interrupted 6-O Dexon sutures and then proceed with the skin closure, using some spacing sutures of 6-O silk and a running intracuticular 5-O Prolene for the final closure. One may take the procedure further and follow the technique of Flowers (anchor blepharoplasty), or of Sheen (supratarsal fixation procedure), both of which are designed to give a deeper upper lid fold and a more contoured upper lid.

Lateral canthus

One of the first signs of aging is ptosis in the lateral canthal area. This may amount to a ptosis of the tissues of the upper lid only or may amount to an actual droop and sag of the external canthus with relaxation in the external canthal ligament itself. Elevation of the external canthus gives the eyes a more youthful appearance and a more happy look. When the external canthus is elevated upward and laterally to a greater degree, one may give the eyes an exotic look, which may be desirable for some patients. Obviously, when the eyes have an upward curve already, the external canthus is located superiorly and there is no need for this type of procedure.

The procedure advocated by Gonzalez-Ulloa uses a triangular flap pulled upward and laterally to repair into the upper lid resection (Fig. 24-8). The upper and lower lid resections are continuous, leaving a single long extension laterally beyond the triangular flap repair. Control of the resection in the lower lid may be difficult with this procedure, and an extension of the incision laterally is frequently necessary. A bowstring contracture of the scar laterally has been described, but I have not seen it. If the flap is adequate, the bowstring effect is very unlikely. However, to avoid the extensive lateral extension of the con-

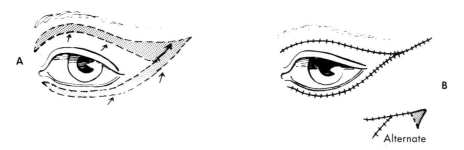

Fig. 24-8. A, Technique of Gonzales-Ulloa combines upper and lower lid resection and pulls triangle of skin at external canthus upward and laterally *(arrows)* to support external canthus. **B,** Repair of combined resection leaves single incision line extending upward and laterally beyond repair of triangular flap. This incision line may extend upward to temple hairline before reaching flat end point unless some type of resection of dog-ear is carried out. I have modified this technique by resecting small dog-ear in line with eyebrow as shown in *alternate.* Although bowstring contractures of scar laterally have been described, I have not seen this complication from this technique.

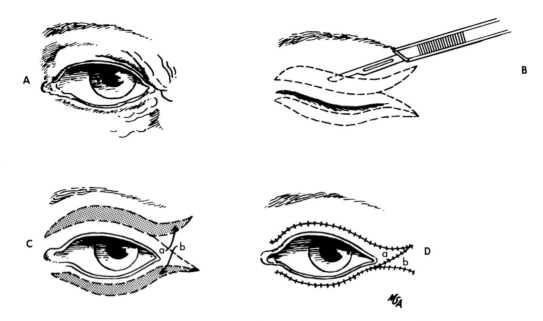

Fig. 24-9. Z-blepharoplasty allows surgeon to do combined upper and lower lid resection and at same time elevate and support external canthus. It uses flap based at external canthus that is to be pulled upward and laterally as natural extension of upper lid repair. Upper lid flap is rotated downward and medially to support external canthus further. This technique uses same principle as technique of elevating external canthus (shown in Fig. 24-8) but avoids long external incision and in addition gives further support to external canthus by laterally based flap that is rotated from upper lid downward to or below external canthus. **A,** Eyelid with marked blepharoptosis and blepharochalasis. Note that external canthus is sagging and soft tissues above and opposite external canthus are drooping badly. **B,** Resection of skin from upper lid is similar to routine upper lid blepharoplasty. Resection of skin from lower lid is similar to routine lower lid blepharoplasty except that less skin is likely to be excised from lateral half of lower lid and opposite lower lid, since lower lid will actually be elevated in position in external canthal area. **C,** Resection of skin from upper and lower lids has been carried out, and flaps *a* and *b* opposite external canthus are ready for rotation and exchange. Proper progression of operation is to perform upper lid blepharoplasty and Z-blepharoplasty and finally to resect from lower lid. Lower lid resection cannot be properly judged until rest of procedure is relatively complete. **D,** Completion of procedure with flap *a* supported upward into upper lid repair and flap *b* being rotated downward for further support to external canthus. (From Lewis, J.R.: The Z-blepharoplasty, Plast. Reconstr. Surg. **44:**301, 1969.)

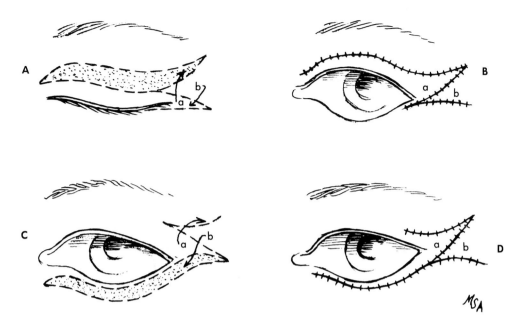

Fig. 24-10. Variations of Z-blepharoplasty allow for partial upper and lower lid blepharoplasty or for support of external canthus alone. **A,** Upper lid blepharoplasty may be carried out with Z-blepharoplasty without lower lid blepharoplasty when there is no need for work on lower lid. **B,** Completion of upper lid blepharoplasty and Z-blepharoplasty to support external canthus but without carrying out usual lower lid blepharoplasty. **C,** When upper lid is relatively normal and there is need for lower lid blepharoplasty and external canthal support alone, Z-blepharoplasty and lower lid blepharoplasty are carried out. **D,** Completion of lower lid blepharoplasty and Z-blepharoplasty for support of external canthal area. NOTE: Z-blepharoplasty may be carried out at external canthus alone without involving main body of upper and lower lids when there is simply an early sag in external canthal area. Usually, however, upper and/or lower lids are repaired at same time as Z-blepharoplasty. Z-blepharoplasty may be used in various modifications for repair following resection of lesion from upper or lower lid or external canthus and for correction of mild to moderate ectropion in external canthal area following injury, irradiation, or overzealous lower lid skin resection. (From Lewis, J.R.: The Z-blepharoplasty, Plast. Reconstr. Surg. **44:**301, 1969.)

joined incision, the dog-ear may be resected downward in line with the natural curve of the eyebrow.*

Z-blepharoplasty

I described the Z-blepharoplasty in 1969 and feel that it has a definite place in this type of case (Figs. 24-9 to 24-12). It not only elevates a triangular flap based at the external canthus into the upper lid repair, but moves a triangular flap based laterally downward to the external canthus to give further support. One may accomplish resections in both upper and lower lids without long lateral incisions. The procedure may be modified to do a complete upper lid blepharoplasty and the Z to elevate the external canthus, or it may be modified to do a complete lower lid blepharoplasty with the simple Z for elevation of the external canthus without doing the upper lid blepharoplasty. Most often, upper and lower lid blepharoplasty is carried out in the usual fashion except that less skin is resected from the lower lid, since the lower lid margin is actually elevated in its lateral half and particularly in the external canthal portion.

Fatty hernias

A resection of the hypertrophic fat pads in the medial and intermediate compartments of the up-

*EDITOR'S NOTE: In reference to the description of Dr. Gonzalez-Ulloa's dealing with the lateral canthus and Fig. 24-8, which refers to his technique of combining the upper and lower lid incisions laterally, it is my experience that this procedure leads to increased edema and postoperative pigmentation of the strip of upper lid skin, the circulation of which is now even more isolated. (G.P.G.)

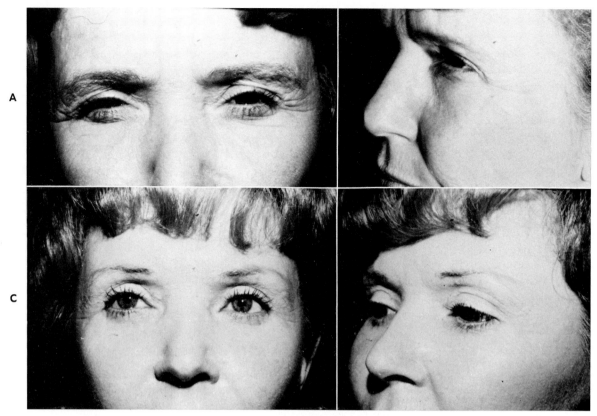

Fig. 24-11. A and **B,** Patient with marked blepharochalasis of upper and lower lids with moderate hernias of upper and lower lids. **C** and **D,** Appearance following upper and lower lid blepharoplasty combined as **Z**-blepharoplasty and performed at same stage as meloplasty and rhytidectomy. Meloplasty and rhytidectomy obviously give further support to upper and lower lids. Muscle resection and tarsal fixation were performed in lateral half of upper lids.

per lid and in the medial, intermediate, and lateral compartments of the lower lid is dictated by their size and by the bulge that occurs into the lids. The true hernias in the medial compartments of upper and lower lids should also be resected in proportion to the need (Figs. 24-13 and 24-14). These may be so extensive as to extend over into the intermediate compartments in some instances, most likely in patients having suffered thyroid disease. When resection of these hernias is carried out, it is advocated that they be clamped, resected, and lightly fulgurated to avoid the possibility of postoperative hematoma. After having one retrobulbar hematoma occur, the plastic surgeon is very likely to follow this technique closely to avoid having a second such case.

The eyelid that is relatively flat and smooth with no obvious bulge probably needs no resection of fatty hernias. By pressing lightly through the upper lid against the globe, one may see any latent protrusions of fat into the lower lid. In a similar fashion, the lower lid may be pushed lightly against the globe and made to show up any latent hernias in the upper lid. Certainly, these latent hernias should be trimmed as needed.

Eyes that are relatively deep set ("sunken") should probably have no resection of hernias, and the resection should be limited to the excess loose skin. Even these eyelids may sometimes have localized herniations of fat that need trimming. However, one should avoid giving the eye a more sunken look by resecting orbital fat that gives no real visible evidence of its existence.

Medial Z-plasty

In the Oriental eyelid (Fig. 24-13), one creates a more Western look by elevating the low or absent upper lid fold to a higher level. This is ac-

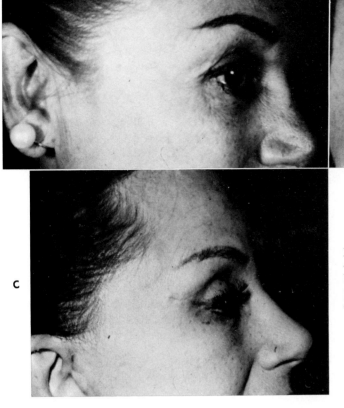

Fig. 24-12. Patient before partial Z-blepharoplasty, **A,** at 4 days postoperatively, **B,** and 6 weeks following lower lid blepharoplasty, Z-blepharoplasty, and repair of lateral portion of upper lid only, **C.** Medial portion of upper lid obviously needs no correction at this time.

complished by resecting the lid hernias and performing a tarsal fixation procedure. However, a medial Z-plasty (or a medial and lateral Z-plasty) may be required to correct the medial epicanthus or medial and lateral epicanthi that are present (Fig. 24-15). The lateral Z-plasty is not the same as the Z-blepharoplasty and is primarily used for correcting the epicanthal fold. Obviously, one would wish the Z-plasty to be performed in such a way as to minimize the resulting scar while accomplishing the correction of the medial and lateral epicanthi. It should also contribute to the elevation medially and laterally of the transverse lid fold* (Figs. 24-15 and 24-16).

———
*EDITOR'S NOTE: Medial and lateral Z-plasties to correct epicanthal folds in Oriental patients should be undertaken with caution. They may result in conspicuous scars. Most often, the patient is only seeking the creation of a distinct fold and the removal of heaviness (protruding fusiform fat). (G.P.G.)

Face-lift and brow lift

Additional procedures that may be indicated for support of the facial tissues may improve the results of the eyelid surgery itself (Fig. 24-17). The coronal forehead lift and brow lift give additional support to the upper lids as well. The combination of the brow lift and upper lid blepharoplasty may achieve a rather remarkable result in the extreme case. My modified brow lift may be of value for the ptotic upper lid associated with brow ptosis (Fig. 24-18).

The forehead lift will obviously give some support also to the eyebrows and the upper lids. Usually upper lid blepharoplasty is still required, but the two procedures may be more worthwhile than blepharoplasty alone when there is brow ptosis of the whole forehead.

Whenever the cheeks have heavy droops and sags, or whenever the lateral eyebrow areas are

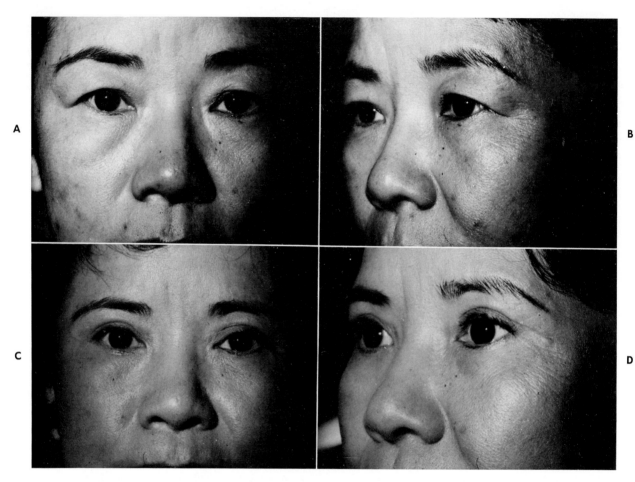

Fig. 24-13. A and **B,** Oriental eyelid with very low upper lid fold and marked redundancy of soft tissues of upper lid indicating large medial hernia and intermediate fat pad extending far laterally. Medial and, to a degree, lateral epicanthi are present. There are also lower lid hernias and relaxation of lower lid skin. **C** and **D,** Appearance following medial Z-plasty to correct epicanthal fold, upper lid blepharoplasty with resection of skin medially and of intermediate hernias, and with muscle resection and tarsal fixation. Lower lid blepharoplasty was carried out at same procedure.

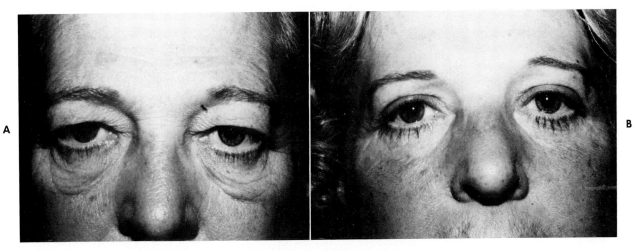

Fig. 24-14. A, Patient with marked blepharoptosis of upper and lower lids with large hernias of all compartments of upper and lower lids. Although contour and heavily hooded fold of upper lid resemble Oriental eyelid, it is quite different in that levator attachment is high. **B,** Appearance following upper and lower lid blepharoplasty and resection of large hernias in medial, lateral, and intermediate compartments of upper lids and medial and intermediate compartments of lower lids. Repair of these hernias is essential to good result in upper and lower lid blepharoplasty when these hernias are present. Light pressure of finger against upper lid will reveal latent hernias in lower lid and vice versa. Resection of large hernias and adequate skin will usually give this kind of lid a pleasing lid fold without resection of muscle or tarsal fixation.

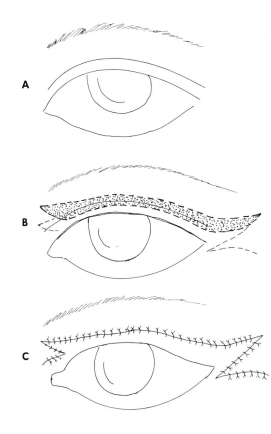

Fig. 24-15. For more marked Oriental-type eyelid, **A,** with absent epicanthal sulcus or very low lying sulcus with medial and lateral epicanthi and markedly hooded fold of upper lid skin, double Z-blepharoplasty may be of value: Z-plasty along medial epicanthus, Z-plasty along lateral epicanthus, and resection of skin in between the two Zs. It is important to adequately excise medial and intermediate hernias of upper lid and to trim strip of orbicularis across whole lid and lateral to external canthus, or at least in lateral two thirds of upper lid and lateral to external canthus, so that tarsal fixation and higher attachment of supratarsal fold are possible. **C** shows appearance following repair of medial and lateral Z-blepharoplasty and intervening skin repair shown diagrammatically in **B.** Actually, there is more gentle curve upward to simulate normal supratarsal fold.

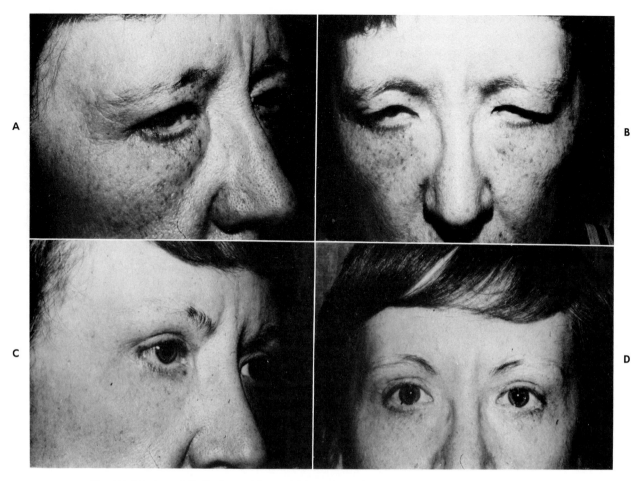

Fig. 24-16. A and **B,** Patient with marked ptosis of brows, ptosis of upper lids, elastosis of soft tissues of forehead, brows, and lids, and marked visual problem. **C** and **D,** Appearance following bilateral brow lift, bilateral shortening of levator expansion to improve actual ptosis of upper lids, and bilateral double Z-blepharoplasty of upper lids with resection of fatty hernias and with tarsal fixation bilaterally.

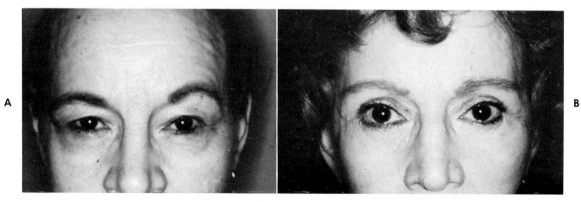

Fig. 24-17. A, Patient with unilateral ptosis of brow, as well as blepharoptosis and blepharochalasis of lids. **B,** Appearance following modified brow lift with incision in eyebrow. Upper and lower lid blepharoplasty were carried out simultaneously.

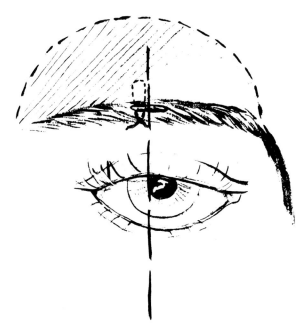

Fig. 24-18. My modified brow lift with short incision in eyebrow, which allows access for securing underside of orbicularis at eyebrow upward to higher level on occipitofrontalis.

ptotic, meloplasty and rhytidectomy of the cheeks and temples contribute more to improvement of of the upper and lower lids than does upper and lower lid blepharoplasty alone. This combination of procedures may be very worthwhile, and the procedures are commonly carried out together; however, some surgeons accomplish them as a two-stage operation during one hospital stay.

CONCLUSION

Upper and lower lid repair may be varied, depending on the indications. The variations are dictated by the objective findings and in some instances by the subjective symptoms. The surgeon should be very careful not to overdo surgery on the eyelids, for ectropion occurs readily when an excess of tissue is resected. This is particularly true for the lower lids, for one must leave enough relaxation in the lower lid skin for the eyelids to follow the globe and not pull away when the eyes look upward. Excessive resection of orbital fat may cause an enophthalmic look and add age to the patient's appearance.

One must also remember that the expression lines, or crinkle lines, which occur about the eyes, are difficult to eradicate and always appear when the patient smiles. These are neither pathological nor signs of aging and must be acceptable to some degree to the surgeon and to the patient. If these lines are excessive despite a blepharoplasty, with or without a meloplasty, a chemical peel of the area may help. If a peel is carried out, it should extend only to the major crease of the upper lid, leaving the lower portion of the lid untouched. For the lower lid the peel is carried to the base of the cilia. Since the eyelid skin is thin and not rich in sebaceous glands as compared with the skin of the cheeks, it behooves one to peel less deeply to avoid scarring, contracture, and ectropion. It goes without saying that one should take great care to avoid endangering the eyes themselves. The Aston procedure may be of value in improving the so-called smile lines (see Chapter 23).

Often a patient's age, weight loss, and unhappiness are reflected more in the eyes than in any other area of the face. This is particularly true in the external canthal area, but is also true in relation to both the upper and lower lids. A correctly performed upper and lower lid blepharoplasty improves the appearance and therefore the self-image of the patient. Hence, it is incumbent on the surgeon to be familiar with variations of blepharoplasty techniques so as to adapt these to the particular need in the individual case.

Editorial comments
Chapter 24

Dr. Lewis describes the indications for resecting a strip of orbicularis oculi muscle from the upper lids to avoid a heaviness or crowding of soft tissue following blepharoplasty. Because of the attenuation of the skin and orbicularis muscle, it seems reasonable that as the skin stretches, the muscle similarly must stretch with it. As Dr. Owsley points out in Chapter 22, most, if not all, of the preseptal portion of the orbicularis muscle can be removed without causing any functional impairment. This simple maneuver gives a better-defined, clean-cut supratarsal fold. This is true of routine blepharoplasty, blepharoplasty in the Oriental, or blepharoplasty in any patient with an indistinct supratarsal fold.

G.P.G.

Chapter 25

A potpourri of blepharoplasty problems

Thomas M. Biggs

A well-done blepharoplasty in a well-selected patient can yield remarkable results that satisfy both patient and surgeon. In many instances the gain in appearance is dramatic. Where there is room for dramatic improvement, however, the situation also exists for striking problems. In a poorly performed operation or in a patient with contraindications for surgery, the complications can create a heavy burden for all parties.

It is not the purpose of this chapter to discuss the extensive list of undesirable effects that blepharoplasty can cause, for these have been amply described before.[2-9] Rather, the chapter is a presentation of my perspective on several of these problems that perhaps either have not been described or have not been discussed sufficiently to be common knowledge in the hundreds of plastic surgery clinics throughout the country.

PATIENTS WHO SHOULD NOT HAVE BLEPHAROPLASTY

Certainly, the most ideal way to avoid complications from any surgery is to not do the operation. This is obviously not an appropriate course of action for a plastic surgeon dedicated to fine aesthetic surgery. The next best thing, however, is to select patients so that the predictability of problems will be as low as possible. In order to do this, we must recognize some unavoidable pitfalls.

In the initial consultation and examination one may recognize a mild asymmetry about the orbit. Often the degree of asymmetry is minimized by folds of skin and fat of the upper lids and possibly of the lower lids. Resection of this redundancy will remove this mask and often increase the perception of asymmetry. Whether the asymmetry is on the orbital rim, nasal root, or from a mild proptosis, the same holds true; alteration to correct soft tissue redundancy can have the reverse effect to enhancing the patient's appearance. In patients with a mild form of ptosis, a surgical correction of the problem can be done, but this may be such a subtle thing that the accuracy of correction may not match the increased reality of the problem. At least, this is a circumstance that should be recognized beforehand and discussed openly with the patient.

Dark circles around the eyes are usually caused by increased pigmentation in the skin. Patients whose main complaint is dark circles and whose fat deposits are not sufficient to create shadows to cause the darkness must be considered poor candidates for blepharoplasty.

Perhaps the most common type of patient who should not have blepharoplasty is the patient with such a minimal problem that surgery would effect no noticeable change. This is frequently seen in my practice and presents a difficult and occasionally somewhat unhappy experience; it is as if the surgeon is holding out on the patient and refusing to give the patient what he or she needs and is eager to pay for. I frequently resort to the "risk-reward ratio" by saying the risk of problems is too great for the little bit of reward, and this in most instances allows postponement of the operation for a few years at least. On occasion this patient will simply go to the nearest alternate plastic surgeon who will perform the operation, but the ultimate result is usually that which was predicted—an unhappy patient.

EXCESSIVE SUPRASEPTAL FAT

Some patients who complain of baggy upper lids and who undergo the standard upper lid blepharoplasty of skin excision and resection of fat beneath the orbital septum have persistent

239

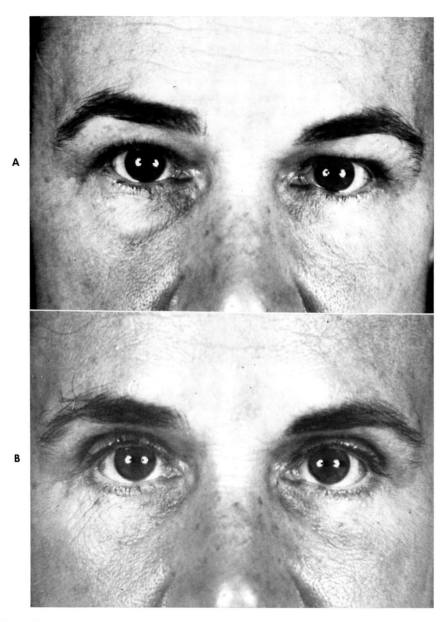

Fig. 25-1. A, Patient with excessive fat in tissues external to orbital septum. **B,** Appearance after upper and lower lid blepharoplasty. In upper lids excess fat external to orbital septum was principal cause of fullness.

bagginess. This may be due to orbicularis oculi muscle or excessive fat outside the septum and beneath the orbital rim. Resection of this fat can be done with no harm (although occasional temporary supraorbital numbness may be observed), and enhancement of the brow may be achieved (Figs. 25-1 and 25-2). The problem may be increased by a low-hanging supraorbital rim, and, if so, resection with an osteotome of a portion of the lateral aspect of the rim may further improve the surgical results.

LOW-LYING FOLD

The patient with a low-lying fold and a "tumbling over" the fold of skin and soft tissue will have no improvement of the problems with simple excision of skin and fat. The remaining tissue will continue to tumble over, and the inexperienced or less-perceptive surgeon will fall into the trap of returning to the operating room and resecting more skin until the patient is short of skin and cannot adequately close the lids, while still

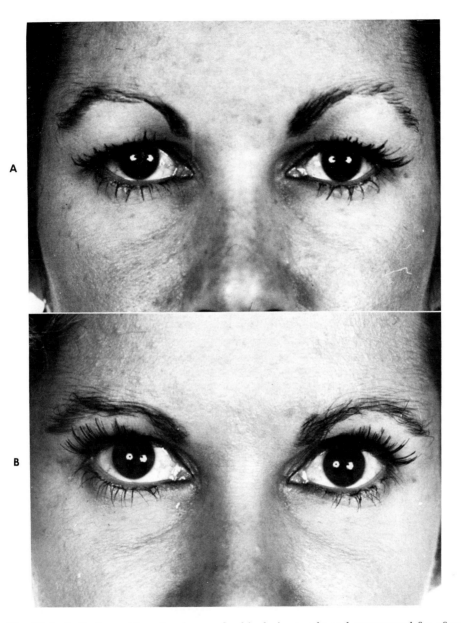

Fig. 25-2. A, Patient with redundancy of orbicularis muscle and supraseptal fat of upper lids. **B,** Appearance 2 years after excision of redundant muscle and supraseptal fat.

having the appearance of needing a blepharoplasty when the eyes are open.

Avoidance of this problem has been amply described by Sheen[10] and expounded on by Flowers.[1] Although I respect the great contributions made by these authors, I prefer a more modest approach. This is accomplished by resection of muscle and fat and the simple suturing of the lower edge of the orbicularis muscle to the orbital septum (Fig. 25-3). This is easier than suturing to the tarsal plate and creates less of a stark look than that resulting from the "anchor blepharoplasty."

Regardless of the technique used to correct this anatomical alteration, the principal challenge is to recognize it as being different from the typical problem of the aging face. In an effort to demonstrate that this is not a problem of excess skin, I have done a series of upper lid blepharoplasties in which no skin was excised, only muscle

Text continued on p. 246.

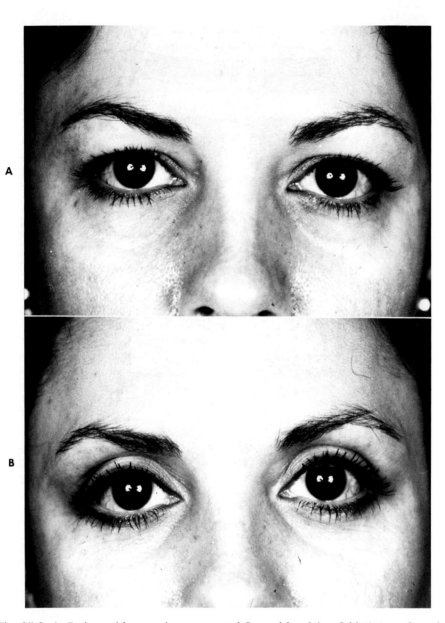

Fig. 25-3. A, Patient with excessive extraseptal fat and low-lying fold (0.4 cm from lash margin). **B,** Appearance 8 months after upper and lower lid blepharoplasty. In upper lids extraseptal fat (as well as fat beneath septum) was removed. A new fold 1.5 cm above lashes was created by suturing lower edge of orbicularis muscle to orbital septum. No skin was excised in this operation.

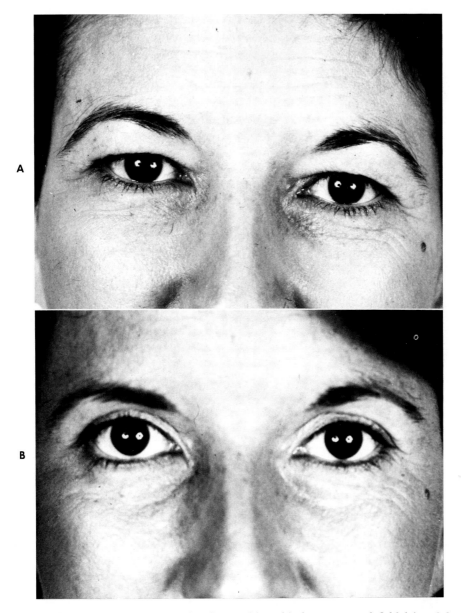

Fig. 25-4. A, Patient with excessive fat outside orbital septum and fold lying 0.3 cm from lashes. **B,** Appearance 9 months after upper lid blepharoplasty in which excess fat and excess orbicularis muscle were resected. Lower edge of orbicularis muscle was sutured to orbital septum. No skin was excised in blepharoplasty.

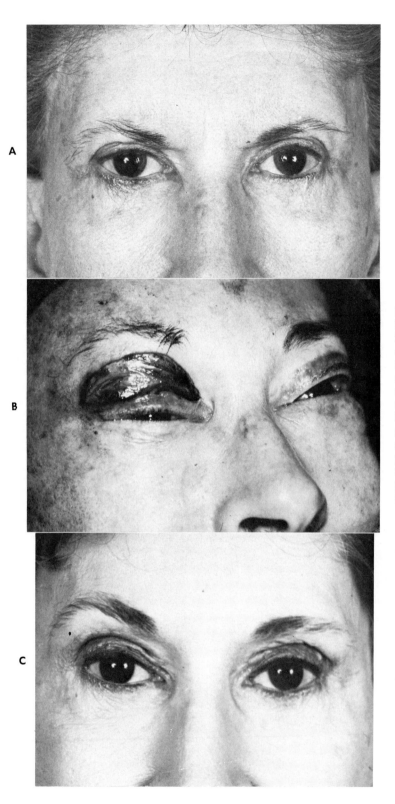

Fig. 25-5. A, Patient who had upper lid blepharoplasty 10 years earlier. Because of inadequate correction of problem of redundancy, more skin was excised 5 years later. Since that time, she was unable to close her eyes completely while sleeping and had to employ taping of her lids to protect against corneal exposure. **B,** Defect on right upper lid was created by incising old scar across lid and allowing tissues to fall into normal position. Left lid has not been incised. **C,** Appearance 4 months after full-thickness graft to defect depicted in **B.** Graft was also placed on left upper lid. Patient no longer needs tape to close her eyes.

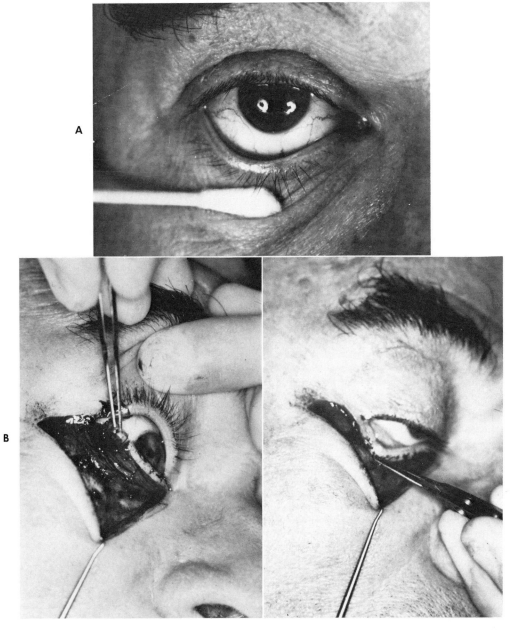

Fig. 25-6. A, Candidate for lower lid blepharoplasty in whom weight of cotton-tipped applicator is sufficient to pull lid away from globe. **B,** Flaccidity of lid is depicted. Area of excision of wedge is in lateral one third. **C,** Excision of wedge 3 to 5 mm in diameter. This tightens lid in transverse diameter and allows lid to lie in contiguity with globe. Closure rarely requires more than one 6-0 plain catgut suture buried and one 6-0 silk suture in lash margin.

and fat, with a suturing of the lower edge of the orbicularis to the orbital septum (Fig. 25-4). In each instance the fold was raised from less than 0.5 cm to 1.5 to 2.0 cm from the lash line. In so doing, the redundancy necessary for the lid to close is forced to fall back above the globe behind the orbital rim rather than tumbling over the fold onto the lash line.*

TOO MUCH SKIN EXCISED

In patients who have the problem of inadequate skin, a full-thickness skin graft should be performed in conjunction with the creation of a fold as previously described. If the fold is placed at least 1.5 cm from the lash line, the amount of skin needed to allow easy closure is often considerable. Because of the fold's placement, the graft does not tumble over, since it is nicely stored in the recesses of the superior orbit and mobilized into view only when needed to close the lids (Fig. 25-5).

FLACCID LOWER LIDS

In many patients, and occasionally young ones, one may often see a flaccid lower lid. This is made more pronounced when the lid is pulled away from the globe, and its return to a position of contiguity with the globe is slow. Blepharoplasty performed on this lid will result in an induration that will pull the lid away from the globe, creating an unpleasant appearance and a series of problems. This is not the result of too much skin excised (although this too can cause a problem in anyone) but the result of pull from induration on a flaccid lid. Avoidance and correction of this complication can be accomplished by a V-shaped full-thickness

excision of a portion of the lower lid. No more than 3 to 5 mm need be removed, and closure can be with one buried 6-O plain catgut and one 6-O silk suture at the lash line. The ideal place for the excision is in the lateral one third of the lid but far enough from the lateral canthus so as not to alter its appearance (Fig. 25-6).

SUMMARY

A potpourri of problems relating to blepharoplasty has been presented. The purpose of this chapter has not been to create an encyclopedia of complications, but to discuss items that are not commonly discussed or referred to. Problems mentioned include patients who should not be operated on, excessive supraseptal fat, the low-lying fold, too much skin excised, and flaccid lower lids.

REFERENCES

1. Flowers, R.S.: Anchor blepharoplasty. In Marchak, D., and Hueston, J.T., editors: Transactions of the Sixth International Congress of Plastic and Reconstructive Surgeons, New York, 1976, Masson Publishing USA, Inc.
2. Graham, W.P., Messner, K.H., and Miller, S.: Keratoconjunctivitis sicca symptoms appearing after blepharoplasty, Plast. Reconstr. Surg. **57:**57, 1976.
3. Huang, T., Horowitz, B., and Lewis, S.: Retrobulbar hemorrhage, Plast. Reconstr. Surg. **59:**39, 1977.
4. Hueston, J.T., and Heinze, J.B.: Blindness after blepharoplasty: mechanism and early reversal, Plast. Reconstr. Surg. **6:**347, 1978.
5. Klatsky, S., and Manson, P.: Numbness after blepharoplasty: the relation of upper orbital fat to sensory nerves, Plast. Reconstr. Surg. **67:**20, 1981.
6. Levine, M.R., et al.: Complications of blepharoplasty, Ophthalmic Surg. **6:**55, 1975.
7. Rees, T.D.: Complications following blepharoplasty. In Tessier, P., et al., editors: Symposium on plastic surgery in the orbital region, St. Louis, 1976, The C.V. Mosby Co.
8. Rees, T.D.: Blepharoplasty. In Courtiss, E.H., editor: Aesthetic surgery: trouble—how to avoid it and how to treat it, St. Louis, 1978, The C.V. Mosby Co.
9. Rees, T.D.: Prevention of postblepharoplasty complications. In Goulian, D., and Courtiss, E.H., editors: Symposium on surgery of the aging face, St. Louis, 1978, The C.V. Mosby Co.
10. Sheen, J.H.: Supratarsal fixation in upper blepharoplasty, Plast. Reconstr. Surg. **54:**424, 1974.

---

*EDITOR'S NOTE: The concept of doing an upper lid blepharoplasty without skin removal is intriguing. The surgical result shown by Dr. Biggs is at least equal to that which could have been achieved with any other approach. The key to obtaining a good fold in this type of patient may be adequate removal of fat and preseptal orbicularis muscle. Any type of "fixation" is rarely necessary. (G.P.G.)

Chapter 26

Blepharoplasty and loss of vision

Donald R. Weis

Of all the ocular complications that occur with blepharoplasty, loss of vision ranks as the most devastating. There have been a total of 58 cases reported, and one could merely speculate as to the number of others that have gone unreported for obvious reasons. In one state alone, a series of five recent cases were reviewed but not reported.[5]

CASE REPORTS

The first case reports of this complication were those of Hartmann, Morax, and Vergez[7] in 1962. These authors observed four cases of visual loss following blepharoplasty, in two of which the patients had persistent total blindness. No other reports appeared until 7 years later, when Morax and Blanck[15] reported a single case. In 1973 Moser, DiPirro, and McCoy,[16] after mailing questionnaires to plastic surgeons, collected 12 additional cases, but complete data were intentionally withheld from them in 5 of these cases. In six of the seven cases they reported the patients had permanent total unilateral blindness. Of significance is the fact that 100 of their surveyed colleagues were totally unaware of the possibility of this complication. In 1973 Hartley, Lester, and Schatten[6] reported a case of blindness that was reversed following treatment of a retrobulbar hemorrhage, and Jafek, Kreiger, and Morledge[11] reported a similar case the same year, also secondary to retrobulbar hemorrhage, which ultimately resulted in optic atrophy and a final visual acuity of 20/70. In 1973 DeMere, Wood, and Austin[3] in a national survey, sent questionnaires to 16,000 ophthalmologists and plastic surgeons and received 3000 responses. They gathered 40 cases of blindness in over 98,000 eyelid operations for an incidence of 0.04%, or 1 in every 2500 operations. Hueston and Heinze[9,10] reported a soli-

tary case in 1974, and another in 1977, 800 blepharoplasty operations later. Both cases resulted in total permanent blindness. Putterman[19] reported a single case in 1975 in which he was able to reverse the blindness. Wiggs[22]; Hepler, Sugimura, and Straatsma[8]; and Waller[21] reviewed the subject, the last adding one additional case to the literature in which the ultimate vision was legal blindness. Rafaty[20] and Planas[18] reported temporary blindness and iridoplegia during blepharoplasty, and the latter noted induced transient strabismus. Kelly and May[13] reported a solitary case in 1980 in which vision recovered from total blindness to 20/20 vision following the institution of precise emergency therapy, whereas in a 1981 report by Miller, Venuat, and Grange[14] the ultimate outcome was blindness because the gravity of symptoms was not recognized and therapy was initiated too late.

CAUSES

Probing investigations have failed to reveal a solitary explanation for loss of vision in blepharoplasty, but the complication has never been documented in the absence of the removal of orbital fat. Furthermore, there has never been a report of a bilateral case.

Hartmann, Morax, and Vergez theorized that a "vascular spasm" of the optic nerve or retinal blood supply resulted secondary to a painful pull on orbital fat. Moser, DiPirro, and McCoy's analysis of their seven cases failed to elucidate any specific cause, and none were associated with excessive bleeding. DeMere and Austin's national survey likewise failed to reveal any causal relationship in most of their cases; neither the type of dressing nor anesthesia could be incriminated. Two cases, however, were directly attributable to retrobulbar hemorrhage, although they were unable to reproduce this experimentally in animals. Likewise, Fredericks[4] was unable to reproduce blindness in rabbits by injecting large amounts of blood into the retrobulbar space. In Gorney's series[5] all five patients had been injected with a local anesthetic containing epinephrine and were not observed in the immediate postoperative period, the blindness being discovered on subsequent examination. The cases of Rafaty and Planas almost certainly represent neurological changes secondary to diffusion of a local anesthetic into the retrobulbar space, and it is surprising that these findings have not been noted more commonly. The ophthalmologist intentionally produces temporary mydriasis, iridoplegia, ophthalmoplegia, and amaurosis every time a retrobulbar anesthetic injection is given. In at least one postoperative case of blindness undergoing litigation, careful investigation revealed that the blindness had existed long before the surgery.[2]

Most authors who have personally been involved in a case have incriminated elevated pressure associated with retrobulbar hemorrhage as the causative factor. In reporting on blindness following orbital floor fracture repair, Nicholson and Guzak[17] likewise thought that increased orbital pressure was the single most important factor. It has been theorized that in most cases the elevated orbital pressure eventually exceeds the systolic blood pressure, interrupting flow either through the central retinal artery or through the small nutrient vessels to the optic nerve. In addition, the elevated pressure could be transmitted directly to the globe, markedly elevating the intraocular pressure to produce an occlusion of the central retinal artery internally. Another conceivable mechanism for blindness is the direct stripping away of the nutrient vessels to the optic nerve from traction on orbital fat, for there is direct continuity between this fat and the short posterior ciliary vessels.[21]

PREVENTION

Wiggs; Hepler, Sugimura, and Straatsma; and Waller have all emphasized many of the important precautionary measures. Preoperatively a patient undergoing blepharoplasty should have had an ophthalmic examination with a documented visual acuity. DeMere, Wood, and Austin found that only 15% of those operated on by plastic surgeons had such documentation. Amblyopia alone has an incidence of 2% in the general population, and a high percentage of these individuals are unaware of their differences in visual acuity. One must know the preoperative acuity in case one is confronted with an unexplainable postoperative decrease in vision.

Some medical conditions are often associated with eyelid abnormalities and should be ruled out before any operation is contemplated. Surgery is contraindicated during the active phase of endocrine exophthalmos and should be postponed until the condition has stabilized. The baggy eyelids associated with myxedema and the periorbital edema of certain renal diseases will often disappear with appropriate medical therapy. Blood dyscrasias, particularly those accompanied by clotting abnormalities, and severe generalized vascular disease are accompanied by a higher surgical risk and should be investigated. Orbital fat removal in a one-eyed patient or one with severe optic nerve disease, such as advanced glaucoma, should not be undertaken.

OPERATIVE PROCEDURE

During the operation the most critical factors are related to fat removal, for this appears to be the final common denominator in loss of vision. It is advisable to remove only that fat which is apparent readily on slight orbital palpation. Undue pressure on the globe is to be avoided, as is reaching through the orbital septum and tugging excessively on fat. Hemostasis must be meticulous. Whether it is best to clamp the fat and cauterize the stump after scissors section or to isolate and cauterize individual blood vessels, avoiding the clamp, is a controversial point. It does seem, however, that it may not always be possible to locate all of the individual blood vessels that should be cauterized, particularly if they have been constricted by epinephrine. The temporary vasoconstriction produced by epinephrine is often followed by a rebound dilatation and bleeding. Barker[1] has shown during rhytidectomy surgery that moderate bleeding can recur 30 minutes after adequate hemostasis has been obtained by cautery and ligation.

Following the operation the patient should be kept under close observation when epinephrine has been used during orbital fat excision. It must be possible to return quickly to the operating room if necessary. Compression dressings are to be totally avoided, for they by themselves can produce marked elevations in intraorbital pressure and loss of vision.[12] The eyes should be left unpatched so that any changes in the ocular status can be readily detected by the patient or observer.

Cold compresses may be used to facilitate hemostasis and reduce swelling.

DIAGNOSIS

A retrobulbar hemorrhage is usually heralded by a sudden increase in the amount of pain. Blepharoplasty is not usually associated with much postoperative pain, and if severe pain develops, the surgeon should be notified immediately. If active retrobulbar bleeding is occurring, it will shortly become manifest by increasing eyelid swelling and ecchymosis. As the orbital pressure increases, decreased motility of the globe and increasing proptosis may become apparent. The intraocular pressure may now rise to high levels, vision may blur, and the pupil may dilate and become sluggish. Meanwhile, pain continues to increase in severity. It is at this point that emergency ophthalmic consultation should be requested so that a thorough ophthalmoscopic examination can be performed. Fundus examination may reveal distended veins and sludging in the arteriolar circulation; total cessation of arteriolar blood flow may be evident, and the entire retina may appear pale and edematous if the orbital pressure has exceeded the systolic blood pressure. At this point the eye may be functionally blind and the pupil maximally dilated and unreactive. The condition, however, is still totally reversible for an indeterminate period of time.

TREATMENT

Therapy is aimed at arresting any active bleeding and decreasing the orbital and intraocular pressures to increase retinal perfusion. An intravenous infusion is started, and 50 ml of a 25% solution of mannitol is injected as a bolus over a 3-minute period. Following this, a 20% solution is allowed to run in rapidly so that a total of 2.0 g/kg is given over a 45-minute period if there are no cardiovascular contraindications. The sudden increase in blood osmolarity will draw fluid from the orbit and eye and immediately lower the intraocular pressure. The blood pressure, however, must be monitored because of the rapidly expanding blood volume. Acetazolamide (Diamox) is used to inhibit aqueous humor formation; 500 mg is given as an initial intravenous dose and 250 mg is given by mouth every 6 hours for four doses. The usefulness of vasopressor or vasodilating drugs has not been established, but the inhalation of Carbogen (5% carbon dioxide and 95% oxygen) or bag breathing is thought to enhance retinal vasodilation. Paracentesis of the globe is a procedure that should not be undertaken, for it is unnecessary and has potentially disastrous complications.*

The patient should be returned to the operating room immediately and a lateral canthotomy performed. This will immediately increase the orbital volume and, in combination with the above, may be all that is necessary to adequately reestablish retinal circulation. Exploration of the operative incisions may allow the escape of trapped, clotted blood or may reveal a source of active bleeding, so that definitive cautery can be employed. After normal blood flow has been restored, the patient's vision, pupillary reactions, motility, and fundus appearance must be monitored carefully over the next 24 hours to ensure that the situation is improving.

SUMMARY

The loss of vision is a rare but devastating complication of blepharoplasty. Its incidence is approximately 0.04%, or 1 in 2500 operations. The principal causative mechanisms appear to be either a sudden, rapid increase in orbital pressure from retrobulbar bleeding or a mechanical tearing of small posterior vessels during fat resection. The elevated intraorbital pressure either occludes small nutrient vessels to the optic nerve or occludes the circulation through the central retinal artery. It is a complication that can be minimized by meticulous dissection of orbital fat coupled with exacting hemostasis. Postoperatively it can be detected by signs and symptoms appearing usually within the first 12 hours after the operation. Increasing pain and diminishing vision are the cardinal symptoms and are caused by increasing pressure from intraorbital bleeding. Therapy is aimed at arresting the hemorrhage, decreasing the orbital and intraocular pressures, and increasing retinal perfusion.

---

*EDITOR'S NOTE: In addition to the procedures to be followed for treatment of retrobulbar hemorrhage (as outlined by Dr. Weis), the immediate removal of sutures may help in evacuation of the hematoma. This can be carried out before returning the patient to the operating room. (G.P.G.)

REFERENCES

1. Barker, D.: Prevention of bleeding following a rhytidectomy, Plast. Reconstr. Surg. **54:**651, 1974.
2. Castañares, S.: Eyelid plasty. In Goldwyn, R.M., editor: The unfavorable result in plastic surgery: avoidance and treatment, Boston, 1972, Little, Brown & Co.

3. DeMere, M., Wood, T., and Austin, W.: Eye complications with blepharoplasty or other eyelid surgery: a national survey, Plast. Reconstr. Surg. **53:**634, 1974.

4. Fredericks, S.: Personal communication, 1980.

5. Gorney, M.: Personal communication, 1980.

6. Hartley, J.H., Jr., Lester, J.C., and Schatten, W.E.: Acute retrobulbar hemorrhage during elective blepharoplasty: its pathophysiology and management, Plast. Reconstr. Surg. **52:**8, 1973.

7. Hartmann, E., Morax, P.V., and Vergez, A.: Complications visuelles graves de la chirurgie des poches paepibrales, Ann. Ocul. **195:**142, 1962.

8. Hepler, R.S., Sugimura, G.I., and Straatsma, B.R.: On the occurrence of blindness in association with blepharoplasty, Plast. Reconstr. Surg. **57:**233, 1976.

9. Hueston, J.T., and Heinze, J.B.: Successful early relief of blindness occurring after blepharoplasty: case report, Plast. Reconstr. Surg. **53:**588, 1974.

10. Hueston, J.T., and Heinze, J.B.: A second case of relief of blindness following blepharoplasty: case report, Plast. Reconstr. Surg. **59:**430, 1977.

11. Jafek, B.W., Kreiger, A.E., and Morledge, D.: Blindness following blepharoplasty, Arch. Otolaryngol. **98:**366, 1973.

12. Jarrett, W.H., and Brockhurst, R.J.: Unexplained blindness and optic atrophy following retinal detachment surgery, Arch. Ophthalmol. **73:**782, 1965.

13. Kelly, P.W., and May, D.R.: Central retinal artery occlusion following cosmetic blepharoplasty, Br. J. Ophthalmol. **64:**918, 1980.

14. Miller, H.E., Venuat, G., and Grange, B.: Amaurose unilaterale irreversible apres intervention "pour poches sous les yeux," Bull. Soc. Ophthalmol. Fr. **81:**295, 1981.

15. Morax, P.V., and Blanck, C.: Un nouveau cas de complication visuelle grave apres chirurgie des poches paepibrales, Bull. Soc. Ophthalmol. Fr. **69:**454, 1969.

16. Moser, M.H., DiPirro, E., and McCoy, F.J.: Sudden blindness following blepharoplasty: report of seven cases, Plast. Reconstr. Surg. **51:**364, 1973.

17. Nicholson, D.H., and Guzak, S.V.: Visual loss complicating repair of orbital floor fractures, Arch. Ohthalmol. **86:**369, 1971.

18. Planas, J.: Transient total blindness during blepharoplasty (letter), Ann. Plast. Surg. **4:**526, 1980.

19. Putterman, A.M.: Temporary blindness after cosmetic blepharoplasty, Am. J. Ophthalmol. **80:**1081, 1975.

20. Rafaty, F.M.: Transient total blindness during cosmetic blepharoplasty, Ann. Plast. Surg. **3:**373, 1979.

21. Waller, R.R.: Is blindness a realistic complication in blepharoplasty procedures? Ophthalmology. **85:**730, 1978.

22. Wiggs, E.D.: Blepharoplasty complications, Trans. Am. Acad. Ophthalmol. Otolaryngol. **81:**OP-603, 1976.

Editorial comments
Chapter 26

Blepharoplasty is performed in outpatient surgical facilities as standard surgical practice today. This automatically limits the duration of postoperative observation. It is, however, important to consider the following precautionary steps:

1. The patient should be observed in the outpatient facility until the periods of vasoconstriction caused by epinephrine and the reflex vasodilatation have ended.
2. The patient should be instructed in writing as to how to contact the surgeon or his office should there be any sudden increase in pain, swelling, bleeding, or diminishing vision.
3. The patient should have someone in attendance at all times the first day following surgery. This person should be able to bring the patient back to the surgical facility or the hospital if necessary.

G.P.G.

Chapter 27

Problems and complications in lower lid blepharoplasty

Gilbert P. Gradinger

PROBLEMS

Problems to be considered prior to lower lid blepharoplasty can be divided into two groups: those that are perceived by the patient and those that are perceived by the surgeon.

When a patient seeks consultation regarding possible lower lid surgery, problems perceived by this person include:

1. Bags
2. Wrinkled, heavy, loose, or swollen skin
3. Dark circles under the eyes
4. A tired look and/or a sad look

Problems perceived by the surgeon may be:

1. Protruding intraorbital fat
2. Redundant, thick, edematous, pigmented, or wrinkled skin
3. Hypertrophied or atrophied pretarsal orbicularis muscle
4. Senile or cicatricial ectropion
5. Increased scleral show
6. Skin lesions that might cause an alteration in the surgical approach to lower lid blepharoplasty

It is the surgeon's responsibility to address the problems expressed by the patient and inform the patient which of those problems can be improved with surgery and which cannot. The patient wants to get rid of the problems. *Rid* implies perfection. The surgeon must stress *improvement*. (Patients may be told that the surgeon's goal is perfection, but realistically this goal is unobtainable.)

The biggest preoperative problem of all occurs when the patient enters into surgery with unrealistic expectations of the result that will be achieved. In that framework, no matter how technically successful the surgery is, the patient is destined to be disappointed. The unfortunate thing about unrealistic expectations is that patient dissatisfaction is a certainty no matter how pleased the surgeon may be with the result. In order to prevent unrealistic patient expectations, the surgeon has a number of responsibilities.

The surgeon's expectations should be reasonable, and he should convey the limit of these reasonable expectations to his patients. He should identify for the patient any of the patient's desires that are unrealistic, and he should inform the patient that postoperative complications can occur and that surgery causes minor transient problems that are to be expected.

Postoperative problems such as pain, swelling and bruising, eye irritation and discoloration of the lower level of the lid margin, awareness of blinking and some initial discomfort, and visible scarring should be reviewed. If patients know that these problems will or might occur, they are much better able to accept them.

COMPLICATIONS

The surgeon also needs to review the complications that may occur following surgery. These can be divided into general, eyelid, and ocular complications.

General complications

General complications include bleeding, infection, delayed healing, and excessive scar tissue formation. These complications can follow any type of surgery.

Bleeding. A small amount of bleeding from

252

the suture line is not unusual. Bleeding in the retrobulbar space can be catastrophic. As Dr. Weis points out in Chapter 26 of this text, retrobulbar hemorrhage can follow injection of a local anesthetic into the retrobulbar space in preparation for cataract and other types of ocular surgery. In the routine performance of blepharoplasty, it is unnecessary to ever direct anesthesia posteriorly. Retrobulbar hemorrhage from injection, then, should be, at the most, rare with blepharoplasty. It must be remembered that as soon as the orbital septum is either penetrated by a needle or opened surgically, an orbitotomy has been performed.

The most likely time for hemorrhage to occur is when the vasoconstrictive effects of epinephrine have worn off and the reflex vasodilatation occurs. It thus makes sense to observe the patient in the recovery room setting throughout this initial postoperative period. The second most likely time for hemorrhage to occur is during a sudden hypertensive episode, which could theoretically occur anytime in the first several postoperative days. It is impractical to consider close observation of the patient throughout this entire period. Patients therefore need to be advised to contact the surgeon immediately if there is a sudden increase in pain, swelling, or visual disturbance.

As soon as the diagnosis of retrobulbar hemorrhage is made, ophthalmological consultation, medical therapy, and usually surgical therapy are indicated. All therapy is directed at decreasing intraorbital and intraocular pressure. The goal of therapy, of course, is preservation of vision.

Infection. Infection following blepharoplasty is rare. Routine perioperative use of antibiotics is not common practice. Minor inflammation may be associated with sutures and disappears shortly after they are removed. Orbital cellulitis and/or abscess requires early diagnosis and vigorous treatment. In spite of prompt diagnosis and appropriate vigorous treatment, blindness may occur (Fig. 27-1).

Delayed healing. Prolonged healing or healing by secondary intention is unusual following blepharoplasty. The healing period varies and depends on the amount of swelling, bruising, and scar tissue formation. It is advisable to tell patients preoperatively that it may be several weeks before their appearance is satisfactory to them for social activities.

Excessive scar tissue formation. Eyelid skin heals kindly, and the scars usually become inconspicuous with time. The closer the lower lid incision is to the lash margin, the less conspicuous the scar will be. The incision extending beyond the lateral canthus should be lower than a horizontal line directed posteriorly from the lateral canthus. This will prevent tethering or hooding of skin

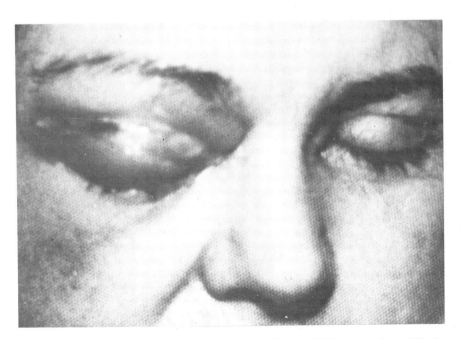

Fig. 27-1. Right orbital cellulitis following upper and lower lid blepharoplasty. Blindness resulted.

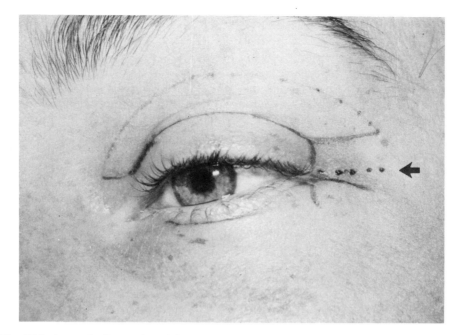

Fig. 27-2. Arrow indicates dotted line extended horizontally from lateral canthus. Lower lid incision is kept below this line.

over the lateral commissure (Fig. 27-2). When upper and lower lid blepharoplasty is done as a combined procedure, it is common to suture the upper lid incision first. This pulls up on the skin of the lower lid lateral to the lateral canthus. The effect of this is to raise the line of the proposed incision on the lower lid in a cephalad direction. This can result in the incision passing above the imaginary line extended from the lateral canthus.

Hypertrophic scars are unusual and fade and flatten with time. Rarely, revision and/or injection with a steroid is necessary. Depressed scars are similarly unusual. If the contour does not improve spontaneously in several months, judicious injection of collagen can be beneficial. (I am indebted to a colleague who, by such treatment, successfully improved the contour of the scar of a patient of mine who had been unhappy with her result.)

Eyelid complications

Ectropion. The two major causes of postoperative ectropion are unrecognized preoperative incipient senile ectropion and overresection of lower lid skin.[3]

Unrecognized preoperative incipent senile ectropion. The cardinal signs of this condition are increased scleral show secondary to lowering of the lid margin (particularly laterally), visible atrophy or absence of pretarsal orbicularis muscle, and loss of elasticity or resiliency of the lower lid as determined by the "snap test."

The performance of a standard lower lid blepharoplasty in such a lid without special effort to shorten and support the lid will most probably result in ectropion. If the ectropion is relatively mild, it may improve satisfactorily with time (Fig. 27-3). If the ectropion is severe, temporizing serves no purpose and only leads to increased frustration on the part of patient and surgeon (Fig. 27-4). A modification of the Kuhnt-Szymanowski procedure is helpful in this situation.[4] Elevation of a skin and muscle flap followed by a tarsal conjunctival triangular resection of the free margin of the lid results in tightening of the lid (Fig. 27-5). Supporting the skin and muscle by suturing to the lateral canthal tendon or orbital periosteum takes the tension off of the free margin of the lid (Fig. 27-6).[7]

Overresection of lower lid skin. Castañares[1,2] and others have cautioned against overresection of skin of the lower lid. Similarly, many have pointed out the importance of transferring the tension of the skin and/or skin-muscle flap to more rigid structures (lateral canthal tendon, periosteum, or orbital bone) (Fig. 27-6). There is no question that more skin and muscle can be resected if the flap is supported laterally, rather

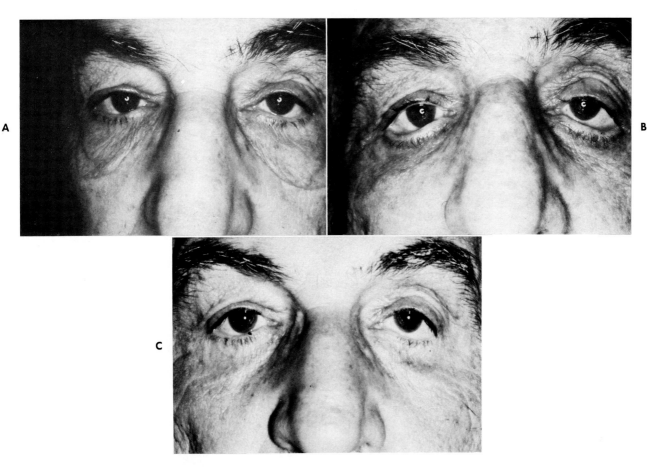

Fig. 27-3. A, Older patient with increased scleral show, atrophy of pretarsal orbicularis muscle, and low festoons of redundant skin. **B,** Bilateral ectropion following conservative skin excision. **C,** Patient 6 months postoperatively with spontaneous improvement but persistently altered lid margins.

than hanging on the free margin of the lid. Once this sutured support is in place, the skin should drape itself in the proper position below the lid margin without alteration of the level of the free margin of the lid. Whereas the amount of skin to be removed from the upper lid is determined as the initial step in upper lid blepharoplasty, the amount of skin to be removed from the lower lid is determined after fat resection and as the final step before closure. The lateral support should include both skin and muscle, whether the surgeon uses a skin-muscle flap or separate skin and muscle flaps.

When surgery is performed with the patient under local anesthesia, the time-honored technique of having the patient gaze directly up at the ceiling with the mouth open as wide as possible to determine the amount of extra skin is still commonly employed (Fig. 27-7). With the patient un-

der general anesthesia, gentle pressure on the globe transmitted through the upper lid results in elevation of the lower lid and therefore assists in judging the proper amount of skin excision.[6]

Scarring has been incriminated as a causative factor in postoperative ectropion. This implies that the ectropion would appear sometime after the initial first several days. This is unusual, but it has been known to occur.

Persistent or recurrent protruding fat. If the orbital septum is opened widely, it is usually very easy to identify the three separate fat pockets (Fig. 27-8). If the skin incision is limited to the free margin of the lid without lateral extension, the lateral-most pocket may be overlooked. Rarely, even when all three pockets have been identified and the protruding fat resected, there may be recurrent protrusion of fat postoperatively (Fig. 27-9). (It is somewhat surprising that this does not

Text continued on p. 260.

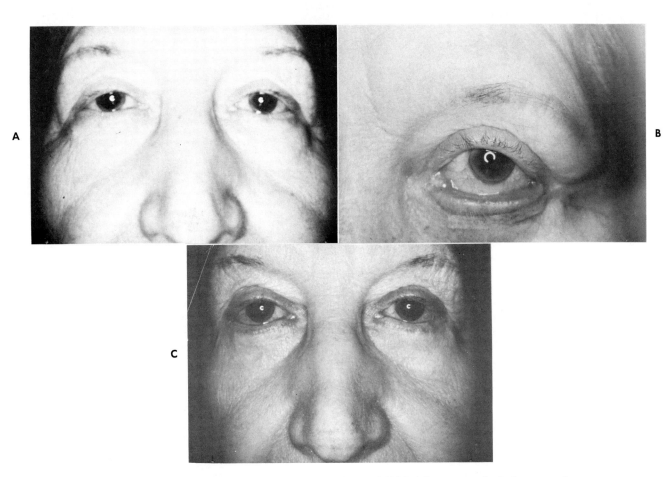

Fig. 27-4. A, Older patient who demonstrates good lid level preoperatively but no evidence of pretarsal orbicularis muscle. **B,** Postoperative ectropion in left eye, aided only slightly by Steri-Strip support. **C,** Appearance 3 months after corrective surgery (see Fig. 27-5).

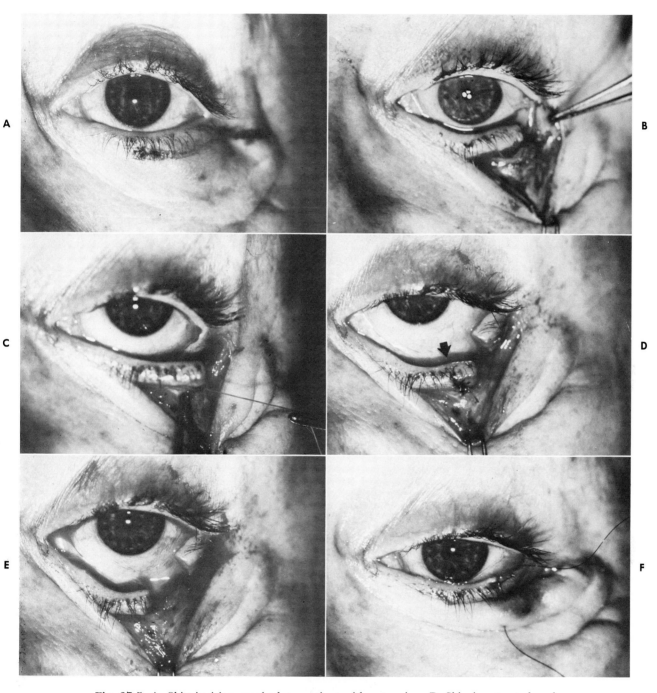

Fig. 27-5. A, Skin incision marked on patient with ectropion. **B,** Skin is retracted and free margin of lid incised vertically. **C,** Overlapping of free margin is done to judge amount to be resected. **D,** Marking ink on free border *(arrow),* indicating amount to be resected. **E,** Appearance of lid margin after full-thickness tarsoconjunctival wedge resection. **F,** Preliminary approximation prior to skin excision. Note improved level of lid margin.

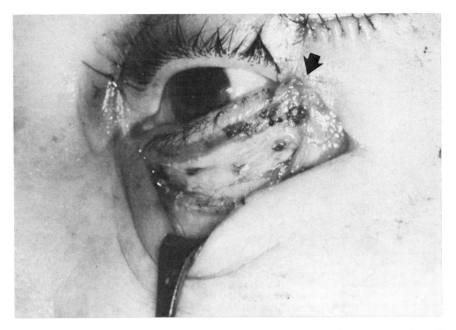

Fig. 27-6. Pretarsal portion of orbicularis muscle ends in lateral canthal tendon (ligament). It is at the point *(arrow)* where it attaches to bone that lower lid flap should be supported.

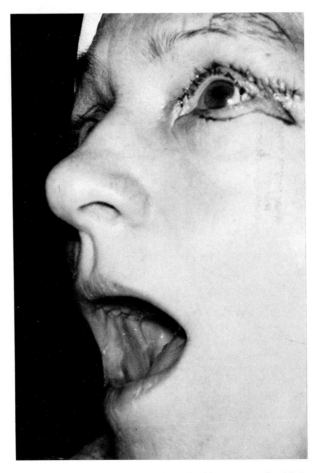

Fig. 27-7. Skin marked for excision with patient looking upward with her mouth open.

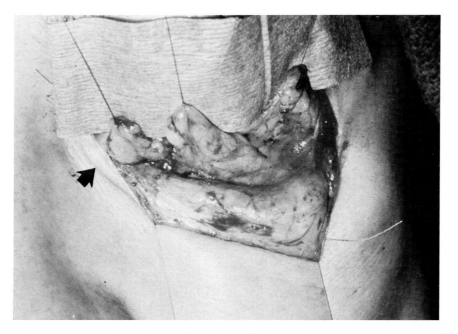

Fig. 27-8. Demonstration of protruding fat in all three pockets. Arrow points to medial pocket.

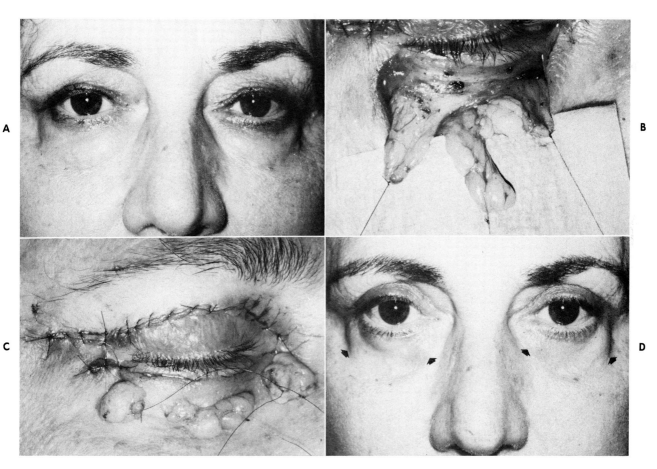

Fig. 27-9. A, Preoperative photograph showing fat in all pockets. **B,** Excess fat in all pockets. **C,** Fat has been resected from all pockets. **D,** Patient 6 months postoperatively with recurrent (or persistent) protrusion of fat in medial and lateral pockets of both lower lids *(arrows)*.

happen more often, since it is not a true mass that is being resected, but only the presenting portion of a much larger amount of intraorbital fat. Also, the surgeon does not reconstitute the orbital septum (for fear of trapping blood within the orbit).

Persistent excess skin. Patients with low bags or festoons are apt to be disappointed with surgery unless special attention is given to skin removal. In my opinion, this condition is the only time separate skin and muscle flaps offer an advantage to the skin-muscle flap.

An alternate approach (particularly in men) is the direct excision of the inferiorly located redundant skin, sometimes referred to as secondary bags (Fig. 27-10). The incision must be directed inferiorly from medial to lateral to avoid persistent edema.

Hyperpigmentation. Many patients complain of darkening of the lower lid skin preoperatively. It is possible for the skin to become darker follow-

ing surgery. This probably occurs less frequently with the increased use of the skin-muscle flap. Separation of the skin and muscle results in more ecchymosis and edema. It seems logical that it would impair venolymphatic circulation to some degree.

Hypesthesia. A patient may indicate that it is more difficult to apply mascara to the lashes because of decreased feeling. This is more common in the upper lid and is temporary, lasting up to several months.[5]

Persistent muscle bulging. Muscle excision may be less than, equal to, or more than the corresponding skin excision. If there is hypertrophied orbicularis oculi muscle, selective excision of strips of this muscle, independent of skin excision, is necessary to prevent the bulging from being visible postoperatively. The desired amount of pretarsal orbicularis muscle prominence seems to be a matter of personal aesthetics. Since the

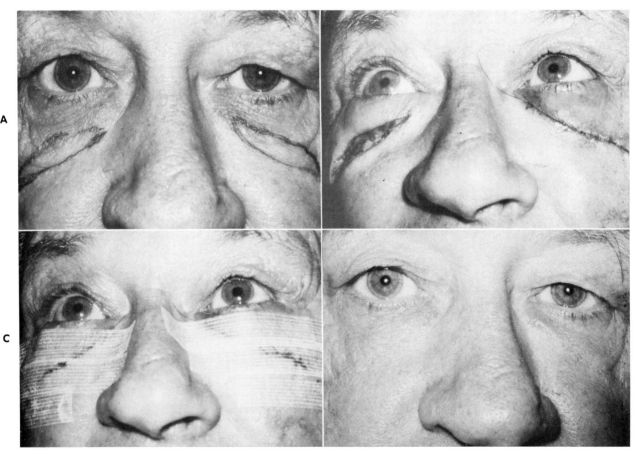

Fig. 27-10. A, Older patient without usual bags but who was unhappy with redundant skin over orbital rim. **B,** Intraoperative photograph. **C,** Steri-Strips are used to help prevent edema. **D,** Result at 3 months.

pretarsal orbicularis becomes, or at least is incorporated in, the lateral canthal tendon, its presence is important for providing support for the free margin of the lower lid. All but a narrow strip of pretarsal orbicularis muscle is elevated with the skin-muscle flap (see Fig. 27-6).

Ocular complications

Ocular complications include:
1. Corneal abrasion
2. Keratoconjunctivitis sicca
3. Diplopia
4. Loss of vision

Corneal abrasion and keratoconjunctivitis sicca. Good preoperative evaluation and meticulous surgical technique are the most important factors in preventing surface irritation of the eye. Swartz, Schultz, and Seaton[8] and others have pointed out how important the preoperative history and examination are in the prevention of corneal disease. Symptoms of dryness, itching, excessive tearing, blurring of vision, and frequent irritation must be evaluated prior to surgery. (See Chapter 21.) The preoperative presence of exophthalmos, proptosis, and increased scleral show makes the likelihood of incomplete postoperative lid closure greater than normal. Diagnosis of a tendency toward dry eye can be made preoperatively and may in fact mitigate against surgery. If

surgery is decided on, special precautions can be taken. In all instances of blepharoplasty, the cornea should be kept from drying during and after surgery. During surgery, frequent irrigation and the instillation of artificial tears are very helpful. The use of soft contact lenses is another valuable aid during surgery as well as postoperatively. Postoperatively, daytime drops and nighttime ointments and taping, along with lenses, act as an effective prophylaxis against corneal ulceration. Avoidance of coarse gauze sponges, which may accidentally rub the eye, and the use of cotton or Weck cellulose sponges help prevent injury. From the moment the blepharoplasty has been completed on one eye, that eye should be protected with drops or ointment and a cold cotton compress, with the eyelid gently maneuvered to the closed position. This is especially important when blepharoplasty is being combined with another facial procedure, such as rhytidectomy, and the blepharoplasty has been performed first.

Familiarity with the Schirmer test, the use of rose bengal and fluorescein dyes, evaluation of extraocular muscle movement, and testing for Bell's phenomenon should be part of one's diagnostic armamentarium and used appropriately.

Minor conjunctival irritations respond quickly to conservative measures. Full-blown keratoconjunctivitis sicca is a debilitating illness that re-

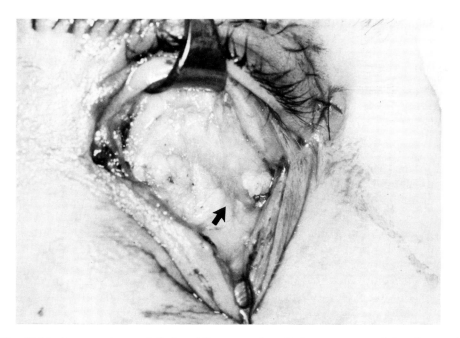

Fig. 27-11. Arrow points to inferior oblique muscle, which separates medial and central fat pads.

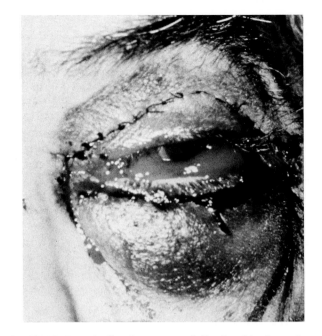

Fig. 27-12. Retrobulbar hematoma following blepharoplasty.

quires ophthalmological consultation and close follow-up. The symptoms frequently persist for many months. Permanent scarring with visual loss and erosion into the eye are the feared long-term complications.

Diplopia. Postoperative diplopia may be due to either mechanical muscle injury or removal of an excessive amount of intraorbital fat.

The inferior oblique muscle is the only extraocular muscle commonly visualized during blepharoplasty. It is between the medial and central fat pads of the lower lid and serves as an anatomical landmark (Fig. 27-11). Fat from these pockets should be removed separately to avoid accidental injury to this muscle.

It is theoretically possible that when lower lid blepharoplasty is being performed, the removal of a greater amount of fat from one side than the other could lead to diplopia (and enophthalmos) on a basis similar to that seen with loss of the orbital contents into the antrum in a blowout fracture. I have seen diplopia in only one of my patients following bilateral upper and lower lid blepharoplasty. This was noted by the patient in superior gaze and noted only when driving while approaching a stoplight and seeing two lights of the same color, one on top of the other. This disappeared spontaneously over a period of 4 to 6 weeks. No interference with extraocular move-

ments could be detected, nor could any discrepancy in eye level be demonstrated.

Loss of vision. Chapter 26 of this book deals with loss of vision following blepharoplasty. The loss may be temporary or permanent. It is the complication that is dreaded by every surgeon performing blepharoplasty. For me, it is the most difficult complication to discuss with patients preoperatively, but I do discuss it.

Retrobulbar hemorrhage. The prevention of retrobulbar hemorrhage and the early recognition of retrobulbar hemorrhage are of paramount importance (Fig. 27-12). Without meaning to seem "Pollyannish," if we are able to perform surgery on a calm, normotensive patient, judiciously inject the local anesthetic so as not to go deep into the orbit, achieve meticulous hemostasis during surgery, apply cold compresses immediately after surgery with a pain-free patient in a semisitting position, observe the patient throughout the period of vasoconstriction and initial reflex vasodilatation, and see that the patient avoids unusual postoperative stress from such things as strenuous activity and smoking, we surely will minimize the incidence of retrobulbar hemorrhage. It is quite clear that reduction of the incidence of retrobulbar hemorrhage will reduce the incidence of postoperative loss of vision. The diagnosis of retrobulbar hemorrhage constitutes an emergency. The onset of loss of vision requires emergency medical and surgical treatment. As Dr. Weis points out in Chapter 26, all medical and surgical treatment is designed to decrease intraorbital and intraocular pressure. All other considerations become secondary to the restoration of vision.

REFERENCES

1. Castañares, S.: Blepharoplasty for herniated intraorbital fat, Plast. Reconstr. Surg. **8:**46, 1951.
2. Castañares, S.: Complications in blepharoplasty, Clin. Plast. Surg. **5:**139, 1978.
3. Edgerton, M.T.: Causes and prevention of lower lid ectropion following blepharoplasty, Plast. Reconstr. Surg. **49:**367, 1972.
4. Fox, S.A.: Modified Kuhnt-Szymanowski procedure for ectropion and lateral canthoplasty, Plast. Reconstr. Surg. **39:**214, 1967.
5. Klatsky, S., and Manson, P.N.: Numbness after blepharoplasty, Plast. Reconstr. Surg. **67:**20, 1981.
6. Rees, T.D.: Technical aid in blepharoplasty, Plast. Reconstr. Surg. **41:**497, 1968.
7. Rees, T.D.: Correction of ectropion resulting from blepharoplasty, Plast. Reconstr. Surg. **50:**1, 1972.
8. Swartz, R.M., Schultz, R.C., and Seaton, J.R.: "Dry eye" following blepharoplasty, Plast. Reconstr. Surg. **54:**644, 1974.

Chapter 28

Secondary blepharoplasty

Charles E. Horton
J. Brien Murphy

We have noted an increasing population of individuals who are seeking and obtaining aesthetic surgery at an earlier age. This in turn has created a second population of patients who, as the years progress, desire revision and secondary operations as the effects of age continue after their primary surgery.

The purpose of this chapter is to review our experience with patients seeking secondary blepharoplasty and to present the differences in evaluation between the patient seeking secondary aesthetic eye surgery early postoperatively and the patient seeking secondary surgery many years later. It is not the intent of this chapter to critique or discuss the complications of the primary blepharoplasty.

ANATOMY

In 1951 Castañares[1] beautifully reviewed the periorbital anatomy as it applied to blepharoplasty. His findings have held up to multiple challenges over the last 25 years and have been further reinforced by the experience of those doing aesthetic eye surgery. Castañares re-presented the findings of Sichel, who described the separate and encapsulated compartments of the eye. In cadaver dissections and clinical studies he demonstrated that the upper lid had central and medial compartments and that the lower lid had lateral, central, and medial compartments of fatty tissue, which caused eyelid bags. Failure to individually identify and isolate each pocket of protruding orbital fat during surgery will result in inadequate correction of the deformity if orbital fatty protrusion is a problem. The lower lateral compartment

is the most frequently missed fat pad, probably as a result of inadequate exposure.*

Our experience has shown that the results of correctly performed aesthetic blepharoplasty are generally long lasting. The patient who is satisfied with the primary operation usually will not seek a secondary operation for 10 to 12 years after the initial surgery. Gravity continues to exert its forces over this time span, but the effects, when compared with those of the face-lift, are usually not as severe when examined against the same time interval. This appears to be true for two reasons. First, the eyelid skin is lighter, and there is less gravitational pull as compared with the general heavy skin of the face. Second, the scarring initiated by the primary operation, especially with an adequate fatty compartment exploration, strengthens the inhibiting septum to retard any protrusion of fat against the septum and muscle. An increase in fine wrinkles and crow's-feet lines may be noted as the skin ages, because of drooping of the skin, loss of elasticity, and continued smiling, which creases the periorbital area, sometimes without accompanying bulges.

UPPER LID

It is important to carefully examine the patient who desires a secondary blepharoplasty to determine the problems that are present. The patient who returns after 2 or 3 years following the initial blepharoplasty usually has problems related to skin redundancy of the upper lid. It does not nec-

---

*EDITOR'S NOTE: And its location—significantly cephalad to the central and medial compartments. (B.L.K.)

essarily mean that an inadequate operation was done initially. The preoperative markings of skin excess of the upper lid are difficult to determine with exactness. We require that the patient sit or stand to determine the influence of ptosis of the brow and forehead, which may demonstrate the true extra upper eyelid tissue on relaxation. Often, 2 or 3 years will allow more brow relaxation, and a previously acceptable position may change to a lower, undesirable level. This may be corrected by simple outpatient skin excision. More commonly, however, in the early-returning patient with upper lid problems, there is true ptosis of the forehead with drooping of the brows, which causes excessive upper lid skin and sagging of the upper lids. This can best be managed by a brow lift. Initially the patient may have been able to manage to give the illusion of a brow lift by simply plucking the lower hairs of the eyebrows and by painting the upper margin of the brow, but significantly increasing brow ptosis can be managed only be appropriate corrective surgery.

The patient who returns late usually also has recurrence of excessive skin wrinkling of the upper lid with or without brow ptosis. Recurrent fat protrusion may not be a problem, and simple skin excision, as in a routine blepharoplasty, is adequate for correction in these patients without brow ptosis. More commonly, however, simple eyelid skin excision will not correct the problem. In these cases a brow lift should be performed first, followed by simultaneous excision of upper lid skin.* Placement of incisions for the brow lift depends on the presence and consistency of the eyebrow hair, the total length of the forehead, and the scalp hair, as well as the quality of the forehead skin. Patients who already have a fair amount of wrinkling in the forehead are better able to disguise direct skin incisions for correction of the brow ptosis. Patients who have no brows and who always paint an artificial brow can have a direct revision in the brow area. Patients with a long vertical forehead should have an incision anterior to the scalp hairline to shorten the forehead. Patients with a short forehead with limited wrinkles should have an incision in the scalp hair approximately 2 to 3 cm behind the hairline. In general, we prefer this incision in most cases. When lateral brow ptosis is present, only lateral incisions are necessary.

---

*EDITOR'S NOTE: Note the order—brow lift *first*, before upper lid blepharoplasty, to avoid possible lagophthalmos. (See section on technique and Chapter 11.) (B.L.K.)

When herniated fat is present, exploration of the pockets and removal of excess fat is required. Usually the fat protrusion does not recur in a previously explored area. Most frequently, the medial pocket has bulged and requires excision. We believe that these patients frequently had no medial pocket protrusion at the initial operation and that the normal septum allowed protrusion with aging. To strengthen the septum, we explore all pockets at the initial operation, even if no fat is protruding. This produces a fibrous septum that contains the fat better over a long period of time.

LOWER LID

In the lower lid, the problems are different in the early-returning patient and in the late-returning one. The most common postoperative problem in the lower lid is the prominent lateral fat pad. This usually represents an unexplored bulging compartment that may not have been prominent at the time of the first operation and therefore was ignored. Exploration and excision will adequately repair this problem. We explore all compartments during the initial operation even if fat pad protrusion is not a problem. This retards the postoperative problem of the missed fat pad and, more important, creates a uniform scar in the divided septum. This scar reinforces the septum and provides a durable barrier against recurrence of the fat pad protrusion.

If excess skin is the only problem in the returning patient, simple excision of skin is adequate therapy. Caution to prevent excessive skin removal is paramount. Occasionally muscle bulging may cause irregular ridges, which can be erroneously attributed to fat protrusion. If fat protrusion is not found, trimming of the excess orbicularis oculi muscle will smooth the lower lid.

The lower lid in the late-returning patient usually presents one of two problems. Fine wrinkling, which may have been present at the time of the first operation, has become more prominent, accentuating the aging of the eye. This wrinkling may be seen in combination with excess skin and can be corrected with a chemical peel or surgical excision, depending on the depth of the wrinkling and the amount of skin redundancy. One should never combine the two procedures at the same sitting, for the peel alone may cause enough tightening that excision is unwarranted and indeed may be contraindicated. A reevaluation after the peel will determine if a surgical excision is necessary.

Previously excised fat pads, as mentioned

above, are usually not a problem in the returning patient. We believe that this is a result of scarring in the previously opened septum, which adds strength to the septum and prevents recurrence of the protrusion. The septum usually shows minimal laxity at the secondary operation because of the durability of the scar. Skin excision or peel is usually all that is necessary in the late secondary lower lid blepharoplasty unless previously untouched compartments are bulging.

TECHNIQUE

There are certain key elements in the timing of eyelid surgery, as well as some points in technique that we wish to emphasize.

When a brow lift is combined with a blepharoplasty, the brow lift should be done before the blepharoplasty, although they may be done at the same surgical sitting. It is important to do the procedures in this order, because the brow lift frequently corrects a fair amount of what appears to be redundant upper lid skin. By doing the brow lift first, one avoids overresection of upper lid skin. Evaluation and correction of the eyelid skin redundancy should be done after the face-lift or brow lift.

In dealing with the lower lid and extensive lateral crow's-feet, one should never hesitate to extend incisions lateral to these lines. The resulting scar, which may be prominent early postoperatively, fades and is well hidden in the final result. In severe cases lateral excision and tightening of the orbicularis muscle may be required. We feel that this technique is a good one, but rarely necessary, since other techniques are capable of correcting the problem in most cases.

In reexploration of the lower lid, damage to the inferior oblique muscle must be avoided. At the second operation there is scarring, which distorts the area, and it is important not to resect the muscle, which may be adjacent to the scar.

SUMMARY

Many patients seek secondary blepharoplasty. Careful examination of the problems is critical. The problems of certain patients can be corrected with simple lid skin reexcision. Others require brow lifts in conjunction with skin excision or in lieu of skin resection. Certain patients can be helped more easily with a skin peel alone, particularly if wrinkling of the skin without excessive tissue sagging is present. Fat pad herniation, a usual finding in primary blepharoplasty, is rare, since the septum is scarred from the primary surgery. The scarred septum appears stronger than the original septal tissue, thereby adding greater strength to resist the fatty protrusion. Fat pads untreated during the primary procedure may protrude and require excision during the secondary operation. By following these simple points, plastic surgeons can create satisfied patients who, if the progress in medicine and extension of life span continues, may allow us to perform tertiary blepharoplasties.

REFERENCE

1. Castañares, S.: Blepharoplasty for herniated intraorbital fat: anatomical basis for new approach, Plast. Reconstr. Surg. **8**:46, 1951.

Part IV

Aesthetic plastic surgery
of the neck

Chapter 29

Anatomical considerations in aesthetic plastic surgery of the anterior neck

Lars M. Vistnes

Apart from the skin and subcutaneous tissue, the main feature of anatomy to consider in the anterior neck is the platysma muscle. The word *platysma* is derived from the Greek word meaning "a plate."[2]

SUPERFICIAL FASCIA

If one looks at the cross-sectional anatomy of the anterior neck, as illustrated in Fig. 29-1, one sees that the platysma is invested on both sides by the superficial cervical fascia. The superficial layer of the superficial cervical fascia is densely an-

chored to the underside of the dermis by multiple fibrous bands, and there is a layer of fatty tissue sandwiched in between.[3,4] The superficial fascia exists throughout the body. In some areas it is less well defined, and in other areas, such as in the abdomen, it is well known by such names as Camper's fascia and Scarpa's fascia.[6] Some areas of the body have a particular tendency toward accumulation of fat in the superficial fascia, such as the breasts and buttocks in women and the abdomen in both sexes. The neck is another area where there is a marked tendency toward such fat

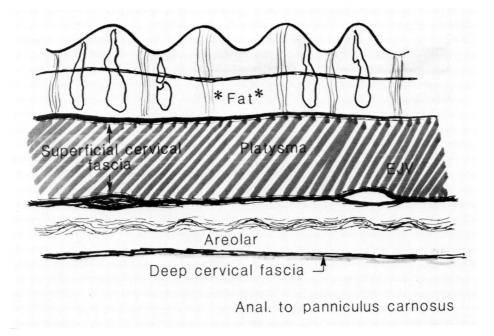

Fig. 29-1. Schematic representation of cross-sectional anatomy from anterior neck showing platysma sandwiched between two layers of superficial cervical fascia.

accumulation, resulting in the so-called double chin.[4] Between the deep layer of the superficial fascia and the deep cervical fascia, a loose areolar layer is found. It should be pointed out that the external jugular vein in the neck is intimately connected with the deep layer of the superficial cervical fascia to the degree that separating it away from that structure requires sharp dissection.[1,3]

The platysma in humans is the only remaining vestige of the panniculus carnosus in animals and is analogous to this structure.[3]

PLATYSMA

As the Greek meaning implies, the platysma is a quadrangular sheet of muscle that completely crosses the first two bones in this area to ossify, namely the mandible and the clavicle.[6] The muscle originates on the fascia of the pectoralis major and ascends upward to its insertion. There are three points of insertion that are noteworthy in this discussion (Fig. 29-2). The anterior fibers tend to decussate below the chin with the anterior fibers of the muscle on the opposite side. The more central fibers insert densely in the periosteum of the body of the mandible, whereas the most posterior fibers sweep forward and blend in-

timately with the fibers of the risorius muscle.[1,6]

Because it is such an important part of the topic, the question of the decussation of the anterior fibers is worthy of more detail. Fig. 29-3 illustrates a cadaver dissection (A) depicted schematically (B). The decussation reliably begins at the level of the hyoid bone. This decussation is a tight and stable one at all ages where such decussation occurs. A cross-section from the area below the decussation shows the two layers of superficial fascia coming together as a single fused layer in the midline. Deep to this single fused layer of superficial fascia, a separate anatomical fat pad can sometimes be found. Otherwise, if there is general distribution of fat in the neck, this fat is found evenly distributed just below the dermis as shown on the cross-sectional anatomy in Fig. 29-1.[5]

Clinical implication

The clinical implication of the foregoing information is the reality that mechanical pull may be exerted on other muscles if the direction of pull on the posterior fibers of the platysma are changed. Thus it is easy to imagine that if the platysma is detached anywhere in the neck and pulled in a different direction, such as laterally,

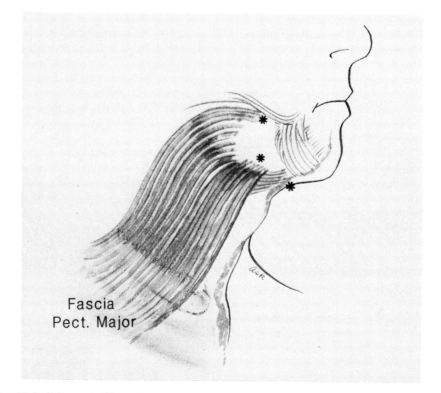

Fig. 29-2. Schematic illustration of right platysma muscle showing origin and insertion as well as extent and direction of fibers. Three asterisks draw attention to three different areas of insertion.

there is not going to be any effect on the most anterior fibers nor on the middle fibers, because the latter are densely attached to the periosteum of the mandible, whereas pull on the posterior fibers that freely cross the mandible without such attachment and attach into the risorius may result in the production of an unpleasant grin.[4]

INNERVATION

The platysma is innervated by the cervical branch of the facial nerve. The main branch emerges from below the lower border of the parotid gland and splits up into multiple branches that innervate the platysma from its deep aspect. It is of special importance to note, however, that there is an intimate intermingling or anastomoses between the upper twigs of the cervical branch and the lower twigs of the marginal mandibular branch, and that these join as single nerve fibers before they pass on to supply the muscles of facial expression that are traditionally thought of as being supplied by the marginal mandibular branch (i.e., the risorius and the depressor anguli oris)[2,6] (Fig. 29-4). The point at which the cervical branch of the facial nerve enters the posterior border of the platysma is roughly one finger's breadth below the angle of the mandible. Thus there is an intimate proximity to other vital structures in the neck, such as the submandibular gland.

Clinical implications

The clinical implications of the foregoing are twofold. First, damage to the cervical branch of the facial nerve cannot be looked at with a cavalier attitude, since it may result not only in denervation to the platysma itself, which may or may not be of great consequence, but, more important, in paralysis of those muscles of facial expression that are very obvious, namely the muscles controlling movement of the corner of the mouth. Furthermore, because of the intimate connection between the external jugular vein and the deep layer of the cervical fascia, bleeding and hematoma become a real possibility when elevation of this muscle is undertaken.

ANATOMICAL VARIATIONS

Normal anatomical variations of what has been described up to now are three in number.[2,6] The first variation, that of absence of one of the platysma muscles, is rare. The second variation, that of absence of both platysma muscles, is also rare. The third variation, however, that of no decussation anteriorly, has been found to be quite common and is seen in as many as 40% of the total population examined.[5] The two vertical parallel bands in the anterior neck between the chin and the clavicular area, so familiar to all plastic surgeons, denotes a failure of decussation in these muscles anteriorly (not as is sometimes referred to

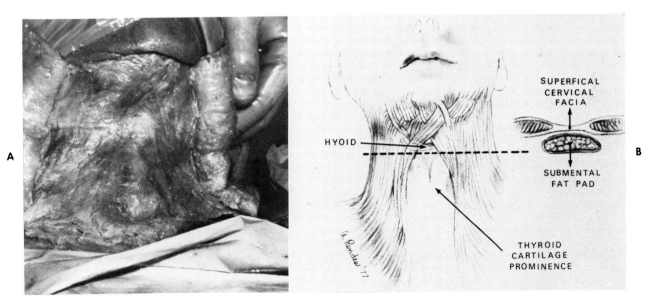

Fig. 29-3. A, Cadaver dissection of superficial structures of anterior neck showing definite decussation of anterior fibers of platysma muscles of both sides beginning at level of hyoid bone. **B,** Schematic illustration of anatomy seen on left with cross-sectional representation showing location of submental fat pad if one is present.

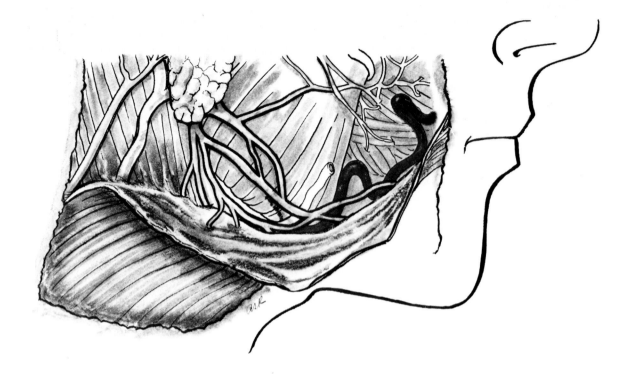

Fig. 29-4. Schematic illustration of innervation of platysma from its deep aspect with cross-innervations to what is traditionally thought of as marginal mandibular territory.

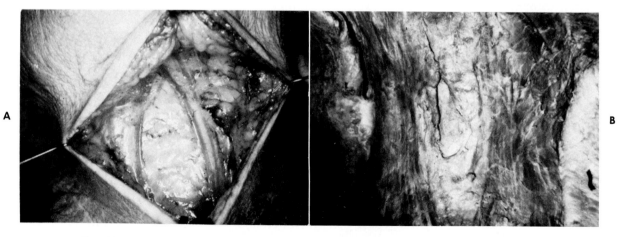

Fig. 29-5. A, Surgical dissection of anterior neck showing failure of decussation. **B,** Cadaver dissection of same area.

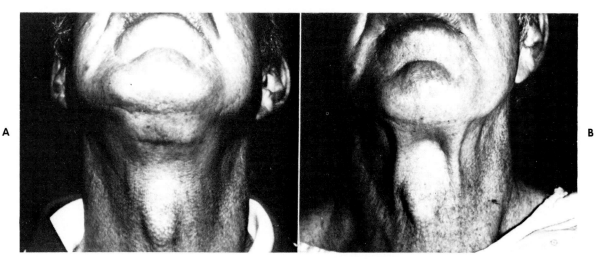

Fig. 29-6. A, Preoperative photograph of 55-year-old man showing two vertical bands representing free border of platysma in congenital failure of decussation in this area. **B,** Appearance 6 weeks following surgery, at which time, in conjunction with face-lift through separate incision in anterior neck, free borders of platysma were reapproximated to recreate decussation that normally occurs.

as dehiscence). Such failure of decussation is illustrated both by cadaver dissection and surgical dissection in Fig. 29-5.

Clinical implication

The clinical implication of this point of anatomy is that the two vertical bands seen in the anterior neck in many individuals represent a congenital failure of the fibers of the paired platysma muscles to decussate between the tip of the chin and the body of the hyoid bone. This becomes an objectionable anterior cosmetic neck deformity for which many individuals seek correction.

If correction of such a deformity is attempted by transecting all or part of the platysma muscle low down in the neck and pulling it laterally, this must be done with the realization that what one achieves is a separation of the free margins, which does not correct the problem. It seems more reasonable to reapproximate the muscles in the midline, thus creating the decussation that is present in the majority of individuals between the tip of the chin and the body of the hyoid. If this is done, it would not seem either mechanically or surgically reasonable to put tension on the suture line by simultaneously pulling the rest of the muscles laterally, which would tend to pull apart the medial suture line.

If such a problem is present, a separate horizontal neck incision can be made halfway between the tip of the chin and the hyoid bone.[5]* This can be done in conjunction with a face-lift, in which the dissection on the cheek and neck flaps must have complete continuity across the midline, so that the platysma can be pulled together in the midline completely independently of the dense fibers that connect to the underside of the skin. This type of dissection makes it possible for the platysma to be pulled independently to the midline where it belongs and for the skin and subcutaneous tissue to be pulled upward and backward where it once was (Fig. 29-6).

---

*EDITOR'S NOTE: Or in the submental crease. (B.L.K.)

REFERENCES

1. Gardner, E., Gray, D.J., and O'Rahilly, R.: Anatomy, Philadelphia, 1965, W.B. Saunders Co.
2. Grant, J.C.B., and Basmajian, J.V.: Grant's method of anatomy, ed. 7, Baltimore, 1965, The Williams & Wilkins Co.
3. Romanes, G.J.: Cunningham's textbook of anatomy, ed. 10, New York, 1964, Oxford University Press, Inc.
4. Schaeffer, J.P., editor: Morris' human anatomy, ed 10, Philadelphia, 1942, The Blakiston Co.
5. Vistnes, L.M., and Souther, S.G.: Anatomical basis for common cosmetic anterior neck deformities, Ann. Plast. Surg. **2:**381, 1979.
6. Warwick, R., and Williams, P.L., editors: Gray's anatomy, Br. ed. 35, Philadelphia, 1973, W.B. Saunders Co.

Chapter 30

Complications of the neck lift

José Guerrerosantos

With the increased popularity of aesthetic plastic surgery, which readily restores good appearance and youthfulness to the face, more and more patients are consulting plastic surgeons for correction of the sagging neck deformity. Its surgical correction, in my personal experience, is one of the most rewarding and gratifying of all aesthetic plastic operations, if all goes well. If serious complications suddenly arise, it may become a veritable nightmare to the patient and to the surgeon alike. Because of this, the highest technical operative refinement must be strived for in order to do everything humanly possible to prevent serious complications, some of which occasionally are unavoidable in spite of the best surgical skill.

Within the past two decades, neck lift surgery has been greatly improved by the development of several new techniques. In the classical operation, the surgeon depends on the cutaneous lift and the pull applied to the flap only. Usually the undermining is limited. Aesthetic results with this type of operation may be good on slender patients with minimal submental laxity. But on patients with fat deposits in submandibular and submental regions and with moderate or severe laxity in the submandibular and submental regions, the results may be poor and short lived. In such patients modern neck lift techniques, including wide cutaneous undermining, cervical lipectomy, platysmaplasties, and submandibular gland lifting, are indicated. The well-performed modern operation gives superior aesthetic results, but we must always keep in mind that the surgical maneuvers are extensive, and complications may be serious.

Complications in the neck lift operation occur in direct proportion to the extent of undermining and in inverse proportion to the adequacy of hemostasis. If undermining and skin resection are kept to a minimum, the possibility of complications is also reduced to a minimum. This type of surgical indulgence, however, will not produce a satisfactory aesthetic result or any degree of gratification for the patient. As the operation is extended in compliance with the aesthetic demands of the situation, the incidence of complications increases in direct proportion. The best treatment for any complication is prevention.

Generally speaking, the causes of failure of the neck lift operation fall into three categories. The first reason for failure is poor patient selection by the surgeon. Unfavorable physical factors in the cheek and neck reduce the chances of achieving a good result. These factors may include (1) a neck that is too short and thick, (2) an unfavorable low position of the hyoid bone in relation to the mandible, (3) the degree of cutaneous flaccidity, (4) the amount and location of accumulated fat in both the submental region and the submandibular region, (5) flaccidity or rigidity of the platysma muscle in both its medial and posterolateral portions, and (6) ptosis or hypertrophy of the submandibular glands.

Another cause of failure is poor planning and the selection of an inappropriate technique by the surgeon. This derives from an incorrect concept of the neck lift operation or from an inadequate application of the techniques. A conservative procedure for a patient with severe neck laxity and very flaccid skin, excess cervical fat, and marked laxity of the platysma muscle will produce an inadequate result. On the other hand, an overly radical procedure for mild deformity could expose the patient to unnecessary risk.

The third reason for failure includes those factors that are beyond the plastic surgeon's control. These may be related to the intrinsic conditions of the tissues that are being operated on, or they may be associated with the patient's habits. Obese patients with fat necks require special care by the surgeon. It is important to control certain factors that modify the normal healing process, such as peripheral circulatory alterations that favor thrombus formation, hinder reabsorption of hematomas and seromas, and facilitate liquefaction of the residual fat of the flaps and fascias, and hematomas caused by high blood pressure and metabolic disorders due to anticoagulants or to other medication. Any candidate with a fat, fallen neck who is under treatment with any of these types of medications or who has hypertension should receive adequate preoperative preparation by appropriate specialists several weeks before the corrective surgery.

The usual complications associated with the face-lift have been noted in detail in the plastic surgery literature.[1,2] Most surgeons are acutely aware of those factors which may produce untoward results.

By all odds, the most frequent unhappy sequela of cervicofacial rhytidectomy is an unsatisfactory result. This is rare in the hands of the skilled plastic surgeon, but it does occur. The surgeon who is improving his skill may encounter numerous problems initially. Some of these, as well as secondary procedures for their correction, are taken up later in this chapter.

The specific purpose of this chapter is to discuss causes, prevention, and treatment of complications of neck lift operations. As in any surgical procedure, complications may and do occur. The material for this chapter was compiled through careful review of consecutive neck lift procedures that I have done over the past 15 years. The complications outlined include those which occurred in my series of cases, as well as some encountered by other members of the staff of the Jalisco Reconstructive Plastic Surgery Institute.

A statistical analysis of 1424 consecutive cervicofacial rhytidectomies is presented. Complications occur in a significant percentage of neck lift operations. The plastic surgeon must be aware of the incidence and significance of these complications, as well as know how to avoid and manage them.

The incidence of major complications is shown in Table 30-1.

Illustrative cases demonstrating complications listed in Table 30-1 are presented below.

EXCESSIVE SUBMENTAL SKIN REMOVAL

In neck lifts it is seldom advisable to remove skin from the submental area, since the apparent surplus skin is needed to cover the neck after the surgeon has completed the cervical lipectomy and has reconstructed the underlying tissues. I believe that it is necessary to remove submental skin in only 5% of patients.

CASE REPORT

A 58-year-old woman underwent cervicofacial rhytidectomy with neck lift emphasis. She also had a blepharoplasty and frontal lift. The neck was corrected by a wide cutaneous lift, discrete cervical lipectomy, lateral platysma plications, and a submandibular gland lift.[3]

After being examined clinically 2 years after surgery, she was found to have a very reasonable aesthetic improvement except for a vertical cutaneous band located at the midline of the neck as a result of excessive submental skin removal (Fig. 30-1).

In my early experience with neck lift cases, I thought that the aesthetic improvement would be better if the supposed surplus skin of the neck were removed. I recommend, especially to those who are less experienced in this type of surgery, that they avoid removing submental skin, and in cases where such removal seems indicated, to consider it carefully and make an accurate assessment of the skin that appears to be in excess. It is easy to do a secondary surgical correction for excess skin, whereas a vertical cutaneous band is very hard to correct.

Table 30-1. Complications in 1424 consecutive cervicofacial rhytidectomies, 1965-1979

	Number	*Percent*
Abnormally sharp submentocervical angle	8	0.56
Lateral "bunching" due to rolling up of divided platysma	52	2.24
Injury to cervical branch of cranial nerve VII	8	0.56
Injury to marginal mandibular nerve	2	0.14
Submental fullness of either side of midline	68	4.62
Postoperative irregularities	56	2.54
Excessive fat removal (central submental depression)	24	1.68
Excessive skin removal	60	4.20
Residual medial platysma fibers	28	1.96
Large hematoma	52	2.24
Large skin necrosis	10	0.70

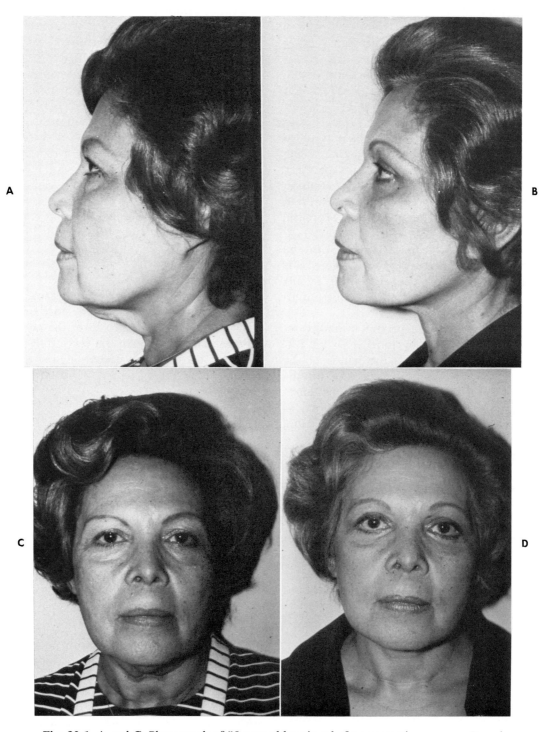

Fig. 30-1. A and **C,** Photograph of 58-year-old patient before corrective surgery. **B** and **D,** Appearance after submental lipectomy and lateral plication of platysma muscle and submandibular gland. Cervicofacial rehabilitation is good except for cervical cutaneous band due to excessive submental skin removal.

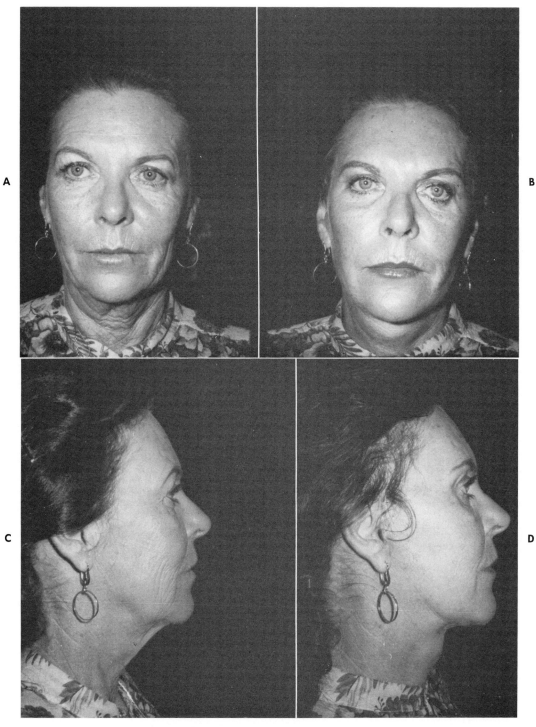

Fig. 30-2. A and **C,** Photograph of 56-year-old patient before surgical correction. **B** and **D,** Appearance after cervicofacial rhytidectomy, blepharoplasty, and forehead lift. Observe abnormally sharp submentocervical angle on profile view.

ABNORMALLY SHARP SUBMENTOCERVICAL ANGLE

An abnormally sharp cervicomental angle is an undesirable result from a neck lift, giving a masculine appearance to female patients. This deformity is due to excessive lifting of the underlying tissues, with too much pull up and backward, or to excessive defatting at the angle.*

In order to avoid this, the surgeon must estimate as accurately as possible (1) the amount of fat to be removed by cervical lipectomy and (2) the traction to be exerted on the lateral plicating sutures to lift the submandibular gland and the platysma muscle.

CASE REPORT

A 56-year-old woman sought correction for cervicofacial flaccidity. She underwent cervicofacial rhytidectomy, blepharoplasty, and frontal lifting. On follow-up a year later, the result in the frontal view was excellent (Fig. 30-2, *B*).

In the profile view (Fig. 30-2, *D*) the integral result was good except for the abnormally sharp submentocervical angle.

I believe that this postoperative deformity bothers the perfectionist surgeon more than the patient. At present there is no reported technique to solve this aesthetic problem.†

POSTOPERATIVE IRREGULARITIES

Following neck lift operations some patients may have postoperative irregularities as a result of inadequate performance of the operation. The most common causes of these deformities include undermining at different levels, producing uneven contours, residual vertical bands of platysma muscle, uncorrected submandibular gland ptosis, and a residual fat pad (Fig. 30-3).

CASE REPORT

A 63-year-old woman sought correction for marked cervicofacial flaccidity (Fig. 30-4, *A*). She underwent total facial rejuvenation with a frontal lift, blepharoplasty, and cervicofacial rhytidectomy.

---

*EDITOR'S NOTE: Additional causes of overly sharp cervicomental angles include (1) dividing the medial platysma bands too high (superiorly) in the neck, (2) carrying the suture line too far posteriorly (if the medial borders of the submental portion of the platysma are sutured), (3) making the postauricular pilot cuts in the skin too deep and causing the skin over the cervicomental angle to be too tight, and (4) pulling up the cheek superficial musculoaponeurotic system (SMAS) too tightly. (B.L.K.)

†EDITOR'S NOTE: Would a dermis graft be of help? (B.L.K.)

Two years later bulging was found in both submandibular regions, which was due to two factors: insufficient fat resection and failure to resuspend the submandibular gland (Figs. 30-4, *B* and *C*). Therefore 2 years after the primary surgery, a secondary neck lift was done that included submandibular lipectomy, placing of plicating sutures, and submandibular gland lifting.[3] When she was seen a year after the secondary neck lift, the result was reasonably good (Fig. 30-4, *D*).

LATERAL "BUNCHING" DUE TO ROLLING UP OF DIVIDED PLATYSMA

Techniques that radically transect the platysma muscle may produce a lateral "bunching" deformity due to a welling up of divided platysma. In the past on our service, we used to see some patients with this condition after using techniques involving platysma muscle flaps made at the midline and then pulled toward the mastoid region (Fig. 30-5). In order to avoid such complications, it is necessary to perform the technique as cleanly as possible after the platysma muscle has been plicated. The surgeon must observe whether any bulge has been formed. It is also advisable to palpate with the fingertips to be sure of what one is seeing.

If there is any bulging, the excess tissue must be removed by beveled excisions, using scissors with serrated blades. If the deformity is observed after the neck lift, it is then advisable to do a secondary operation several months later, beveling the cut muscle edges with serrated blade scissors to make the surfaces smooth and even.

GENERAL COMMENTS

To avoid complications with neck lifting, the causes of such complications should be recognized, patients should be properly selected, and the correct surgical techniques should be chosen for each patient.

In my series, most of the complications and problems I had occurred during my first 5 years of frequent neck lift experiences. In recent years the complications have been only minor.

I have listed the complications I have found in performing neck lift procedures. Even in the hands of the best plastic surgeons, complications will occur. I hope that by my pointing out the troubles I have witnessed, others will be aware of the dangers and will be prepared to recognize and handle them.

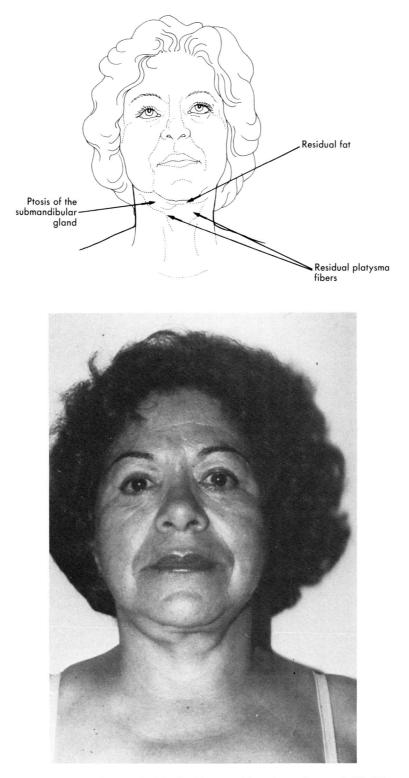

Residual fat

Ptosis of the
submandibular
gland

Residual platysma
fibers

Fig. 30-3. Severe cervical irregularities in 53-year-old patient after neck lift. These were caused by residual platysma bands, submandibular gland ptosis, and residual fat pad.

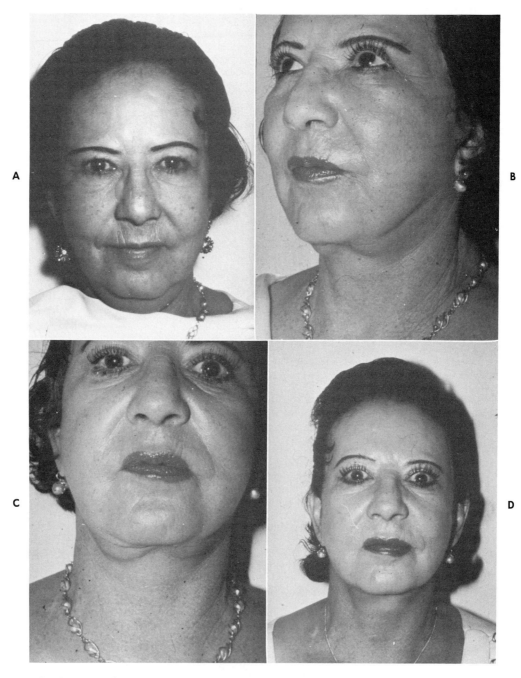

Fig. 30-4. A, Photograph of 63-year-old patient with marked cervicofacial flaccidity. **B** and **C,** Two years after primary neck lift, patient has very noticeable bulging due to residual submandibular fat pad and submandibular ptosis that was not corrected at primary operation. **D,** Appearance 1 year after secondary neck lift that included submandibular lipectomy and submandibular gland lifting.

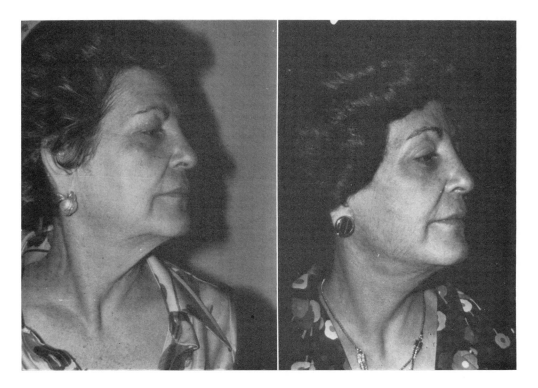

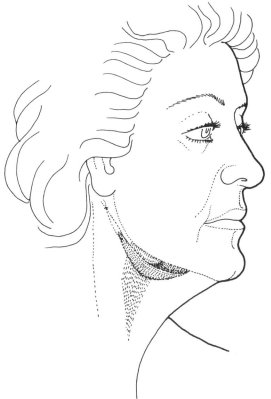

Fig. 30-5. Sixty-one-year-old patient before and after cervicofacial rhytidectomy. Cervicofacial rehabilitation was good, but lateral "bunching" can be seen on neck as result of rolling up of divided platysma.

REFERENCES

1. Adamson, J.E., Horton, C.E., and Crawford, H.H.: Surgical correction of the "turkey gobbler" deformity, Plast. Reconstr. Surg. **34:** 589, 1964.
2. Castañares, S.: Facial nerve paralysis coincident with or subsequent to, rhytidectomy, Plast. Reconstr. Surg. **54:**637, 1974.
3. Guerrerosantos, J., et. al.: Correction of cervicofacial wrinkles, Rev. San. Guad. **4:**97, 1971.

SUGGESTED READINGS

Baker, T.: Sectioning and plication of flaccid cervical bands, Presented at the First Congress of the Ibero-Latin-American Federation of Plastic and Reconstructive Surgery, Quito, Ecuador, August 1976.

Baker, T.J., and Gordon, H.L.: Complications of rhytidectomy, Plast. Reconstr. Surg. **40:**31, 1967.

Baker, T.J., Gordon, H.L., and Mosienko, P.: Rhytidectomy: a statistical analysis, Plast. Reconstr. Surg. **59:**24, 1977.

Baker, T.J., Gordon, H.L., and Whitlow, D.R.: Our present technique for rhytidectomy, Plast. Reconstr. Surg. **52:**232, 1973.

Barker, D.F.: Prevention of bleeding following a rhytidectomy, Plast. Reconstr. Surg. **54:**651, 1974.

Connell, B.F.: Cervical lifts: the value of platysma muscle flaps, Ann. Plast. Surg. **1:**36, 1978.

Connell, B.F.: Contouring the neck in rhytidectomy by lipectomy and a muscle sling, Plast. Reconstr. Surg. **61:**376, 1978.

Dingman, R.O.: Severe bleeding during and after face-lifting operations under general anesthesia (letter to the editor), Plast. Reconstr. Surg. **50:**608, 1972.

Gallozzi, E., Blancato, L.S., and Stark, R.B.: Deliberate hypotension for blepharoplasty and rhytidectomy, Plast. Reconstr. Surg. **35:**285, 1965.

Guerrerosantos, J.: The role of the platysma muscle in rhytidoplasty, Clin. Plast. Surg. **5:**29, 1978.

Guerrerosantos, J.: Surgical correction of the fatty fallen neck, Ann. Plast. Surg. **2:**389, 1979.

Guerrerosantos, J., Spaillat, L., and Morales, F.: Muscular lift in cervical rhytidoplasty, Plast. Reconstr. Surg. **54:**127, 1974.

Kaye, B.L.: The extended facelift with ancillary procedures, Ann. Plast. Surg. **6:**335, 1981.

Leist, F.D., Masson, J.K., and Erich, J.B.: A review of 324 rhytidectomies, emphasizing complications and patient dissatisfaction, Plast. Reconstr. Surg. **59:**525, 1977.

McGregor, M.W., and Greenberg, R.L.: Rhytidectomy. In Goldwyn, R.M., editor: The unfavorable result in plastic surgery: avoidance and treatment Boston, 1972, Little, Brown & Co.

Millard, D.R., et al.: Submental and submandibular lipectomy in conjunction with a face lift, in the male or female, Plast. Reconstr. Surg. **49:**385, 1972.

Millard, D.R., Pigott, R.W., and Hedo, A.: Submandibular lipectomy, Plast. Reconstr. Surg. **41:**513, 1968.

Peterson, R.: Cervical rhytidoplasty—a personal approach, Presented at the Annual Symposium of Aesthetic Plastic Surgery, Guadalajara, Mexico, October 1974.

Rees, T.D.: Face-Lift. In Rees, T.D., and Wood-Smith, D.: Cosmetic facial surgery, Philadelphia, 1973, W.B. Saunders Co.

Rees, T.D., Lee, Y.C., and Coburn, R.J.: Expanding hematoma after rhytidectomy, Plast. Reconstr. Surg. **51:**149, 1973.

Rogers, B.O.: The seagull or "movette" incision for correction of double chins. In Marchak, D., and Hueston, J.T., editors: Transactions of the Sixth International Congress of Plastic and Reconstructive Surgeons, New York, 1976, Masson Publishing USA, Inc.

Skoog, T.: Plastic surgery: new methods and refinements, Philadelphia, 1974, W.B. Saunders Co.

Stark, R.B.: A rhytidectomy series, Plast. Reconstr. Surg. **59:**373, 1977.

Webster, G.V.: The ischemic facelift, Plast. Reconstr. Surg. **50:**560, 1972.

Weisman, P.A.: Simplified technique in submental lipectomy, Plast. Reconstr. Surg. **48:**443, 1971.

Chapter 31

Complications in the neck following rhytidectomy

Norman E. Hugo

In the past, the complications seen in the neck after face-lifting were essentially dependent on the extent of undermining, the subsequent ability to obtain hemostasis, and the tension applied to the flaps in order to create cervical definition. More recently, the entire concept of face-lifting has undergone dramatic changes in which the cutaneous undermining is often more extensive (except perhaps in the superficial musculoaponeurotic system [SMAS]) lift. Cutting and realignment of the platysma is done, and cervical lipectomy is extensive. In addition, increasing numbers of patients are taking a variety of medications that can create problems.

HEMATOMA

Historically, the most common complication following a face-lift was hematoma, averaging slightly over 8% (Table 31-1). Complete and long-term studies are not presently available to ascertain the incidence of hematoma with the present methods, but it appears to be at least as high. This no doubt is due to the extensive undermining, the muscle sectioning, and the cervical lipectomy, as well as the previously-mentioned germane reasons.

It is important to take a detailed medical history to determine the medications being taken by patients. The chief offender is acetylsalicylic acid (aspirin), found in numerous over-the-counter preparations. Patients should be free from this drug for at least 10 days before undergoing any elective surgery. All patients should have the following tests done: a bleeding time (to evaluate platelet function) and a partial thromboplastin time (to assess the integrity of blood clotting and the intrinsic pathway). In addition, many patients with hypercholesterolemia will be taking clofibrate. Interaction of this drug with lidocaine results in a severe depression of platelet function and should be avoided.

The best treatment of hematoma is prevention, and this requires absolute hemostasis. The "second look" introduced by McDowell[7] has been

Table 31-1. Complications following rhytidectomy

Author	No. of patients	Infection	Facial nerve injury	Hematoma	Slough
Baker et al.[1]	137 (men)	0	0	26 (18%)	0
Rees, Lee, and Coburn[9]	806	0	0	23 (2.8%)	0
Conway[4]	325	2 (0.6%)	2 (0.6%)	21 (6.5%)	1 (0.3%)
Baker, Gordon, and Mosienko[2]	1500	15 (1.0%)	8 (0.5%)	234 (15.6%)	17 (1.1%)
Thompson and Ashley[12]	922	17 (1.8%)	6 (0.6%)	44 (4.7%)	3 (0.3%)
Singer and Lewis[10]	100	1 (1%)	1 (1%)	5 (5%)	0
McDowell[7]	105	0	2 (1.9%)	3 (2.9%)	1 (0.9%)
McGregor and Greenberg[8]	524	0	14 (2.6%)	42 (8.0%)	16 (3.0%)
Stark[11]	500	4 (0.8%)	2 (0.4%)	30 (6%)	1 (0.2%)
Leist, Masson, and Erich[6]	324	0	1 (0.8%)	19 (5.9%)	7 (2.1%)
TOTALS	5243	39 (1.0%)	36 (0.8%)	447 (8.5%)	46 (1.0%)

effective in reducing hematomas by allowing the vasoconstriction induced by epinephrine to subside, revealing noncoagulated vessels capable of hemorrhage. My present approach is to inject both right and left sides of the face and neck simultaneously so that there will be equal time for the vasoconstrictive effects on both sides to subside. In addition, if blepharoplasty is to be done, I do this before the second look and closure, to provide sufficient time for the vasoconstrictive effect to subside. I also have the patient cough and strain (i.e., perform the Valsalva maneuver) to provoke any further hemorrhage.

In my experience, the cervical vessels most likely to hemorrhage late are the branch of the facial artery near the submaxillary gland and the cluster of vessels over the mastoid head of the sternomastoid muscle. While suction drains and pressure dressings are also used separately or in combination, their ability to prevent cervical hematomas has not been proved.

Late-developing hematomas can be aspirated with an 18-gauge needle if they are situated low in the neck. When it appears as if the hematoma has been completely evacuated, I instill 1 to 2 ml of triamcinolone (Kenalog 10) into the area to discourage nodular formation. Hematomas near the mastoid area can be manually pressed out after introduction of a hemostat in the retroauricular fold or scalp-mastoid area if a track has been established.

The effects of subcutaneous hematoma with current techniques are more severe than those previously encountered. Hematomas seen after wide undermining but without lipectomy form hard nodules, which are treated by massage and/or triamcinolone injections. The hematomas encountered after lipectomy seem more cordlike and dense and are firmly attached to the dermis. They are not as easily treated, and some require reoperation for their release from the dermis even after prolonged conservative treatment (Fig. 31-1).

NERVE DAMAGE

Nerve damage is a significant but infrequent complication (Table 31-1). It has an incidence of less than 1%, and many of these injuries are tem-

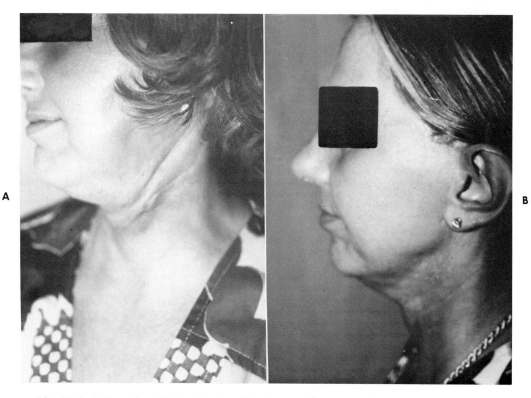

Fig. 31-1. A, In spite of triamcinolone injections and massage, dense cordlike structure persists after hematoma. **B,** Result after surgical release.

porary. Because of the newer and extensive SMAS procedures and cervical lipectomy with or without sectioning and tightening of the platysma, the incidence of nerve damage may increase. Certainly, with deeper and more extensive dissection around the ramus mandibularis, it is not unreasonable to anticipate this. Ellenbogen[5] has described an apparent seeming paralysis of the ramus mandibularis that he attributes to severance or stretching of the rami of the cervical branch of the facial nerve supplying the playtsma. Function of the platysma and return of the smile is apparent in a few weeks. A similar patient is presented in Fig. 31-2. Castañares[3] reviewed the causes of facial palsy seen after rhytidectomy. If the paralysis is evident during surgery, it is wise to identify the severed ends and repair them under magnification. Paralysis seen during the course, or at the conclusion, of surgery can be caused by the injection of a local anesthetic. Otherwise, exercises in front of a mirror, consultation with a neurosurgeon, and conservative treatment for 6 months are indicated. A significant number will have return of function. Good patient rapport is estab-lished by frequent visits and continued interest on the part of the surgeon.

CUTANEOUS COMPLICATIONS

Cutaneous complications occur (Table 31-1) and invariably are the result of inadequate blood supply for whatever reason. They may be manifested as simple blisters or as areas of frank necrosis. It has long been obvious that excessive tension from either too vigorous a pull or that exerted by a hematoma can obliterate blood flow. As a consequence, hematomas must be anticipated, examined for, and immediately evacuated. Slough of postauricular skin is usually a result of too much tension in an effort to tighten the neck (Fig. 31-3). With lipectomy and platysma lifting this should be a less-frequent complication, since these procedures provide greater cervical definition with less tension.

An infrequently mentioned problem is the cutaneous slough caused by smoking. It is seen in patients in the absence of hematoma or tension and develops a few days postoperatively. First, one sees dark, punctate areas, which gradually co-

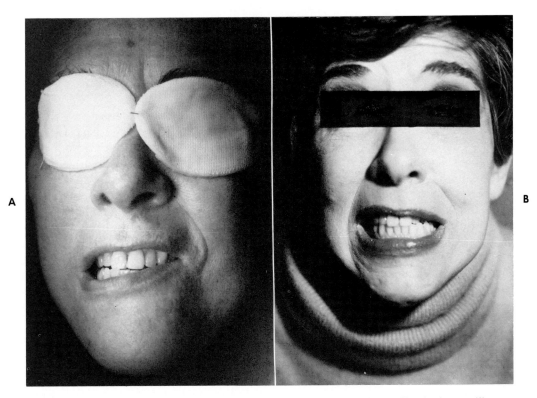

Fig. 31-2. A, Patient with intraoperative inability to depress lower lip during smiling. **B,** Resolution 3 months later. (From Hugo, N.: Rhytidectomy with radical lipectomy and platysmal flaps, Plast. Reconstr. Surg. **65:**199, 1980.)

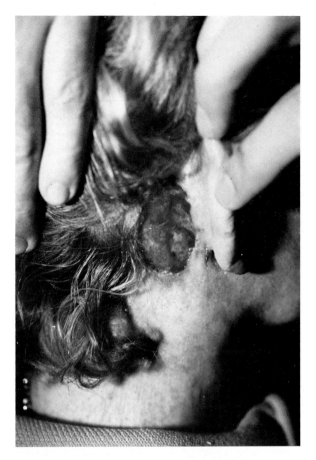

Fig. 31-3. Postauricular slough following excessive tension. Area healed spontaneously. Treatment consists only of wound toilet.

alesce and form larger areas of slough (Fig. 31-4). It is imperative to stop people from smoking tobacco; if they must continue smoking, they should substitute a vegetable cigarette (Fig. 31-5).

Whatever the cause of the skin slough, conservative management is the keystone to success. The area in question should be kept clean with gentle cleansing and protected by antibiotic ointment (usually bacitracin), which not only offers protection against infection but keeps the area soft and pliable. Mechanical debridement should not be done. The eschar is allowed to separate spontaneously, after which healing takes place by wound contraction and epithelialization. A period of 3 to 6 months should then pass before the patient is evaluated for secondary surgery. Fortunately, further surgery is often not required.

INFECTION

Infection is infrequent, because these are clean cases and the areas involved have superior blood supplies. Most series report less than a 1% incidence (Table 31-1). The usual offending organism is *Staphylococcus aureus,* and it generally presents after 3 or 4 days as an enlarging, tender mass. My treatment of this has been to introduce a hemostat from behind the ear into the infected area, express as much purulent exudate as possible, and then irrigate with a saline-peroxide mixture.* This is done on an outpatient, twice-daily basis. Within a week the infection has subsided and no permanent side effects remain. Rarely, one encounters a β-hemolytic streptococcal infection characterized by sudden pain in the area and malaise on the part of the patient. I have had two such patients. Treatment requires hospitalization,

---

*EDITOR'S NOTE: Direct irrigation with appropriate antibiotic solution is also helpful. If the patient is given one of the penicillins systemically, the serum level can be increased by concomitantly administering probenecid (Benemid) to decrease renal excretion of the penicillin. (B.L.K.)

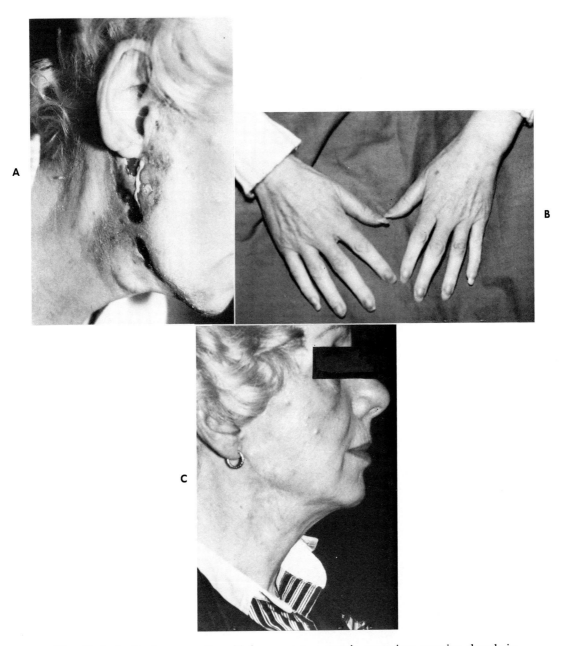

Fig. 31-4. A, Coalescence of multiple punctate necrotic areas into massive slough in chain smoker. **B,** Severity of condition may have been intensified by Raynoud's disease, as demonstrated by digital blanching on exposure to cold. **C,** Resolution with simple wound care. (From Hugo, N.: Rhytidectomy with radical lipectomy and platysmal flaps, Plast. Reconstr. Surg. **65:**199, 1980.)

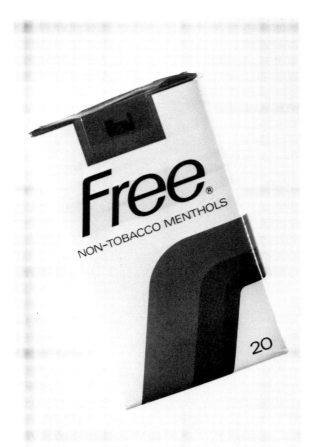

Fig. 31-5. Nicotine-free cigarette substitute.

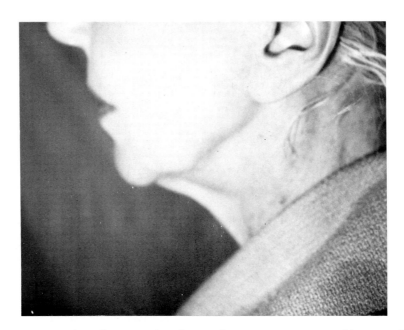

Fig. 31-6. Overzealous lipectomy has flattened area over ramus, making mandibular angle prominent and mimicking jowl when none exists.

intravenous antibiotics, and warm packs applied to the area. Vigorous treatment must be given to prevent tissue slough.

OTHER COMPLICATIONS

Incision and tightening of the platysma can also result in a subluxation of the submaxillary gland, which appears to recreate a jowl. Although it is an infrequent complication, it is distressing to the patient.

Overzealous lipectomy may result in a peculiar deformity in the mandibular area (Fig. 31-6). The SMAS lift should precede the cervical lipectomy, so that the lipectomy will remove fat only up to the mandibular border. If it goes above that, the characteristic deformity will occur.

SUMMARY

While the cervical complications following rhytidectomy are most commonly hematomas and nerve damage, infection and slough remain important considerations. Fortunately, most of these complications are amenable to treatment and, after the passage of time, do not adversely affect the result. Newer methods of face-lifting produce their own special problems. It remains to be seen how they will change the more classic complications.

REFERENCES

1. Baker, D.C., et al.: The male rhytidectomy, Plast. Reconstr. Surg. **60:**514, 1977.
2. Baker, T.J., Gordon, H.L., and Mosienko, P.: Rhytidectomy—a statistical analysis, Plast. Reconstr. Surg. **59:**24, 1977.
3. Castañares, S.: Facial nerve paralysis coincident with, or subsequent to rhytidectomy, Plast. Reconstr. Surg. **54:**637, 1974.
4. Conway, H.: The surgical face lift—rhytidectomy, Plast. Reconstr. Surg. **45:**124, 1970.
5. Ellenbogen, R.L.: Pseudo-paralysis of the mandibular branch of the facial nerve after platysmal face-lift operation, Plast. Reconstr. Surg. **63:**364, 1979.
6. Leist, F.D., Masson, J.K., and Erich, J.B.: A review of 324 rhytidectomies, emphasizing complications and patient dissatisfaction, Plast. Reconstr. Surg. **59:**525, 1977.
7. McDowell, A.J.: Effective practical steps to avoid complications in face lifting, Plast. Reconstr. Surg. **50:**563, 1972.
8. McGregor, M.W., and Greenberg, R.L.: Complications of face lifting. In Masters, F.W., and Lewis, J.R., Jr., editors: Symposium on aesthetic surgery of the face, eyelid, and breast, St. Louis, 1972, The C.V. Mosby Co.
9. Rees, T.D., Lee, Y.C., and Coburn, R.J.: Expanding hematoma after rhytidectomy, Plast. Reconstr. Surg. **51:**149, 1973.
10. Singer, R., and Lewis, C.M.: Rhytidectomies in office operating rooms, Plast. Reconstr. Surg. **63:**173, 1979.
11. Stark, R.B.: A rhytidectomy series, Plast. Reconstr. Surg. **59:**373, 1977.
12. Thompson, D.P., and Ashley, F.L.: Face-lift complications, Plast. Reconstr. Surg. **61:**40, 1978.

Editorial comments
Part IV

Sagging and drooping of the neck, usually accompanied by loose bands and often associated with fullness due to excess fat, are deformities that frequently bring the patient to the plastic surgeon. The straight skin face-lift helped some with the deformity, but, because of early recurrence of drooping skin, as well as residual fullness, additional procedures were needed. Submental lipectomy and the various manipulations of the platysma muscles that have been developed in recent years appear to be helpful additions to our methods of improving these neck deformities.

What to do with the platysma and where to do it are questions that have been given different answers by different surgeons. Dr. Vistnes makes an excellent case for reconstruction of the medial platysma decussation, which is absent in 40% of the population. Dr. Guerrerosantos, on the other hand, gets excellent results by excising the medial platysma bands and slinging the rest laterally. Another method is to transect and rotate the upper half of the platysma superolaterally, suturing the medial borders together. I prefer to partially transect the medial bands, as does Dr. Aston (see Part II, Chapter 16), and suture the medial borders together to create a sling. I also partially transect the lateral border of the platysma to allow for upward rotation of combined lateral platysma-SMAS flap and suture the lateral platysma borders to the underlying sternocleidomastoid muscle. This last maneuver goes against the theory of medial slinging suggested by Dr. Vistnes, but clinically and anatomically it seems to work well for my patients. In treating necks as in skinning cats, there is more than one way.

Dr. Hugo makes many significant points in his discussion of complications of neck lifting. Hematoma remains a problem, especially with more extensive dissections and various platysma manipulations. I thoroughly believe in going back repeatedly to all operated areas to look for bleeders. In face-lift surgery, "a second look and second cook" is more than just an Isaac Bashevis Singer aphorism. I also believe in drains. Although drains will not prevent large hematomas due to arterial bleeding, I firmly believe that they reduce or prevent accumulations of blood that may occur as a result of capillary or venous bleeding. I feel the same way about compression dressings (compression—not pressure), although I only leave them on overnight.

Marginal mandibular and cervical motor nerve injury can be avoided by keeping one's surgical manipulations superficial to the platysma. When defatting the platysma, one should do it after the muscle is put on a stretch by fixing it in its new, transposed position first. Also, as Dr. Hugo points out, defatting platysma after it is repositioned allows the surgeon to see the results of his fat sculpturing directly; he is unlikely to sculpture himself "into a hole," an unhappy circumstance in which he might find, after shifting the platysma secondarily, that he has taken out too much fat and created a contour deformity.

I strongly agree that smoking introduces a significantly increased risk of complications in neck lifts and face-lifts, for at least two reasons. Smoking reduces skin circulation and increases the risk of necrosis. A smoker whose skin has also been damaged by chronic exposure to the sun is at a still greater risk. In addition, smokers tend to cough, increasing the risk of hematoma (and secondary necrosis), and if the procedure is done with the patient under general anesthesia, the patient is subject to all of the increased postanaesthetic problems that smokers may incur. Solutions to the problem are not easy. Long-term abstinence is difficult to achieve. Recent evidence suggests that even stopping for a day or two may help prevent circulatory problems to some extent. Vegetable cigarettes may be an answer provided they are available. One could refuse to operate on smokers; however, they probably would quickly find another surgeon who would be willing to undertake the risk.

One reasonable approach is to strongly impress on these patients, on more than one occasion, the importance of cutting down radically or abstaining from smoking for at least a short time before the operation, citing in simple but direct language the reasons why they should do so. It does not hurt to also have some warning in writing, or at least to have a member of one's staff present as a witness when educating smokers. If problems arise postoperatively, one may at least invoke the old admonition, "You were warned."

B.L.K.

Aesthetic plastic surgery of the earlobes and chin

Chapter 32

Problems and complications related to the earlobes

Verner V. Lindgren

In the standard rhytidectomy procedure it is important to pay special attention to the size and shape of the earlobes. It should be kept in mind that the best time to change the shape of a patient's earlobes, if such a change is warranted, is during a rhytidectomy.

Basically, there may be three preoperative problems concerning earlobes:

1. Lobes that are extremely large[6] (Fig. 32-1)
2. Lobes that are too small (Fig. 32-2)
3. Lobes that are webbed or pixielike[3] (Fig. 32-3)

These three conditions should be looked for during the preoperative examination and if present, pointed out to the patient. When discussing the incision location and resultant scars with a patient desiring a rhytidectomy, one should carefully explain that the appearance of the earlobe attachment will be changed slightly postoperatively. The patient's preference for earlobe size should be determined. Patients with very large earlobes should be advised of the feasibility of reduction if this seems advantageous. Similarly, many patients with small earlobes have difficulty wearing earrings and may wish to have them enlarged. In the case of attached or webbed earlobes—the so-called pixie ears—it will usually be desirable to free them up and at the same time reshape them into a pleasing size and form.

Postoperatively, there may be three basic complications:

1. Lobes that become too small as result of surgery[6] (Fig. 32-4)
2. Lobes that become pixielike and pulled down secondary to previous surgery[6] (Fig. 32-5)

3. Scars from a previous face-lift that may be clearly visible below the earlobes (Fig. 32-6)

When the scars of a previous face-life are located at the area of the earlobe attachment, the normal stretch that occurs with time and gravity may pull the lobe down into a deformed webbed position, or the lobe may remain normal in shape and position, but the scar itself may become visible below it, thus being conspicuously indicative of previous surgery.

Stark,[7] Gurdin,[5] Carlin,[2] and others approached the problem by carefully freeing up the lobe from its attachment almost to the cartilage.[1,4] The initial neck skin was then advanced in the usual manner, and after the surplus skin was removed, the edge was sutured in place approximately 5 to 10 mm higher than the original attachment of the lobe. The anteroposterior edges of the lobe were then closed primarily with sutures.

Stark illustrated a fixation at the anterior edge of the lobe (Fig. 32-7), whereas Gurdin and Carlin advanced the skin high up behind the earlobe in such a way that when normal contracture took place, the scar was well hidden and above the edge of the lobe (Fig. 32-8). This technique has proved useful for the majority of patients with average-size lobes. Again, bear in mind the necessity of informing the patient that the lobes may look a little different postoperatively if they are freed up, but that the higher attachment will hide the scar and prevent its descent below the ear.

A few patients with extremely small lobes present an entirely different problem. They may have

Text continued on p. 301.

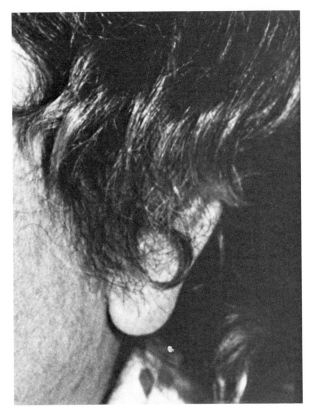

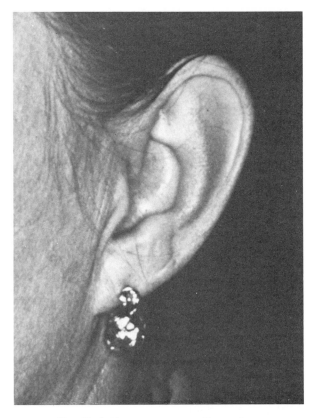

Fig. 32-1. Preoperative extremely large earlobes.

Fig. 32-2. Preoperative small earlobes.

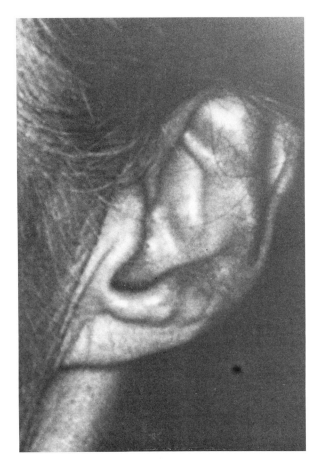

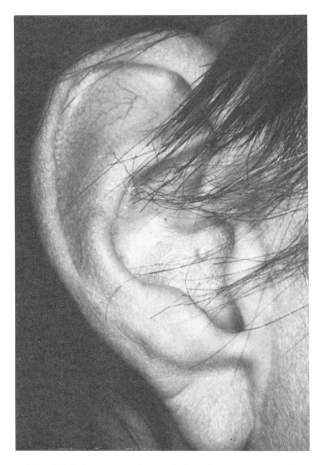

Fig. 32-3. Preoperative earlobes that are webbed or pixielike.

Fig. 32-4. Postoperative earlobes that are too small.

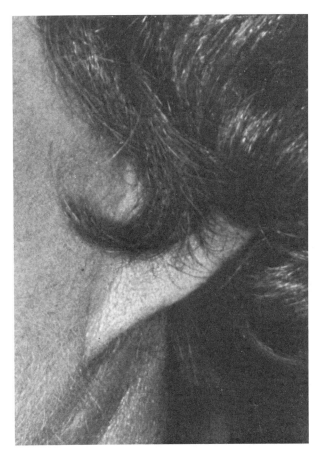

Fig. 32-5. Postoperative pixielike earlobes.

Fig. 32-6. Postoperative scars that are visible below earlobes.

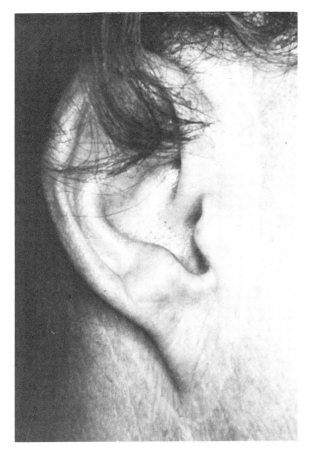

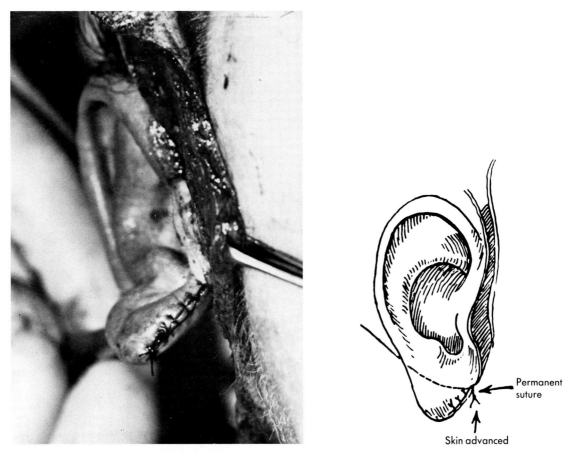

Fig. 32-7. Technique of fixative suture by Stark.

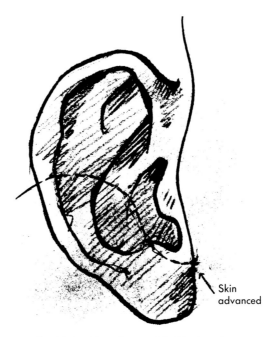

Fig. 32-8. Skin advanced behind earlobe.

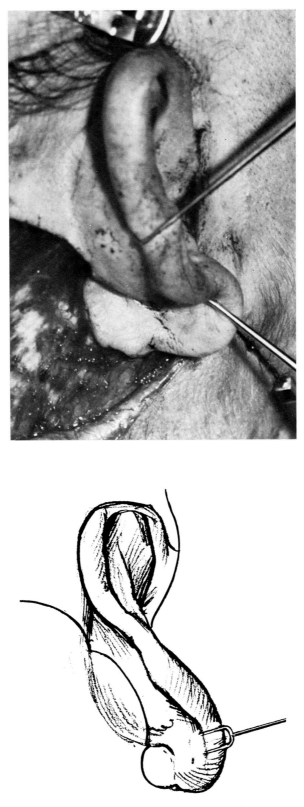

Fig. 32-9. Small flap posterior to earlobe.

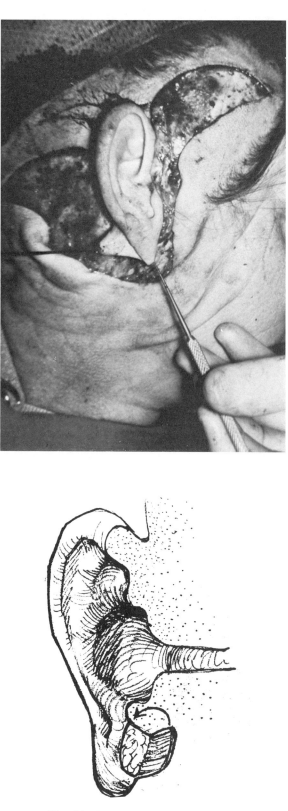

Fig. 32-10. Rotation of earlobe flap.

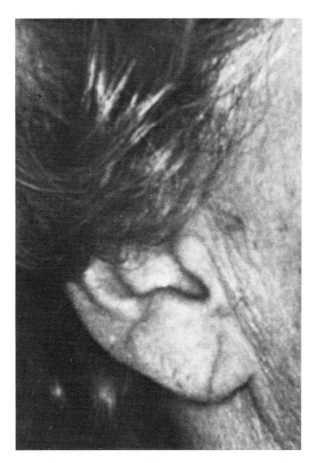

Fig. 32-11. Crease or fold in earlobe preoperatively.

difficulty wearing earrings unless the lobes have been pierced and frequently are dissatisfied with their appearance. The technique demonstrated for such enlargement involves freeing up the entire lobe, as done by Stark, Gurdin, and others, and also creating (at the time of the initial marking) a small flap posterior to the earlobe (Fig. 32-9 and 32-10). If the posterior skin is inadequate, the flap could extend as a pancake type, including the inferior portion of the lobe and some of the skin anterior to it. (This adjacent skin is normally discarded anyway.) When the lobe is completely freed up, one can adjust the size of these flaps until what appears to be an aesthetic-looking lobe has been created. When these adjacent flaps are being used, it is frequently necessary to trim off a small dog-ear on the inferior posterior border of the lobe. This produces a better way to attach the skin to the ear. The usual stretching that takes place along with gravity will

cause most scars to descend, but it will remain above the inferior edge of the lobe and will not be visible.

All plastic surgeons have had other lobe or scar problems. Occasionally a crease formed across the central portion of the lobe will be seen, but usually this same crease will be seen on preoperative photographs. Because patients normally are not aware of this fold until they examine their ears after the operation, it is always advantageous to point out the crease preoperatively, informing them that the condition may remain or even become slightly more conspicuous (Fig. 32-11). Patients can be told that this fold may be corrected at a later date, if necessary, with a Z-plasty or similar procedure.

I routinely form a posterior auricular flap at the level of the earlobe on all patients undergoing rhytidectomy except those who have extremely large lobes. All of the flap, or whatever part might

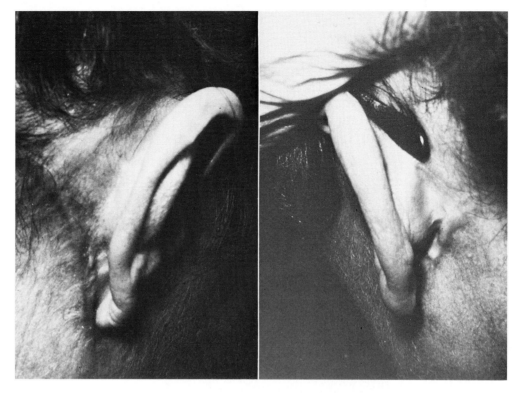

Fig. 32-12. Hypertrophic scars posterior to ear.

be beneficial, may be used for reconstructing the lobe. (In most instances, with an average-size lobe, the majority of the adjacent skin is trimmed off anyway.) This technique, in most cases, has been a useful adjunct for forming an acceptable lobe. Rarely has there been any hypertrophic scarring beneath the lobe or anterior to the ear with this higher attachment; however, the posterior aspect of the neck and ear is the area where there is the greatest amount of tension, and it is the most frequent site for hypertrophic or excessively wide scars to develop (Fig. 32-12).

In summary, one should not hesitate to reduce the size of the earlobes if necessary when doing a rhytidectomy and should consider using the technique of freeing up the lobe and employing a postauricular flap. These simple and easy techniques can produce very satisfactory results in the creation of an aesthetic, attractively shaped earlobe, and are relatively free of complications.

REFERENCES

1. Aufricht, G.: Surgery for excess skin of the face and neck. In Transactions of the International Society of Plastic Surgeons, Second Congress, Edinburgh, 1960, E. & S. Livingstone, Ltd.
2. Carlin, E.: Personal communication.
3. Carver, G.M.: Reconstruction of the earlobe, Plast. Reconstr. Surg. **12:**203, 1953.
4. Converse, J.M., editor: Reconstructive plastic surgery, ed. 2, Philadelphia, 1977, W.B. Saunders Co.
5. Gurdin, M.: Personal communication.
6. Loeb, R.: Earlobe tailoring during facial rhytidectomies, Plast. Reconstr. Surg. **49:**485, 1972.
7. Stark, R.B.: Plastic surgery, New York, 1962, Harper & Row, Publishers, Inc.

SUGGESTED READINGS

Baker, T.J., and Gordon, H.L.: Complications of rhytidectomy, Plast. Reconstr. Surg. **40:**31, 1967.
Spira, M., Gerow, F.J., and Hardy, S.B.: Cervicofacial rhytidectomy, Plast. Reconstr. Surg. **40:**551, 1967.
Subbra Rao, Y.V., and Venkateswara Rao, P.: A quick technique for earlobe reconstruction, Plast. Reconstr. Surg. **41:**13, 1968.
Zenteno Alanis, S.: A new method for earlobe reconstruction, Plast. Reconstr. Surg. **45:**254, 1970.

Editorial comments
Chapter 32

The elongated earlobe attached to the cheek is the most obvious telltale sign of a rhytidectomy having been performed. Just as we try to prevent the skin from pulling down the free margin of the lower lid in blepharoplasty, so should we prevent the skin from pulling down the earlobe. The surest way to do this is to suture the skin to the fascia superior and posterior to the lobe (Fig. 1).

G.P.G.

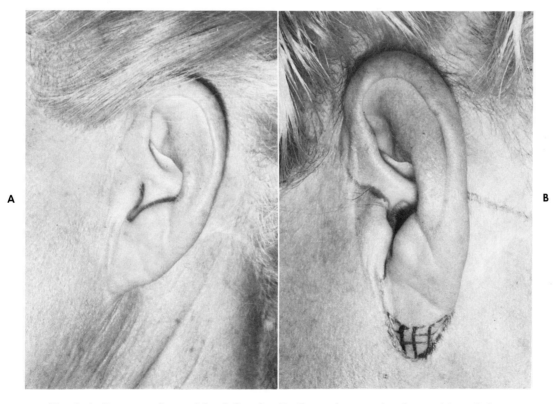

Fig. 1. A, Postoperative earlobe deformity. **B,** Correction may involve excision of elongated portion of lobe.
Continued.

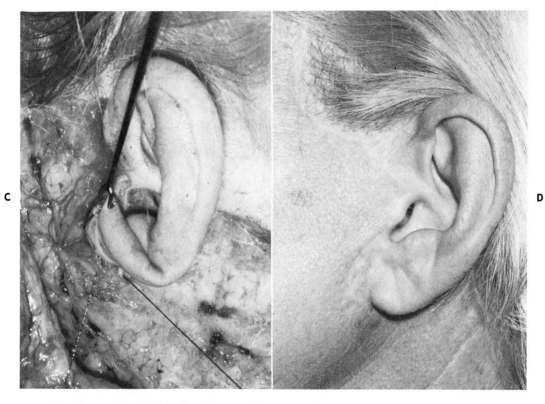

Fig. 1, cont'd. C, Skin flap is sutured to parotid fascia. **D,** More normal-appearing earlobe is achieved.

Chapter 33

Aesthetic plastic surgery of the chin

Matthew C. Gleason

The chin is that part of the face below the lower lip formed by the prominence of the jaw. Leonardo da Vinci determined that the arc of a circle centered on the auditory meatus should touch the forehead, nose, and finally the chin. Other artists have determined that a line (perpendicular to the Frankfort plane) should touch the glabella, lower lip, and tip of the chin (Fig. 33-1), A person whose chin fails to meet this rigid test may be looked on as being "weak" chinned. The fictional hero is usually portrayed as square jawed with a "determined" chin and a will to match.

Hence it is not unusual that individuals with a receding chin would want to improve their self-image with surgery.

When confronted with a chin problem, it is essential that the plastic surgeon start with a plan of accurate diagnosis.[3] The chin and nose should be viewed as a single complex. The size and projection of one directly affects the other. If the nose is large, the chin will appear correspondingly small. In some instances, a patient will seek a reduction rhinoplasty when in fact what is really required is an augmentation mentoplasty (Figs.

Text continued on p. 310.

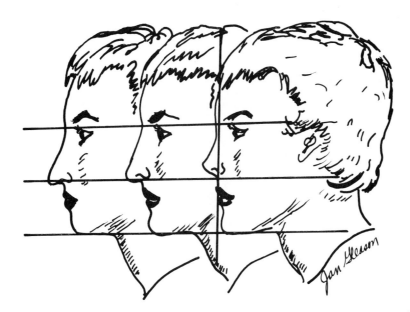

Fig. 33-1. Chin and lower lip should closely approach vertical line. Horizontal lines divide face into thirds. Forehead third is not important, because hairline styles can be changed. Nose is entitled to one third of face, as is distance from nose to inferior border of chin. Long nose *(center)* makes chin look smaller than it is. Receding chin and long nose combine to give bird-beak appearance *(left)*.

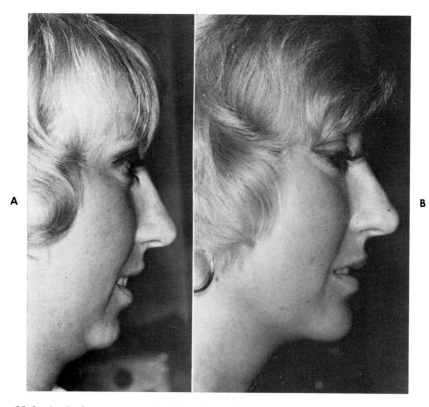

Fig. 33-2. A, Patient requested rhinoplasty. **B,** However, intraoral chin implant restores vertical balance to face. No rhinoplasty was done. It is important that surgeon analyze and diagnose problem.

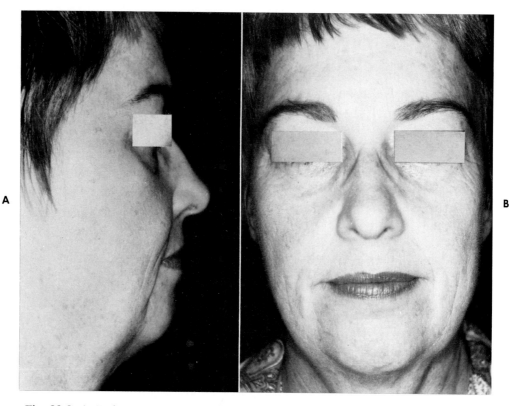

Fig. 33-3. A, Patient requested chin implant. Diagnosis shows that chin is not recessive but that submentum is nonexistent. **B,** Frontal view. Normal chin projection is partially masked by absence of submentum.

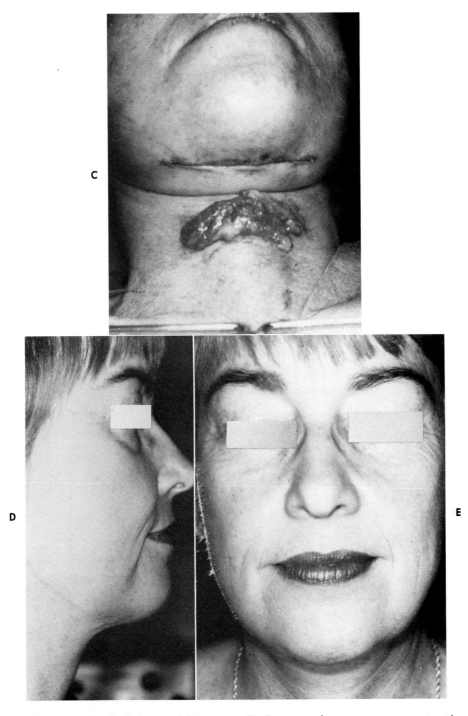

Fig. 33-3, cont'd. C, Submental lipectomy, **D,** Postoperative appearance; restoration of submental angle demonstrates that mentum is normal and needs no chin implant. **E,** Postoperative frontal view.

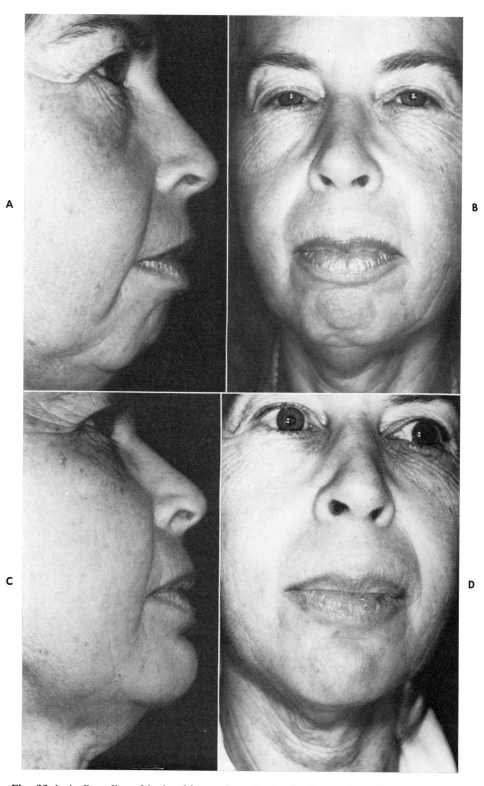

Fig. 33-4. A, Receding chin in older patient. Lack of submental angle is secondary to submental fat. Patient also thought nose was too large. **B,** Preoperative frontal view, with typical pursed lips. **C,** Postoperative appearance. Patient did not want rhytidectomy; therefore generous-sized implant was used to augment chin. It must be made clear that augmenting chin will not take up any of slack beneath chin. **D,** Postoperative frontal view showing correction of pursed appearance of lips.

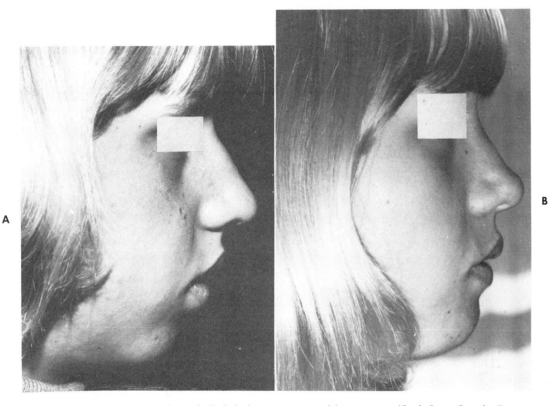

Fig. 33-5. A, Microgenia and slightly large nose combine to magnify defect of each. **B,** Reduction in size of nose and small chin implant combine to reestablish nose-chin symmetry. Note that large correction of chin is not required.

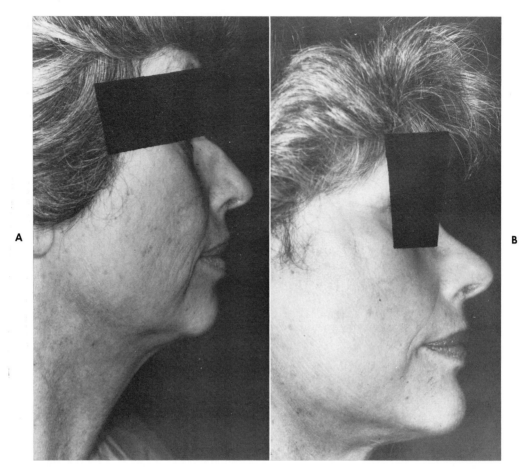

Fig. 33-6. A, Moderate microgenia and moderate nasal dorsum convexity. **B,** Too much surgery was done. Submental defatting plus too-large chin implant have produced too-prominent chin. In addition, too much nasal dorsum was removed. These problems can be avoided by careful preplanning.

33-2 to 33-4). This relationship needs to be carefully explained to the patient.[5] When performing a combination rhinoplasty-mentoplasty, I do the mentoplasty first for the following reasons:

1. The mentoplasty is faster and quieter than the rhinoplasty. Some patients are made apprehensive by the noise during a rhinoplasty bone reduction, even though they are well anesthetized.

2. Even more important is the fact that the surgeon can better observe the nose-chin relationship when the chin has been augmented first and more easily visualize the small reduction that the nose requires (Figs. 33-5 and 33-6).

TECHNIQUE

Anesthesia is obtained by first injecting 1 ml of lidocaine hydrochloride (Xylocaine) with epinephrine near each mental foramen. This opening is easily palpated beneath the skin over the mandible inferior to the second bicuspid tooth. An intraoral injection is made in the mucosa of the lower lip sulcus, and 2 ml is infiltrated into the soft tissues over the mentum. This further anesthetizes the area and provides better hemostasis.

I sit at the patient's head, retract the lip to expose the lower sulcus, and make a 2-ml long horizontal incision in the lip mucosa just superior to the frenulum. It is important to leave a generous amount of mucosa attached to the gingiva for ease of wound closure.[5] The scalpel incision continues distalward over the mentum, leaving a thin layer of muscle attached to the bone. I believe that healing is faster and less painful if the periosteum is not exposed, and that there is less bone resorption.[4] The wound closure is also easier because soft tissue can be approximated to soft tissue. When the inferior border of the mentum is reached, a horizontal pocket is made toward (but not to) the mental foramen. The pocket is formed by gentle spreading of Mayo scissors and use of a peanut dissector. Hemostasis is secured with an electrocautery. A headlight provides good illumination.

The chin implant is then inserted and checked for fit and size. If the implant does not sit correctly, it is removed, and either further tailoring is done to the pocket or the size of the implant is changed. When one is in doubt as to what size looks better, one should always select the smaller. I use a single suture of 5-0 nylon to secure the superior center edge of the implant to the soft tissue over the mentum. This keeps the implant in the midline (of the central incisors) until the capsule forms. The soft tissues are closed with a layer of 5-0 nylon superior to the implant and the mucosa with a 5-0 chromic or 5-0 Vicryl. Since the implant lies accurately and securely in a pocket, no external taping is necessary.

Postoperative care includes a liquid diet for the first day, a soft diet the second day, and a regular well-cooked diet for 10 days. No raw vegetables or foods that require biting with the incisors are allowed during this period. A mouthwash is used after each meal in place of brushing the lower incisors. Tetracycline, 250 mg., 4 times a day, is started 24 hours before surgery and continued for 4 days.

PROBLEMS

Most problems are due to poor assessment in planning or failure to recognize problems that exist. We should bear in mind that our western aesthetic values are based on Caucasian standards and that many races have less-prominent chins as a normal genetic characteristic. If they live in a western society, they may seek chin augmentation, which will not fit in with the rest of their physiogomy. This must be carefully explained, and if augmentation is done, a smaller than usual size should be used. Furthermore, a flatter nasal bridge will be emphasized. While the nasal bridge may be raised with either autogenous grafts or a silicone implant, additional surgery is now being undertaken, which may lead to further problems.

A chin recession may be due to retrognathia and may require mandibular advancement rather than simple augmentation. A marked overbite with a pseudoappearance of hypomentum may better respond to orthodontia.

Asymmetry[2] is present in all faces, and if it is not carefully noted prior to surgery, an implant placed over the midmandible, in its usual position, may exaggerate this asymmetry. When asymmetry is recognized prior to surgery, augmentation implants may then be tailored to lie on one side or the other of the midline and thus help correct the asymmetry (Fig. 33-7).

The skin texture, whether thick and oily, or thin, and the substance of the underlying muscle must be noted, since these structures will overlie the implant and affect the external appearance.

A chin implant is frequently done in conjunction with a rhytidectomy (Fig. 33-8). If a submental incision accompanies the rhytidectomy, the implant may be done via the external approach, but even here I prefer the intraoral technique because of accuracy of implant placement. However, a submental incision invites the use of a submental fat flap to supplement the chin, and I do this whenever needed.

The "witch's chin" (ptosis of chin muscles) is more easily corrected with a submental advancement fat flap[1] than with a chin implant. Indeed, a chin implant may only magnify the problem of chin ptosis (Figs. 33-9 to 33-12).

CHOICE OF MATERIAL

The implant may be either autogenous or synthetic. Bone, while long used, has the disadvantage of requiring a donor site and difficulty in shaping. Furthermore, because of the problems of infection, an external approach is preferred. A dermal fat graft, while easily obtained, has the problem of resorption. Fat flaps from the submental area may be successfully used.[6]

The synthetic materials are more popular because of their ease of insertion and their generally good results. The synthetic material may be a solid block, which is carved by the surgeon at the time of surgery, or preformed and packaged. Most surgeons prefer the preformed implants. They come in such a variety of sizes that the necessity of further carving is obviated. Some come with a Dacron backing for fixation. However, I have found that the Dacron backing sometimes leads to excessive scar formation, which attaches to the skin and produces an external dimpling. The Dacron backing is no longer used in breast implants, and I believe for the same reason need not be used in chin implants (Fig. 33-8, *E*). A solid implant or a gel-filled implant may be used. I use the solid implant, although some surgeons prefer the softer gel-filled implant.

The problem of the protruding chin, whether due to hypertrophy of the mentum or true prognathia, is not covered here. The surgical procedures are more extensive and, of course, need exact planning. *Text continued on p. 318.*

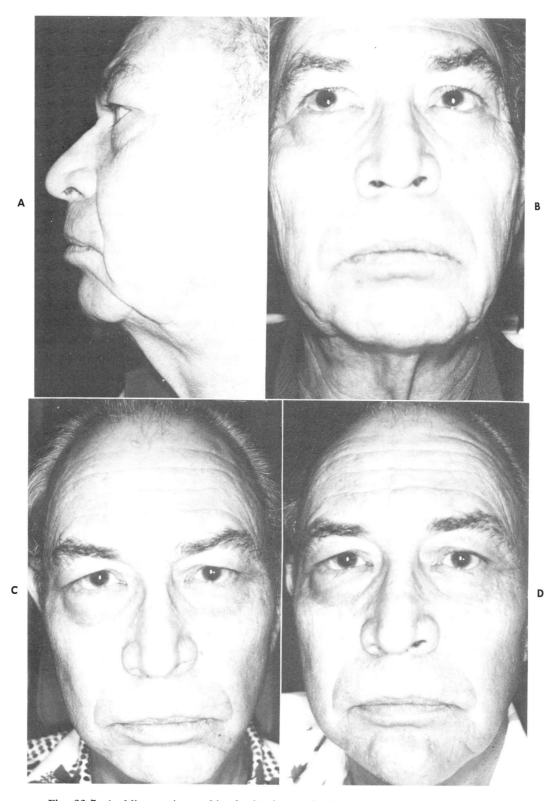

Fig. 33-7. A, Microgenia combined with lax neck skin and submental fat. Diagonal crease extends from lateral chin to upper neck. Patient did not want chin implant at time of rhytidectomy. **B,** Frontal view showing asymmetry—chin deviates to left. This was not noticed because of lax subcutaneous tissues. **C,** Postsurgical appearance. Left chin asymmetry is readily apparent but was still not noticed. **D,** Following chin implant, deviation is now obvious. Chin implant had to be removed.

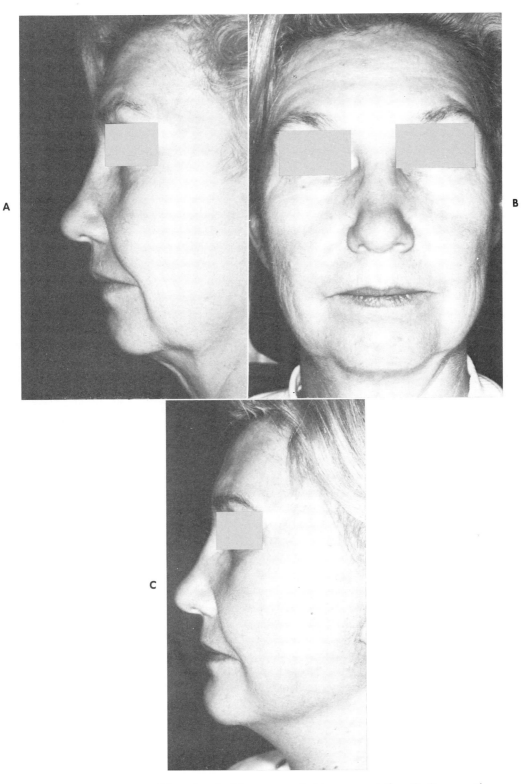

Fig. 33-8. A, Good candidate for rhytidectomy and chin augmentation. **B,** Preoperative frontal view. **C,** Postoperative appearance following chin implant and rhytidectomy.
Continued.

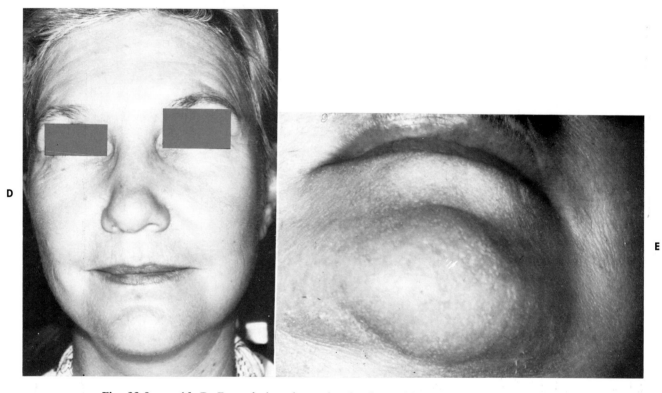

Fig. 33-8, cont'd. D, Frontal view shows that implant adds to balance of face. **E,** Six years later, Dacron backing of chin implant formed dimpled contracture. Implant was removed. I no longer use Dacron backing.

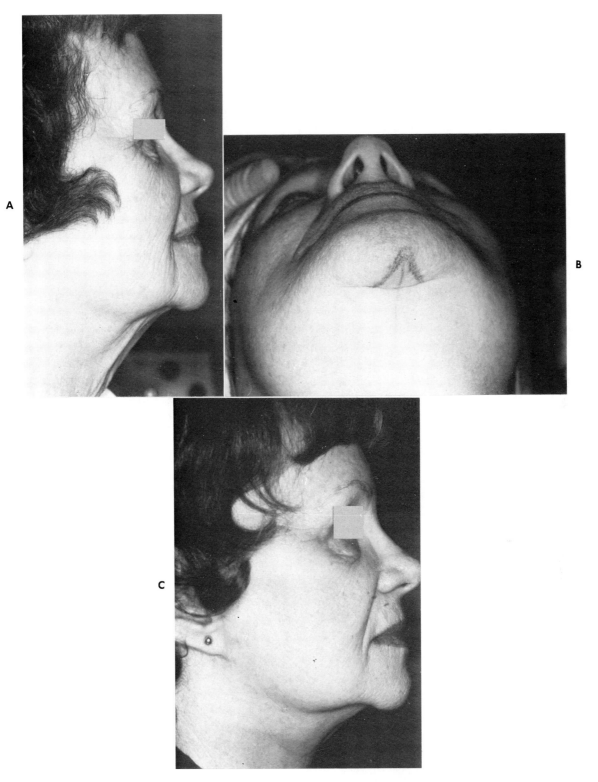

Fig. 33-9. A, Edentulous mandible results in ptosis of chin (witch's chin). **B,** Preoperative outline of Viñas fleur-de-lis incision. **C,** Postoperative appearance. Patient still has ptosis of chin. Better to have "filler" in concavity of submental crease.

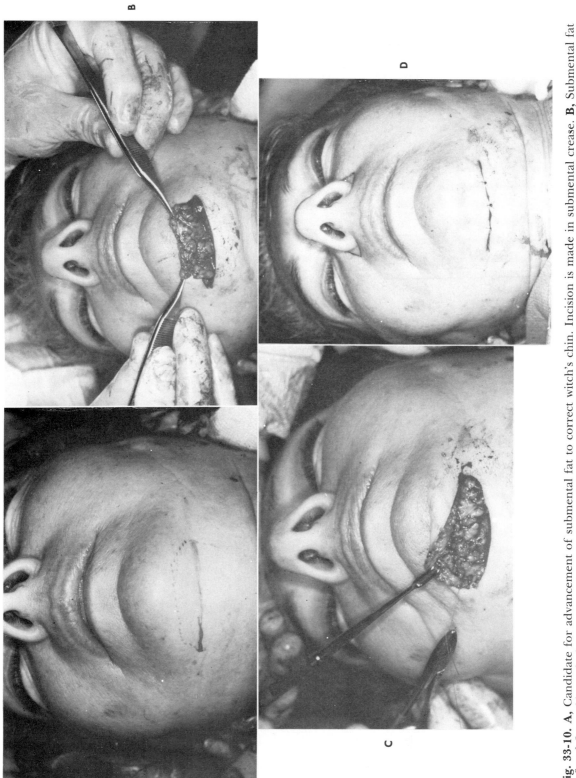

Fig. 33-10. A, Candidate for advancement of submental fat to correct witch's chin. Incision is made in submental crease. **B,** Submental fat is freed from skin and platysma muscle and advanced distalward. **C,** Skin distal to submental crease is undermined to border of mandible, and fat flap is sutured to mentum. **D,** Immediate postoperative photograph.

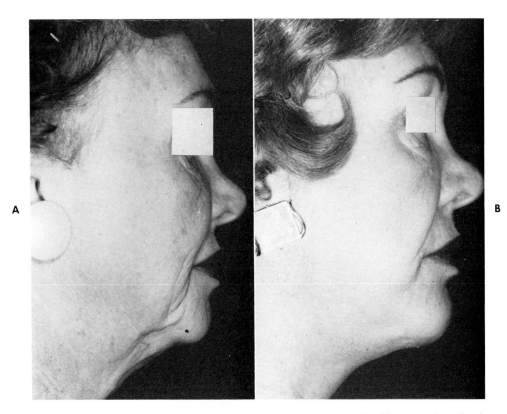

Fig. 33-11. A, Ptosis of chin. **B,** Advancement of submental fat fills concavity of submental crease.

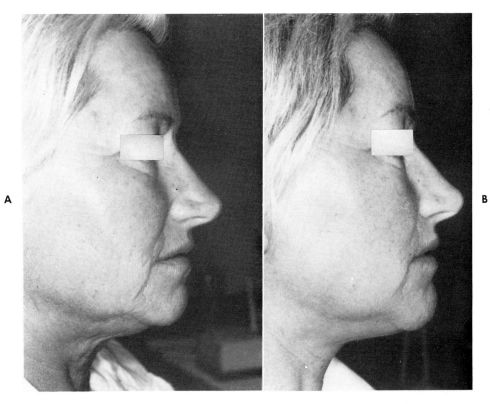

Fig. 33-12. A, Moderate ptosis of chin. **B,** Too much of a good thing!

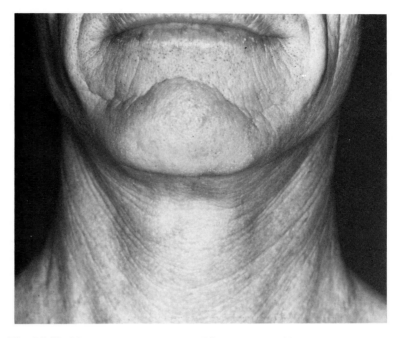

Fig. 33-13. My senescent transverse chin crease. Problem as yet unsolved!

REFERENCES

1. Gleason, M.C.: Videotape discussion: the male rhytidectomy. In Goulian, D., and Courtiss, E.H., editors: Symposium on surgery of the aging face, St. Louis, 1978, The C.V. Mosby Co.
2. Gomez, M., and Harrits, T.: Preoperative and postoperative consideration of natural facial asymmetry, Plast. Reconstr. Surg. **54:**187, 1974.
3. Gonzalez-Ulloa, M.: The role of chin correction in profileplasty, Plast. Reconstr. Surg. **41:** 477, 1968.
4. Jobe, R., Iverson, R., and Vistnes, L.: Bone deformation beneath alloplastic implants, Plast. Reconstr. Surg. **51:**121, 1973.
5. Kaye, B.L.: Mentoplasty. In Courtiss, E.H., editor: Aesthetic surgery: trouble—how to avoid it and how to treat it, St. Louis, 1978, The C.V. Mosby Co.
6. Robertson, I.G.: Chin augmentation by means of rotation of double chin fat flaps, Plast. Reconstr. Surg. **36:**471, 1965.

Editorial comments
Chapter 33

In the Preface to this book, the difficult problem of the "witch's chin" is mentioned. In the past 2 years Drs. Leon Burke and Rex Peterson have independently presented procedures to improve this condition. These procedures fill the depression or cleft between the chin and the cervical region. They represent a significant advance.* In certain cases an additional approach may be beneficial (Fig. 1).

G.P.G.

---

*See also Editorial Comments for Part V, p. 337.

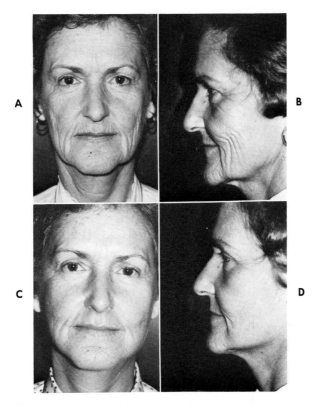

Fig. 1. A, Frontal view of patient. **B,** Profile. **C** and **D,** Type of improvement that can be achieved using variation of Burke or Peterson procedure in conjunction with rhytidectomy and upper lip dermabrasion. This still did not correct chin soft tissue ptosis.

Continued.

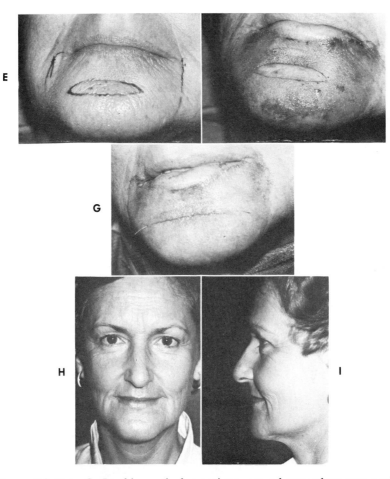

Fig. 1, cont'd. E to **G,** In this particular patient, second procedure was undertaken that involved excision of ellipse of tissue including and just below mentolabial crease. This was carried out in conjunction with dermabrasion. Resultant scar fell in normal mentolabial crease and was no more apparent than original crease. **H** and **I,** Final frontal and profile views with improvement of soft tissue chin ptosis.

Chapter 34

Chin problems

Ivo Pitanguy

This chapter is a description of my technique for correction of hypomentonism. Techniques are also described for correcting deformities of the submental region, depending on specific indications, by means of musculofascial plications and defatting. A raphe flap is described for improvement of the senile, drooping chin. Postoperative care and complications are reviewed.

Since the chin is the main structure of the lower third of the face, it contributes greatly to the whole appearance of the patient. Since its anatomy is based on hard and soft tissue, possible deformity in both of these components should be evaluated.

Hypermentonism and hypomentonism are the most frequent results of abnormalities in underlying hard tissue. When these two entities coexist with functional and more complex disturbances, such as maxillary retrusion or "open bite," multiple techniques, each acting on specific aspects of the abnormality, may be required to solve the problem. On the other hand, when microgenia is a result of insufficient growth of the chin and no other underlying pathological abnormality exists, the insertion of a silicone prosthesis will provide an important aesthetic improvement.

CHIN AUGMENTATION

My technique for chin augmentation grew out of recognition of the embryological development of the region. The configuration of the chin evolves from the union of the two mandibular processes; each process contributes equivalent quantities of mesoderm, from which originate the lateral muscle groups. The fusion of the two processes results in the approximation of these muscle groups, marked by a median raphe.

In certain individuals, at the midline of the chin there is an external depression or dimple that may represent incomplete muscle union. There may be adherence of the skin to the deep plane, because of a minimal local mesodermic deficiency, accentuating the contour of the lateral muscle masses. This dimple, graceful in appearance and desired by a number of patients, can be obtained (along with an improved labial sulcus and a better-proportioned chin) by the following technique. The implant is inserted through an intraoral incision in such a way as to accentuate, rather than diminish or erase, the labial sulcus contour.

A transverse intraoral incision is made 1 or 2 cm above the lower labial sulcus, and dissection is carried downward (Fig. 34-1). A small posterior ridge containing some of the orbicularis oris muscle and remnants of the superior insertion of the median raphe is preserved, and the remaining musculature is separated in the subperiosteal plane. At the midline junction of the two lateral muscle groups, the median raphe is exposed and marked. It is whitish in color and fibrous in consistency. A flap, which will aid in centering and fixing the graft or prosthesis, is made by detaching the raphe from its anterior, inferior insertion and elevating it nearly 180 degrees* (Fig. 34-2). Any fat between the two muscle groups surrounding the raphe is removed; the muscles are pushed slightly laterally to accentuate the contours of the inclusion. A dimple can be obtained in this fashion that simulates the embryological features of the congenital dimple.

While the raphe is held up, the graft or im-

---

*EDITOR'S NOTE: See Pitanguy, I.: Augmentation mentoplasty, Plast. Reconstr. Surg. **42**:461, 1968 (Fig. 2, *E*) for a saggital drawing of this maneuver. (B.L.K.)

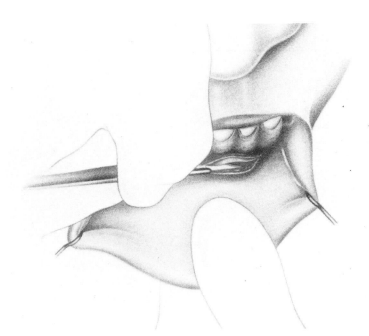

Fig. 34-1. Transverse intraoral incision is made 1 or 2 cm above lower labial sulcus, and dissection is carried downward.

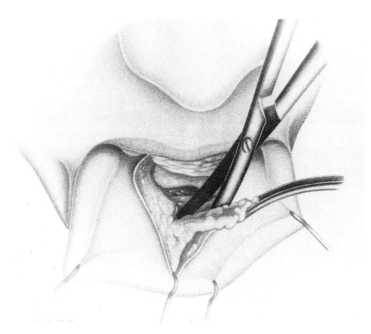

Fig. 34-2. Flap is made by detaching raphe from its anterior inferior insertion and elevating it nearly 180 degrees.

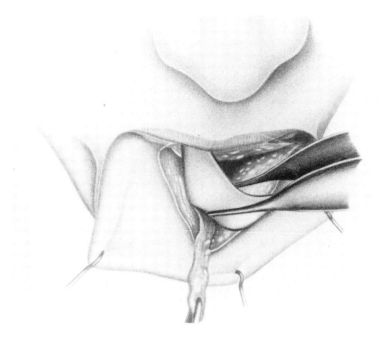

Fig. 34-3. While raphe is held up, graft or implant is introduced into space created posterior to raphe.

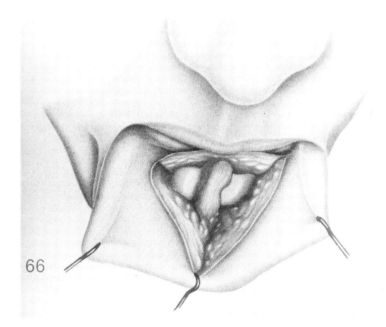

Fig. 34-4. Raphe flap is sutured to small posterior ridge of orbicularis oris muscle and remnants of its own superior insertion, left by dissection at beginning of procedure. This securely fixes and centers implant or graft in case external dimple is desired.

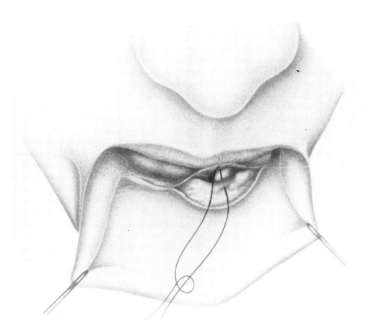

Fig. 34-5. Undermined muscles and mucosa are sutured in separate planes.

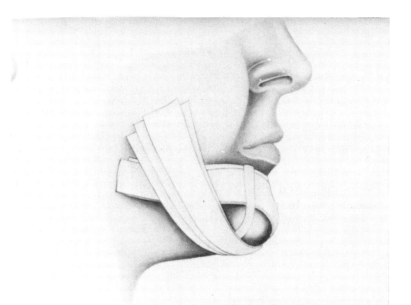

Fig. 34-6. Dressing, made entirely of adhesive tape and maintained for minimum of 10 days, is applied.

plant is introduced into the space created posterior to the raphe (Fig. 34-3). Once the implant (which has a small vertical medial sulcus anteriorly) is in place adjacent to the bone, the fibromuscular flap (obtained from the raphe) is brought over the implant snugly within the carved vertical sulcus. The raphe flap is then sutured to the small posterior ridge of the orbicularis oris muscle and remnants of its own superior insertion, left by the dissection at the beginning of the procedure; this securely fixes and centers the implant or graft in case an external dimple is desired (Fig. 34-4).

With the suturing of the raphe flap, traction is exerted on the cutaneous insertion of the musculature, creating the desired dimple externally and curving the mentolabial sulcus more harmoniously. The undermined muscles and mucosa are sutured in separate planes (Fig. 34-5). A dressing, made entirely of adhesive tape and maintained for a minimum of 10 days, aids fixation and impedes the formation or collection of serosanguineous secretions (Fig. 34-6).

TECHNIQUES FOR CORRECTING SOFT TISSUE DEFORMITIES

Concerning soft tissue deformities, the chin cannot be considered separately from the submental area. Most of these problems are related to three main factors: fat accumulation, weight loss, and aging.

1. *Fat accumulation.* The submental and submandibular regions of the neck are the prime sites for accumulation of fatty tissue, giving the face a typically rounded appearance and deforming the concavity of the cervicomandibular profile. When fat deposition is marked, a characteristic double chin is formed. This is a common trait of the aging face, frequently linked with hereditary or familial factors. In the latter case such a deformity can be seen in the younger subject.

2. *Weight loss.* In patients who have, over the years, suffered repeated gains and losses in weight, there is a gradual loosening of the neck tissue due to stretching and relaxation, resulting in the formation of excess skin and sagging of the neck. The subjacent musculoaponeurotic system is also affected. Relaxation and fibrosis of these structures, particularly the platysma, leads to the formation of vertical bands hanging down from the lower border of the mandible to the clavicle.

3. *Aging.* The skin, subcutaneous tissue, platysma, and other vital structures undergo the usual changes that occur with aging. The end result is an accentuated drooping and flaccidity of the chin, known as the "senile" chin. Sometimes vertical folds of skin and fat appear; this is a particularly objectionable feature of the aging process in male patients and is referred to as the "turkey gobbler" deformity.

There is no single technique that can deal with the various degrees and types of chin deformity. These factors must be assessed clinically prior to the operation and should also be reevaluated at the time of surgery. A suitable operative technique is then employed to correct the specific deformity. In some cases simple resection of submental fat associated with good traction of the face and neck flaps in a standard rhytidectomy is sufficient to obtain an adequate profile. As many other authors have suggested, when there is abundant fat in the submandibular regions, particularly in cases of double-chin deformity, an extensive defatting is performed. Abnormalities in the platysma, such as weakness or absence in the midline or laxity, can be corrected by surgery. Excess loose skin can be trimmed as required, and, when present, the receding chin may be augmented.

It is important, therefore, to adopt a flexible attitude at the time of surgery, so that the techniques required for correction can be chosen appropriately.

The operation is performed with the patient under general anesthesia. It may be carried out separately or in combination with a standard rhytidectomy.

The patient is placed on the operating table with the head extended, and the midline is carefully marked. By flexing the neck temporarily, the redundant tissue becomes evident. It is marked and infiltrated with lidocaine 0.5% and epinephrine 1:200.000.

A 3 to 4 cm transverse incision is made at the submental fold (Fig. 34-7). The skin is undermined down to the level of the hyoid bone (Fig. 34-8). An even depth should be maintained so as to avoid direct fixation of the skin to the subjacent muscular plane, which produces irregularities following lipectomy. Resection of the submental fat is commenced from below, upward, with special curved scissors (Fig. 34-9). Care should be taken to avoid protrusion of adipose tissue through the aponeurosis at the level of the digastric and geniohyoid muscles. Simple resection of submental fat,

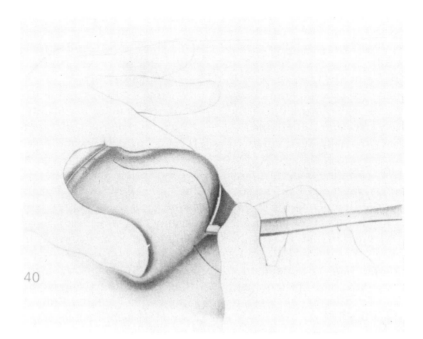

Fig. 34-7. Transverse incision (3 to 4 cm) is made at submental fold.

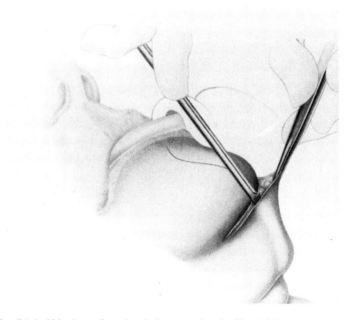

Fig. 34-8. Skin is undermined down to level of hyoid bone.

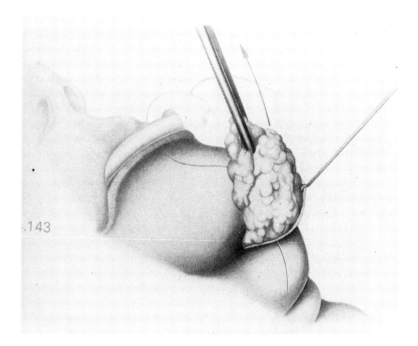

Fig. 34-9. Resection of submental fat is commenced from below, upward with special curved scissors.

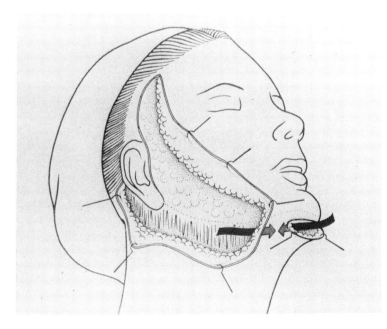

Fig. 34-10. In more severe cases of fatty depositions or when large quantity of redundant tissue is present at submandibular region, undermining is extended so that facelift pocket connects freely with submental region.

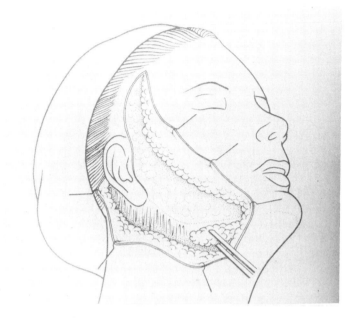

Fig. 34-11. Defatting can extend to submandibular region.

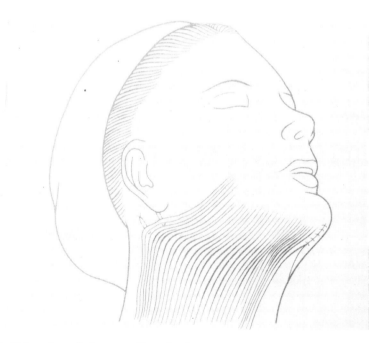

Fig. 34-12. If junction of platysma fibers is absent or very thin in midline, resulting in vertical cervical bands, approximation of medial margins of muscles becomes necessary.

associated with good traction of the face and neck flaps in standard rhytidectomy technique, is often sufficient to reconstruct the contour of the cervical mandibular line and obtain a good profile.

In more severe cases of fatty depositions (e.g., as found in the double-chin deformity, or when a large quantity of redundant tissue is present at the submandibular region), undermining is extended so that the face-lift pocket connects freely with the submental region (Fig. 34-10). With this increased exposure, defatting can extend to the submandibular region (Fig. 34-11). Resection of the fat commences a few centimeters below the submandibular rim, extending posteriorly to the point where the jugular vein crosses the sternocleidomastoid muscle. All the fat is removed evenly. This controlled excision can be extremely time consuming and demanding. When performed carefully, a complete removal of fat exposes an intact platysma, which protects the branches of the facial nerve lying deep to this muscle. Care should be taken when reaching the area anterior to the parotid, where the branches

of the facial nerve are more superficial. This danger area can be identified by the point where the facial artery crosses the mandible.

Once the platysma is exposed, it can be examined. If the junction of its fibers is absent or very thin in the midline, resulting in vertical cervical bands, then suturing of the medial margins of the muscle becomes necessary (Fig. 34-12). Suturing is performed from the mandibular symphysis to the hyoid bone, using interrupted polyglycolic acid sutures (Fig. 34-13). If the platysma and aponeurosis are found to be very lax, then fixation of the posterior margin of the platysma to the sternocleidomastoid muscle, associated with medial approximation, provides firm support.

Following correction of the cervicomandibular contour, traction of the facial rhytidectomy flaps is performed to permit evaluation of the degree of improvement. Any irregularities are corrected. Before closure, any remaining fat can be removed and the skin in the submandibular region shaped to the new contour. Excess skin is marked and removed. In practice, removal of skin in the sub-

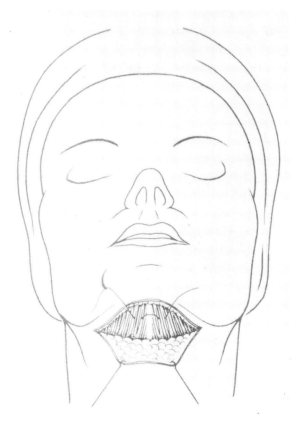

Fig. 34-13. Suturing is performed from mandibular symphysis to hyoid bone, using interrupted polyglycolic acid sutures.

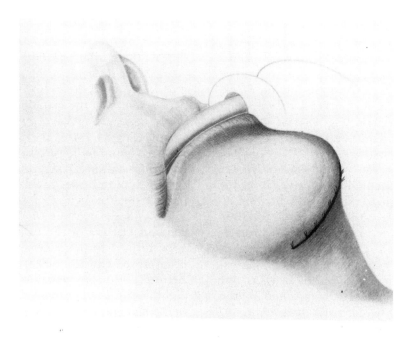

Fig. 34-14. Removal of skin in submental region is generally minimal or nil. Skin can be closed without tension, and formation of hypertrophic scarring or vertical contracture lines is lessened.

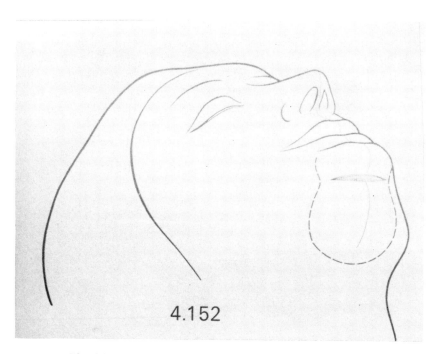

Fig. 34-15. Excess submental fat is used to augment chin.

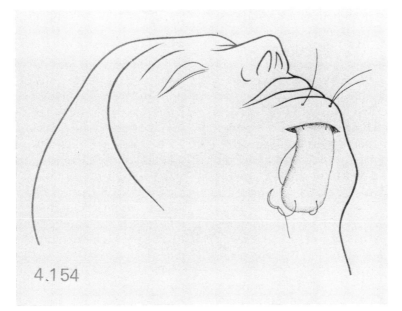

Fig. 34-16. Submental fat is exposed and elevated from below, upward, thus isolating fat flap on superior pedicle.

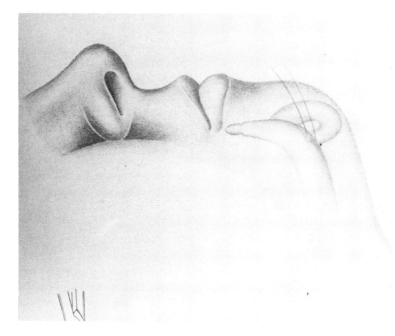

Fig. 34-17. Flap is transposed through 180 degrees and its distal extremity fixed to anterior region of chin.

mental region is generally minimal or nil, because the concavity of the neck is increased by lipectomy and plication, and the area for which cutaneous coverage is needed is thus equally increased. This allows closure of the skin without tension and lessens the formation of hypertrophic scarring or vertical contracture lines (Fig. 34-14). In cases in which the submental and submandibular areas have not been defatted, cutaneous resection is mandatory. Experience has shown that minor defects can be satisfactorily improved by means of a simple excision of an ellipse of skin and a wedge of fat in the submental area. Suction drains (Hemovac) are placed under both flaps and along the submental pocket. This allows for drainage of any blood or serum; in addition, the negative pressure aids the accommodation of the flaps to their bed.

The wound is closed in two layers using polyglycolic acid sutures in the deep dermis and nylon sutures for the skin. A compressive dressing is applied.

In cases of senile chin deformity, in addition to correcting fatty deposition in the submental and submandibular areas, the ptotic characteristics of the skin should also be evaluated, and the surgical procedure should vary according to the local conditions. One method is to use the excess submental fat to augment the chin, thus correcting the ptosis and hypomentonism (if present) and conferring a youthful aspect to the face (Fig. 34-15).

The submental fat is exposed as previously described and is elevated from below, upward, thus isolating the fat flap on a superior pedicle (Fig. 34-16). This flap is transposed through 180 degrees and its distal extremity fixed to the anterior region of the chin (Fig. 34-17). This method may be used when microgenia is associated with the senile chin, but with time the fat has a tendency to be absorbed. A Silastic implant is preferable for correction of the receding chin, the fat flap being reserved for patients who do not wish to have any kind of prosthesis. A Silastic implant can be inserted via the submental approach into a supraperiosteal pocket. The implant is fixed by sutures and the overlying fascia closed directly. An intraoral approach can also be employed, as described previously.

In the case of a drooping chin, when it is a consequence of a soft tissue deformity and is not associated with excess submental fat, a technique that has given me satisfactory results under certain indications consists of an inferiorly based medial raphe flap made through an intraoral approach after adequate undermining of the soft tissue, as for augmentation mentoplasty. The mobilized soft tissues are pulled in a slightly more cranial position with the help of the flap, which is tractioned upward and sutured in the midline.

POSTOPERATIVE CARE

Antibiotics are routinely administered for 5 postoperative days. The first dressing change is performed on the first postoperative day, when a lighter dressing is applied. Submental sutures are removed on the fifth postoperative day.

In cases in which an implant has been used and an adhesive dressing applied to the chin, the splint is kept in position for 7 days. Patients are maintained on a liquid diet for the first 3 days following surgery and then begun on a semifluid diet, which is continued until the eighth postoperative day. Thereafter, a normal diet is permitted.

Patients are advised to avoid exaggerated movements of the head and to restrict exposure to sun and heat for approximately 1 month postoperatively.

RESULTS AND COMPLICATIONS

Results of the techniques described are presented in Figs. 34-18 to 34-20.

In my experience, contouring the neck by submandibular and submental lipectomy appears to be the best way to achieve an ideal cervicomandibular angle. Complications that occur are essentially the same as those following standard rhytidectomy. Irregularities of contour in the neck result from puckering of the skin and localized bulging. The latter occurs if the lipectomy is not carried out in a uniform way. It is important that the adipose tissue included in the submental skin flap is of sufficient thickness and uniformity that puckering of the skin does not occur. This latter complication will inevitably appear if the submental skin flap is too thin or if hemostasis is inadequate. Localized small hematomas that resolve by fibrosis can lead to puckering of the overlying skin.

In my series there was no evidence of damage to the submandibular branch of the facial nerve, since this branch is largely protected by the platysma.

Hypertrophy of the submental scar occurred in four cases and was always associated with removal of submental skin. If no submental skin is excised, the wound edges fit well and no traction is exerted on the wound margins, so that the re-

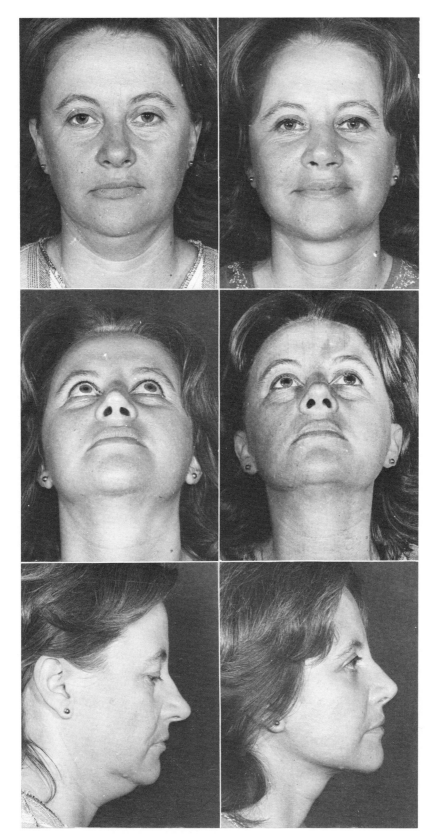

Fig. 34-18. Thirty-nine-year-old patient with neck flaccidity and double-chin deformity underwent face and neck lifting with direct excision of submental fat. Blepharoplasty and rhinoplasty were also performed.

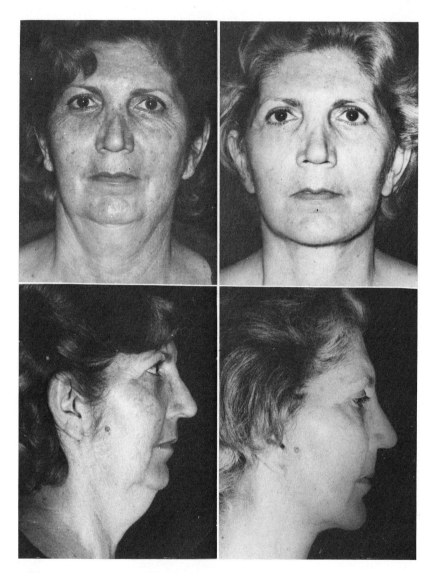

Fig. 34-19. Fifty-six-year-old patient with marked neck deformity underwent cervicofacial rhytidectomy that included submental and submandibular lipectomy and platysma lifting with midline and lateral plication.

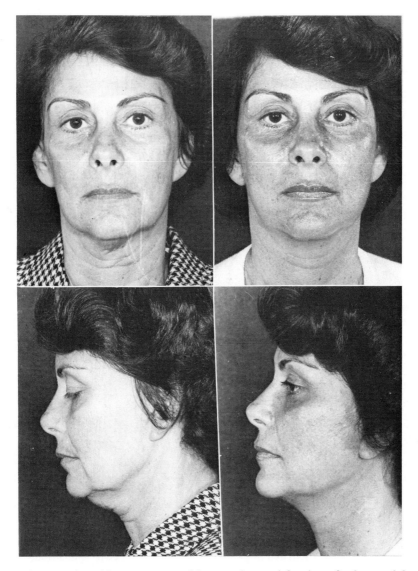

Fig. 34-20. Drooping chin was corrected by eversion and fixation of submental fat flap. Rhytidectomy and blepharoplasty were also performed.

sultant scar is generally of good quality.

As in any fat flap, the fat flap used to augment the chin suffers a certain degree of absorption, and I therefore tend to overcorrect the deformity at the time of the surgery.

I have experienced no cases of infection or fat necrosis.

With regard to the use of Silastic implants, if the pocket is made to fit the implant exactly, complications such as hematoma, infection, and displacement are minimized. The use of the median raphe fibrous flap avoids displacement of the prosthesis. Many of the patients in this series have been followed up to 10 years. In some of these cases, slight bone resorption has been noted on x-ray examination, but the overall cosmetic result has not been significantly altered. I have not noted any difference in the complication rates using either the intraoral or extraoral route. I prefer the extraoral route in cases in which there is already an approach through a submental incision and believe it is unnecessary to add an intraoral incision. On the other hand, I give preference to the intraoral approach for the correction of hypomentonism or a senile chin without associated submental deformity. There have been no cases of extrusion of Silastic implants in this situation in my series to date.

SUGGESTED READINGS

Adamson, J.E., Horton, C.E., and Crawford, M.M.: The surgical correction of the "turkey gobbler" deformity, Plast. Reconstr. Surg. **34**:598, 1963.

Cannon, B., and Pantazelos, M.: W-plasty approach to submandibular lipectomy. In Hueston, J.T., editor: Transactions of the Fifth International Congress of Plastic and Reconstructive Surgeons, Melbourne, 1971, Butterworths, Pty., Ltd.

Connell, B.F.: Contouring the neck in rhytidectomy by lipectomy and a muscle sling, Plast. Reconstr. Surg. **61**:376, 1971.

Couly, G., Mureau, J., and Vaillant, J.M.: Le fascia superficialis chephalique, Ann. Chir. Plast. **20**:171, 1975.

Cronin, T.D., and Biggs, T.M.: The T-Z plasty for the male "turkey gobbler" neck, Plast. Reconstr. Surg. **47**:534, 1971.

Davis, A.D.: Obligations in the consideration of meloplasties, J. Int. Coll. Surg. **24**:568, 1955.

Dingman, R.O., and Grabb, W.C.: Surgical anatomy of the mandibular ramus of the facial nerve based on the dissection of 100 facial halves, Plast. Reconstr. Surg. **29**:266, 1962.

Guerrerosantos, J., Espaillat, L., and Morales, F.: Muscular lift in cervical rhytidoplasty, Plast. Reconstr. Surg. **54**:127, 1974.

Johnson, J.B.: The problem of the aging face, Plast. Reconstr. Surg. **15**:117, 1955.

Johnson, J.B., and Hadley, R.C.: The aging face. In Converse, J.M., editor: Reconstructive plastic surgery, Philadelphia, 1964, W.B. Saunders Co.

Marino, H., Galeano, E.J., and Sandolfs, E.A.: Plastic correction of the double chin, Plast. Reconstr. Surg. **31**:45, 1963.

Millard, D.R., Pigot, R.W., and Hedo, A.: Submandibular lipectomy, Plast. Reconstr. Surg. **41**:513, 1968.

Millard, R.R., et al.: Submental and submandibular lipectomy in conjunction with face lifts in the male and female, Plast. Reconstr. Surg. **49**:385, 1972.

Mitz, V., and Peronie, M.: The superficial musculoaponeurotic system (SMAS) in the parotid and cheek area, Plast. Reconstr. Surg. **58**:80, 1976.

Morel Fatio, D.: Cosmetic surgery of the face. In Gibson, T., editor: Modern trends in plastic surgery, Woburn, Mass., 1966, Butterworth Publisher, Inc.

Owsley, J.R., Jr.: Plastysma fascial rhytidectomy: a preliminary report, Plast. Reconstr. Surg. **60**:843, 1977.

Padgett, E.C., and Stephenson, K.C.: Plastic and reconstructive surgery, Springfield, Ill., 1948, Charles C Thomas, Publisher.

Pangman, W.J., and Wallace, R.M.: Cosmetic surgery of the face and neck, Plast. Reconstr. Surg. **27**:54, 1961.

Pitanguy, I.: Augmentation mentoplasty, Plast. Reconstr. Surg. **42**:460, 1968.

Pitanguy, I., Mentoplastia, O Hosp. (Brasil) **73**:1745, 1968.

Pitanguy, I.: Aesthetic plastic surgery of head and body, Heildelberg, 1981, Springer-Verlag, p. 239.

Pitanguy, I., et al.: Hipermentonismo, Rev. Bras. Cir. **61**:119, 1971.

Pitanguy, I., et al.: Hipomentonismo, Rev. Bras. Cir. **61**:213, 1971.

Pitanguy, I., et al.: Prognatismo, Rev. Bras. Cir. **62**:445, 1972.

Pitanguy, I., et al.: Tratamento das deformidades submentonianas, Rev. Bras. Cir. **69**:291, 1979.

Skoog, T.: Plastic surgery, Stockholm, 1974, Almquist & Wiksell.

Snyder, G.B.: Cervicomentoplasty with rhytidectomy, Plast. Reconstr. Surg. **54**:404, 1974.

Snyder, G.B.: Submental rhytidectomy, Plast. Reconstr. Surg. **62**:693, 1978.

Testut, L.: Traité d'anatomie humaine, Paris, 1904, Doin.

Tipton, J.B.: Should the subcutaneous tissue be plicated in a face lift? Plast. Reconstr. Surg. **54**:1, 1974.

Viñas, J.C., et al.: Surgical treatment of double chin, Plast. Reconstr. Surg. **50**:119, 1972.

Weisman, P.A.: Simplified technique in submental lipectomies, Plast. Reconstr. Surg. **48**:443, 1971.

Editorial comments
Part V

Rejuvenative surgery of the face cannot be confined just to those procedures that elevate and remove the excess skin and fat brought on by time and gravity. Study of aging faces shows other changes that take place with time. Those occurring in the eyelids and brows are well recognized, and most plastic surgeons will include operations for these areas in their treatment plans for facial rejuvenation.

Time also effects changes in other features, including the earlobes, chin, and nose, and ancillary procedures to rejuvenate these features are also important in the total facial rejuvenative program. To use the analogy of redecorating a room, one may redo the basic components, such as wallpaper, carpeting, furniture, and draperies, but smaller items, such as lamps, vases, and artwork, are no less important. Despite their lesser area or volume in comparison with the four basics, they may play a major role in setting off or highlighting the motif of the design. Likewise, treatment of the more subtle but nonetheless significant manifestations of aging can add a great deal to the surgical result.

We know that earlobes can change with time, usually undergoing enlargement. Reduction of large earlobes is a worthwhile ancillary procedure for face-lift surgery. Of course, the opportunity to correct other problems, as discussed by Dr. Lindgren, including previous surgical deformities and pixie earlobes, often presents itself in patients requesting face-lift surgery.

The nose is an obvious feature that undergoes continuous changes with age (see Part II, Chapter 15), including broadening and drooping of the tip, increased hump deformity, and enlargement of the nostrils. Treatment of these changes by partial or complete rhinoplasty can provide a gratifying enhancement of the facial rejuvenative operation.

The chin is a feature that offers an opportunity for aesthetic improvement of the face because of possible congenital deformities as well as changes due to aging. A deficient or retruded chin may contribute somewhat to the accumulation of excess skin in the neck, and augmenting such a chin not only enhances the general facial appearance, but may help a bit to correct the sagging neck (although it is certainly not a substitute for other neck procedures). The external submental incision provides convenient access for both anterior neck procedures and chin augmentation. I have given up the straight submental crease incision for the anterior-pointing gull wing submental incision described by Rogers* because it provides an opportunity for extending the incision laterally and still keeping it within the shadow of the chin without creeping up on the face.

One caution in augmentation mentoplasty in the older female patient: be conservative. Too much chin projection can give the patient a sharp, Punch-and-Judy profile, which in itself can give the appearance of aging. If in doubt, undercorrect.

The drooping or "witch's" chin is a frequent characteristic of facial aging. So far, there has not been any single or universally popular method of treating this problem. External incisions, such as Dr. Gonzalez-Ulloa's triangular excision with V-Y shifting or the fleur-de-lis incision, have been suggested. Dr. Pitanguy's suggestion of mobilizing and shifting upward the medial raphe of the chin is intriguing because of its simplicity.

---

*Rogers, B.O.: The seagull or "mouette" incision for correction of double chins. In Marchac, D., and Hueston, J.T., editors: Transactions of the Sixth International Congress of Plastic and Reconstructive Surgeons, New York, 1976, Masson Publishing USA, Inc.

At the 1982 meeting of the American Society for Aesthetic Surgery in Las Vegas, two intriguing papers were presented. Dr. Leon Burke described filling out the deep submental crease accompanying the drooping chin by advancing the posterior edge of an elliptical derma-fat flap anteriorly, anchoring it on to the mentum. Dr. Rex Peterson treated the problem by advancing an elliptical derma-fat flap posteriorly, along with augmentation mentoplasty and platysma plication. A modification of the latter method that I have used with some success is to deepithelialize a small, transversely oriented submental derma-fat flap based anteriorly and advance it posteriorly, attaching it to the underlying platysma muscles. This procedure tends to draw the inferiorly drooping chin tissues posteriorly and helps reduce the depth of the submental crease. I hope that by the time this volume is published, both of these papers will also have been published.*

B.L.K.

---

*See also Editorial Comments for Chapter 33, p. 319.

Surface surgery

Chapter 35

Chemical peel

Simon Fredricks

The chemical peel was brought to the attention of plastic surgeons by Litton[2] and further popularized by Baker, Gordon, and Seckinger.[1] It appears to be a modality more favored in the Sun Belt region of the country and rarely employed in northern climates. This probably relates to solar damage and the associated dry, wrinkled skin of individuals living in the more arid regions, coupled with the fact that many of these persons are fair-skinned, being descendants of the Welsh, English, and Irish who originally populated the great Southwest of this country.

As a result of the work of the above-mentioned authors, phenol has become the most widely used agent for producing such chemical burns. Others have employed trichloracetic acid, but it is considered by many to be more prone to produce hypertrophic scarring. I have no personal experience with trichloracetic acid and do not know of any scientific comparative study.

Cosmetic manufacturers employ milder skin irritants (e.g. resorcinol or salicylic acid) to produce the variety of so-called face-lift creams. All such creams merely produce mild erythema and edema of the skin, which gives the false illusion of wrinkle removal as the swelling plumps out the wrinkles. These, of course, rapidly return as the edema resolves, generally within 48 hours.

The most frequently imployed formula for a phenol chemical peel is as follows:

	4.5 ml	Supersaturated phenol (88% USP)
	5.0 ml	Sterile water
	0.2 ml	Croton oil
	0.3 ml	Septisol
TOTAL	10.0 ml	Emulsion

One always mixes a total of 10 ml of the solution. Of this, 4.5 ml is the supersaturated phenol, the active agent; 5.0 ml of sterile water serves as the vehicle; 0.2 ml of croton oil serves as a vesicant to produce blistering, and 0.3 ml of septisol (Hexachlorophene Surgical Scrub) is added to create an evenly dispersed emulsion.

I recommend mixing it fresh each time it is used and discarding it after use. Storage of the components is best done in dark, air-conditioned environments. Otherwise, deterioration and chemical alteration can occur with subsequent unpredictable results.

PATIENT SELECTION

A chemical peel is an emotionally demanding experience for the patient. Only stable, well-motivated patients are good candidates. The resulting massive swelling and tight eschar, the initial redness of the skin when the eschar separates, and the final permanent pigment change can be a frightening experience for a patient who has not been well informed about the procedure beforehand.

Therefore it is not a modality to be undertaken lightly and requires complete understanding by the patient of the implications of accepting this mode of treatment. I find that words alone are inadequate to describe the treatment to the inexperienced potential patient. Photographic examples of the pigment change and of the eschar in place and separating are recommended to help select those patients prepared to accept the treatment with reasonable equanimity.

Patients are cautioned that they cannot expose themselves to sunlight (e.g., they should avoid beach and outdoor pool activities, tennis, or golf) for 3 to 6 months, or hyperpigmentation of the skin will occur (Fig. 35-1). Of course, normal everyday outdoor movement is not precluded, but I do recommend that a good sunscreen filter be

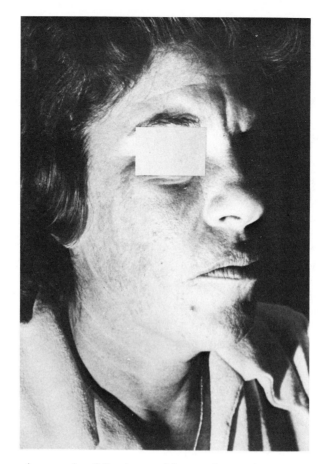

Fig. 35-1. Hyperpigmentation following total face peel secondary to early sun exposure.

used beneath the makeup as a safety net.

Antipregnancy medications similarly should not be employed for 3 to 6 months; otherwise chloasma may occur. Therefore other precautions against pregnancy are recommended, such as spermicides or an IUD.

If hyperpigmentation does occur, the pigment is usually superficial and can be removed by light dermabrasion.

Darkly pigmented, olive- or muddy-complexioned people are poor candidates for this procedure. In view of the severe pigment change and contrast that results in comparison with the untreated areas, such candidates are rejected out of hand in my practice.

Although others have peeled the lower neck and dorsum of the hands successfully, I believe that these areas are prone to hypertrophic, dysfunctional scarring and carry a high degree of calculated risk. Therefore I do not accept patients for a peel to these areas.

Patients who do not use makeup or who do not want to be obliged to use foundation makeup are not good candidates, because without makeup, camouflage of the treated areas becomes difficult.

Freckled patients are problematical, because the peel will remove the freckles, and the transition line between treated and untreated areas becomes very obvious.

Patients must be informed that moles will become more obvious as their pigment darkens. Also, skin pores of the treated areas frequently appear larger and more obvious after treatment. In addition, patients should be aware that the skin tone will be shiny and ultimately bleached.

The aging face with redundant skin and underlying musculature is best treated by surgical intervention; a chemical peel is not a substitute for surgery (Fig. 35-2). The chemical peel is exclusively a complexion or skin tone procedure, improving the quality of the overlying skin but not the quantity thereof. Occasionally one does see patients with excessive solar wrinkling without significant redundancy, for whom a chemical peel alone is the only treatment required (Fig. 35-3).

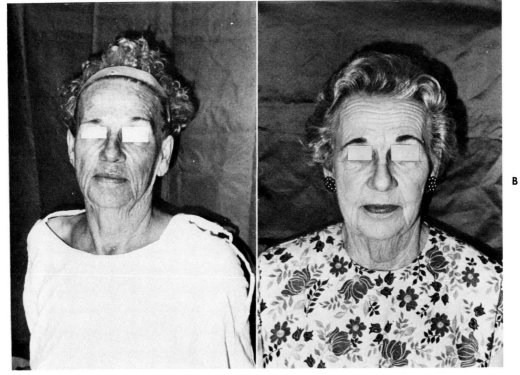

Fig. 35-2. A, Patient with marked redundancy and wrinkling. **B,** Appearance following peel only: inadequate result.

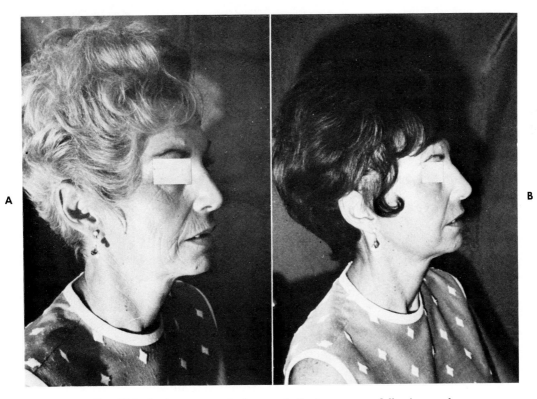

Fig. 35-3. A, Appearance before peel. **B,** Appearance following peel.

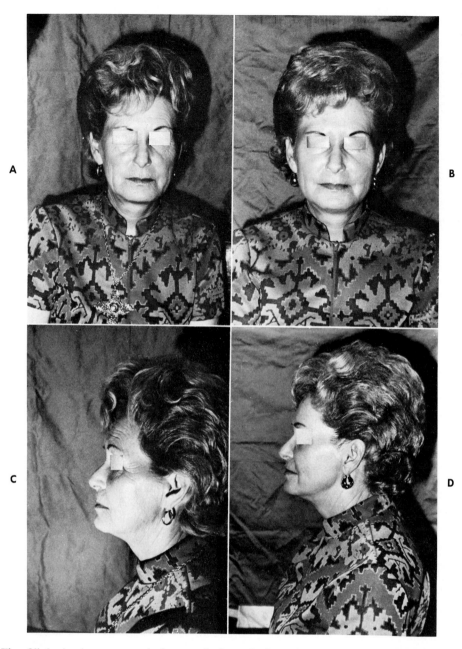

Fig. 35-4. A, Appearance before peel, frontal view. **B,** Appearance following peel, frontal view. **C,** Appearance before peel, profile. **D,** Appearance following peel, profile.

These usually achieve superb results (Fig. 35-4). Finally, patients with known kidney dysfunction should not undergo this procedure, since phenol is specifically excreted by the kidney.

PLAN OF TREATMENT

The plan of treatment may encompass a two-stage rehabilitation. The first stage consists of the surgical improvement with removal of excess skin and fat and muscle tightening. The second stage

is the chemical peel treatment, which is undertaken no earlier than 6 to 8 weeks after the surgical lift and when all wounds are well healed and supple (Fig. 35-5, *A* and *B*).

This is the method that I frequently prefer. After the surgical lift alone, many patients will be satisfied and reconsider having the peel done. This two-stage plan affords them further opportunity to think about the peel.

Most patients readily accept the surgical im-

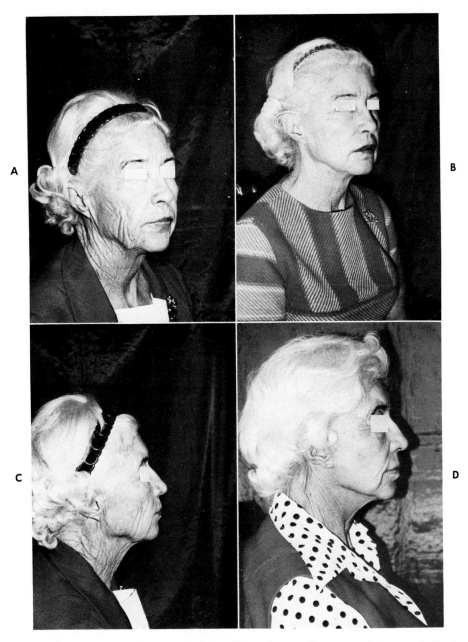

Fig. 35-5. A, Patient before surgical face-lift and second-stage total face peel. **B,** Appearance after surgical face-lift and second-stage total face peel. **C,** Patient before surgical face-lift and second-stage total face peel at age 72. **D,** Appearance 10 years following surgical lift and second-stage total face peel at age 82.

provement plan but mentally wrestle with the implications of the peel. Offering to do it as a second stage puts their minds at ease, and acceptance of the plan is more easily implemented, since nothing is lost and the options remain open. Of course, the effects of the peel are not permanent, but usually they are long lasting (Fig. 35-5, *C* and *D*).

Spira et al.[4] have astutely pointed out that one cannot undermine and peel tissue simultaneously

without a high preponderant risk of skin slough. Insulting both sides of the flap is foolhardy and should be universally condemned. Therefore the areas capable of being peeled at the time of the surgical lift are limited.

Perioral peel

Certainly, the perioral area may be done, and indeed the upper lip alone is the most commonly done area to minimize those vertical fine wrinkle

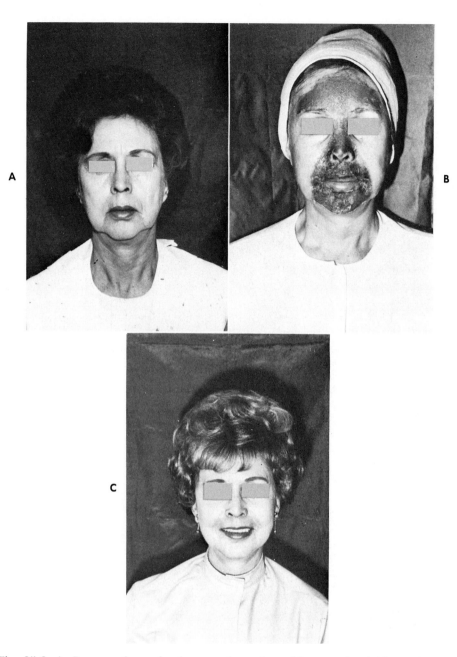

Fig. 35-6. A, Preoperative redundancy and sagging with central wrinkling of upper and lower lips and forehead. **B,** Surgical face-lift and central one-third peel, one stage. Eschar is in place. **C,** Appearance following surgical face-lift, blepharoplasty of all four lids, and central one-third peel, one stage.

lines into which the lipstick bleeds and that are so depressing to patients. This may be extended laterally as far as the nasolabial fold with safety. In the lower lip it may extend from the lateral descending crease lines of the commissure to the highest mentocervical crease.

Central one-third peel

If the forehead has not been undermined, a peel at the time of the face-lift can be done from the frontal hairline, encompassing the intact entire forehead on through the glabella, across the nose from one nasolabial line to the other, and down through the perioral area. Caution must be exercised not to peel the forehead too far laterally over previously undermined temporal scalp (Fig. 35-6).

The advantage of the central one-third peel is that it avoids the potential searchlight appearance of some solitary perioral peels by giving a uniform color and texture to the skin as the observing eye views the face in full vertical direction from the hairline to the chin. It represents the most that can be done in one sitting for patients who cannot accept a two-stage program for whatever reason.

Total face peel

The total face peel is the procedure that I prefer, since it gives a uniform color and texture to the skin of the entire face, with the transition line more easily hidden by the inferior shadow of the concavity of the jawline.

Spotting peel

The spotting peel is a procedure favored by some where the glabella and upper lip are done together with the surgical lift. It represents minimal use of the modality.

TECHNIQUE

Patients may have a chemical peel done as an outpatient procedure if they are stoic, very emotionally stable, and/or have good home support. Patients who require considerable tranquilization or who do not have calm, stable help at home are best admitted to the hospital or support facility (motel or clinic with supervisory personnel) the morning of the peel and discharged when the tape is removed. The procedure should be done in a sterile, well-ventilated, air-conditioned, environment.

The chemical peel is essentially a controlled partial-thickness chemical burn. Therefore any potential superimposed infection should be scrupulously avoided. For that purpose the hair is shampooed, and the face and neck are similarly prepared. I prefer a povidone-iodine scrub if the patient is not allergic to iodine. For the same reason, the usual precaution of gowning and draping is employed.*

I believe it to be of significant importance that the occlusive tape be sterilized prior to use.* If steam sterilization is to be used, this must be done the evening before and the tape adherred to Mayo trays, giving it an opportunity to dry. Otherwise, gas sterilization may be used, and the tape may be left in roll form in the appropriate packet.

To obtain a uniform peel, it is essential to use

an effective degreasing agent after soapy preparation. Otherwise, the dried lipids of the cleanser and natural oils form a protective barrier against the peeling agent and result in a nonuniform peel, with a bizarre geographical pattern of unpeeled skin, much like a miniature of the soap pattern seen on drying window panes. It is therefore also important to use the defatting agent in the depths of the creases of the wrinkles if effective treatment is to be obtained. This is best accomplished by holding the skin taut and stretching the wrinkles and/or using a pointed, fine cotton-tipped applicator.

Ether, acetone, and, more recently, Freon will serve as effective defatting agents. The former are frowned on by fire marshalls. I prefer to go over the area to be peeled twice to be sure that no areas have been skipped. The sponges should not be discarded into plastic bags until they are well evaporated.

Phenol can be rapidly absorbed via the respiratory tract. For that reason, a well-ventilated room is used. Also, one does not dally in the nostril area when applying the emulsion.

Truppman and Ellenby's study[5] confirmed that cardiac irregularity leading to arrest can occur if the phenol is rapidly applied over a large area. For that reason, I use tight, well-stripped cotton-tipped applicators and apply the emulsion over anatomical aesthetic units, pausing between areas to minimize blood levels of phenol absorption. I do not recommend the use of large proctological pledgets for the same reason.

It is appropriate, therefore, that all patients having a phenol face peel done have ECG monitoring and an intravenous infusion. If cardiac arrhythmia occurs, the procedure should be stopped and immediate prophylactic measures taken. I recommend 60 mg of 2% lidocaine bolus intravenously. If normal rhythm is not restored, following with 0.5 mg of propranolol (Inderal) is almost always successful.

The small, tight applicators serve well to ensure that the depths of the creases are treated with the emulsion while the skin is held taut (Fig. 35-7). To avoid skip areas, I recommend treating all areas twice in the same sitting.

Once the skin shows frosting, indicating denaturation of the keratin, absorption is minimal and the area has been appropriately covered (Fig. 35-8). I peel to the upper border of the tarsal plate in the upper lid and never below (Fig. 35-9). Exposure keratitis frequently accompanies peeling below this mark in my experience. In the lower lid I peel to within 2 or 3 mm of the ciliary

---

*EDITOR'S NOTE: These steps are more the individual choices of Dr. Fredricks rather than the standard of care in this country. (B.L.K.)

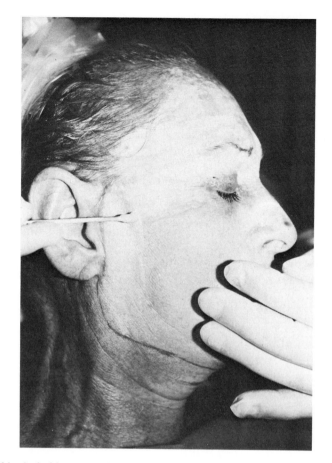

Fig. 35-7. Skin is held taut and treated with emulsion on tight, small cotton-tipped applicators.

margin (Fig. 35-9). I always protect the cornea with ointment, but I exercise care in the instillation so that ointment does not extend out onto the lid area to be treated.

Phenol, of course, will produce instant clouding of the cornea. If phenol should enter the eye, immediate copious flushing with balanced salt solution (BSS) should be done. Therefore balanced salt solution should be open and available on the Mayo stand.

I always insist that the Mayo stand be lowered below the level of the face to avoid someone accidentally tripping over it and causing spillage over the facial area. Furthermore, I insist that all solutions be carried around the face and never over it.

I personally always move the applicators laterally and never across the central eye area. The eyelids are always done with very well stripped applicators from which phenol solution cannot run off.

Operating room lights are not permitted to shine directly into the patient's face, or uncontrollable tearing will, of course, result.

One should always peel directly into the hairline and into the vermilion mucosal junction to avoid unsightly transition areas around the lips. These are notoriously known as the Al Jolson look. I take precautions not to peel into the pinna, which is keloid prone, and instead peel right up to the preauricular crease line. Most frequently, I peel to the highest submental crease line but am willing to go as low as the hyoid level.

The hyoid is my "never go below" line. I do not wish to risk burning over a concave surface that could subsequently tether (Fig. 35-9). It is wise to ink in the inferior peel line to be sure that it is symmetrical in appearance on either side of the neck (Fig. 35-10). Furthermore, this avoids slavishly following the inframandibular line laterally, which invariably rises too high to permit easy disguise of the transition line. The lateral inferior

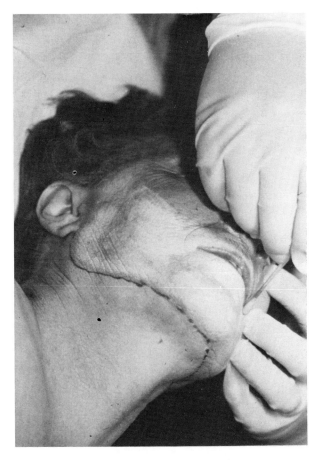

Fig. 35-8. Frosting of keratin.

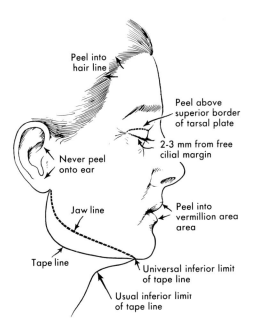

Fig. 35-9. Drawing illustrating extent and limitation of peeled areas.

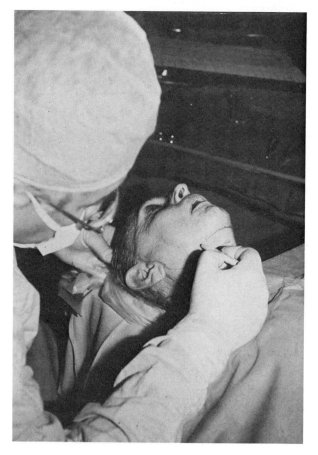

Fig. 35-10. Inking in inferior peel line.

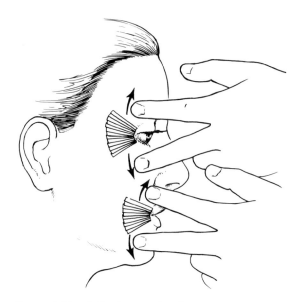

Fig. 35-11. Spreading wrinkles following peel and tape applied in fan pattern at lateral commissures.

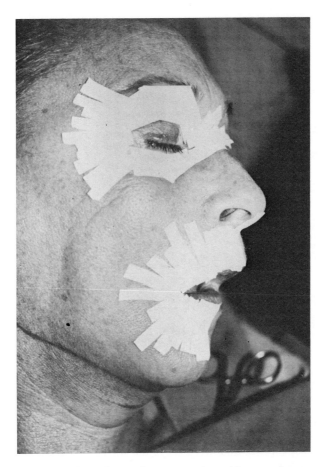

Fig. 35-12. Eyes are taped first where edema onset is rapid; commissures are taped next.

peel line is therefore drawn lower than the lower border of the mandible to better disguise the transition in the shadow of the submaxillary hollow (Figs. 35-7 to 35-10). Gloves are used to mix and apply the emulsion to protect the operator from frequent fingertip chemical burns, which can reduce tactile sensibility. When ready for taping, gloves should be removed and the hands carefully washed of all adherent powder, which might become a barrier to the taping.

The eyelids are the shock organ of the face and swell first. They are therefore taped first, when it is easier to do it. I think it is important to fan out the tape at the lateral canthus of the eye, where the smile lines occur, and at the lateral commissure of the mouth, spreading the wrinkles as one tapes (Figs. 35-11 and 35-12).

Taping should be carried into the hairline across the brows and across the vermilion line (Fig. 35-13). The procedure should always be done with an intravenous "life line" in place, and it is advantageous to flush the kidneys with intra-

venous fluid during and at the conclusion of the procedure. As mentioned previously, the patient should be carefully monitored with a cardiac monitor. Arrhythmias, particularly premature ventricular contractions, as well as auricular extra systoles, are clear indications for stopping the procedure immediately and instituting appropriate therapeutic measures. All necessary personnel, equipment, drugs, and expertise should be available before the treatment is begun in the event that resuscitation of the patient becomes necessary.

I like to give intravenous antibiotic coverage in the form of an initial intravenous bolus followed by an intravenous drip during the procedure, to produce a satisfactory intratreatment blood level. This treatment is then maintained orally for 5 days postoperatively.

Many surgeons prefer dermabrasion as the modality for removing wrinkling of the upper lid. Based on my experience, I do not believe that dermabrasion is as effective. Certainly, there is

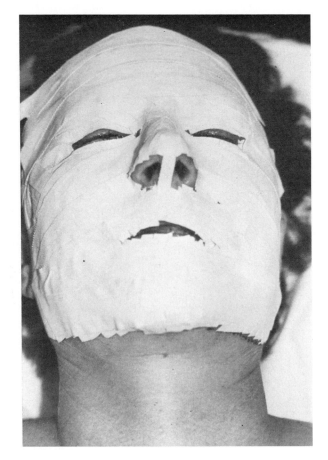

Fig. 35-13. Final total taping into hairline, across vermilion, and over brows.

ample scientific confirmation that chemical peeling stimulates the development of elastic fibers in the treated area of skin, which dermabrasion does not do. I find that the chemical peel is a much easier procedure, particularly in technically difficult areas where dermabrasion is virtually impossible (e.g., the eyelids).

Horton and Fleury (see Chapter 37) suggest chemical peeling followed by immediate dermabrasion. I have not found that this combined method has significantly reduced any morbidity of the procedure, nor has it enhanced the effectiveness of the end result.

POSTOPERATIVE CARE

Intravenous fluids are continued until the patient is able to take fluids by mouth without nausea. I do not permit smoking, excessive talking, or the use of a drinking straw until the tapes are off, to avoid their premature dislodgment. Instead, patients drink directly from a glass or cup, and fluid oral intake is encouraged. Patients are cau-

tioned preoperatively that their eyelids may swell shut. Every patient is encouraged to bring a small pocket radio, which is useful as a vehicle to maintain a conduit to reality. Otherwise, this sudden loss of visual contact could precipitate emotional instability. Postoperatively, patients deserve tranquilization and appropriate analgesics or narcotics as required to keep them comfortable. The initial burning sensation can be relieved by the use of ice packs. Patients should be encouraged to ambulate early with assistance in the postoperative period.

I do not permit patients to have a pillow in the normal horizontal position. Otherwise, the neck will flex, and the inferior tape line can begin to abrade the underlying dermis, particularly with the massive swelling that frequently occurs. If occlusive taping is not done, a satisfactory result will not be obtained. The skin will redden and swell and subsequently return to the pretreated state, but peeling does not result.

It requires 24 hours of occlusive taping to obtain the maximum result. The tape can be removed at the end of 24 hours if it comes away easily. However, in most instances, if one waits 48 hours, sufficient serum production will have occurred to have loosened the tape so that it may be removed less painfully and more easily. As has already been indicated, occlusive taping is necessary for a satisfactory result. Without taping, the skin will redden and swell, but peeling does not result. Spira et al. have advocated peeling without taping to feather the demarcation line. I have been unable to confirm this clinically.

Patients should be instructed to recline with the head elevated above the heart level at an angle of approximately 30 to 35 degrees. The uppermost pillow should be positioned vertically from the head to well beneath the shoulders to prevent neck flexion.

The patient should be checked at 24 hours to see if there is a tendency for the lower edge of the lower tape to cut into the skin because of excessive swelling. If so, this tape should be removed to prevent loss of the underlying dermis, despite the known increased discomfort to the patient in removing the tape at 24 hours.

Mild diuretics are also useful to reduce the massive swelling. Patients should be cautioned against handling the tape and dabbing at the jawline. Once the tape was been removed, it is urgent that the patient cooperate by not touching the raw wound. The serum runoff is annoying to patients, particularly to elderly women, who tend to constantly dab at the chin and jawline with paper tissues and/or handkerchiefs with the same dominant hand with which private parts are handled. This attendant risk of superimposed infection must be guarded against. It is my considered opinion that such superimposed infection and/or tape abrasion are the most common causes of dermal loss and subsequent hypertrophic-keloidal scarring, the complication most feared by practitioners of this modality.

Seropian,[3] who has had extensive experience with the chemical peel, believes that there are two types of reactions to chemical peeling. On the one hand there are those patients who are not extensively swollen and who in fact show little swelling. They do, however, exhibit marked serum runoff exuding from the tape dressing. When these patients have their tape removed, even at 24 hours, they demonstrate punctate hemorrhages and clean, reddened wounds. He believes that these patients, if clinically recognized, should have their tape removed at 24 hours. They will not tend to hyperpigment if exposed to sunlight early, but

will only exhibit erythema of the treated skin.

On the other hand, those patients who exhibit massive facial swelling when the tape is removed at 24 or 48 hours have little or no punctate hemorrhages and do not exhibit clean underlying red dermis. Instead, they are covered with grayish debris. Seropian believes that these patients are more prone to hyperpigmentation, because the pigment-forming cells of the stratum malpighii are still inadequately treated. He suggests that for these patients the tape mask should be maintained for a longer time: 3 or 4 days or until the edema begins to resolve.

I have also noted these two distinctly different types of reactions under the tape wounds but have not as yet drawn the same conclusions.

Premature separation of the eschar, either iatrogenic or traumatic, is the primary cause of localized scarring due to injury of the thin underlying tender epithelium. When the tape is removed, the underlying muck and debris should be carefully and scrupulously cleaned. I favor soft, saline cotton balls for this purpose, used gently with a gloved hand until clean dermis is present everywhere. Occasionally, underlying thick purulence is encountered. The worst case I saw was in a patient who permitted her cat to lick the serum exuding from the face tape mask.

If purulence is present, I recommend removing it with povidone-iodine foam cream (Betadine Helafoam). Cleansing can be carried out daily, if necessary, until all purulent production is controlled, to avoid loss of underlying dermis by superimposed infection. If the dermis is clean without any significant purulence, I dust the area with powdered thymol iodide unless the patient is allergic to iodine (Fig. 35-14). In that latter instance Neosporin powder has been used satisfactorily. Others have advocated using antibacterial ointments instead (e.g., Polysporin ointment) to minimize eschar formation. The hair should be kept out of the wound during the period of eschar formation to avoid its becoming enmeshed in the drying serum. Gauze, sweatbands, ribbons, or even paper tape are useful for this purpose. If the hair is excessively long, it should be placed in a pony tail. Thymol iodide powder is most easily applied with a shaker can device. Care should be exercised to prevent the powder from going into the nasal passages, where it is very irritating. Furthermore, the patient's eyes should be closed during powdering, since the material is painful to the conjunctiva. Once cleansed and uniformly dusted, the patient is placed in the sitting position with

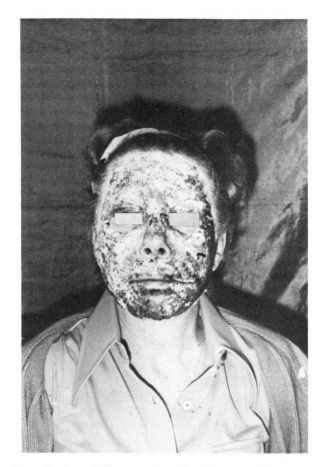

Fig. 35-14. Patient allergic to iodine was dusted with Neosporin powder. Eschar is dry and intact on third day following peel.

the eyes still closed and educated to snort by expiring forcefully once or twice. Then, with the head flexed, the patient opens and closes his or her eyes several times, permitting excessive powder to fall away. The ensuing firm eschar that forms over the next 24 to 48 hours is left intact for a total of 5 days. Itching is controlled with antipuretic agents. I favor trimeprazine tartrate (Temaril Spansules) taken every 12 hours and ice packs. Crisco application is advocated for tightness of the eschar.

After 5 days hydrolization of the eschar is begun with warm, moist turkish towels applied for 10 minutes four times a day, followed by cotton ball washing with povidone-iodine soap using a circular motion. This gently removes the eschar. Loosely hanging eschar may be gently cut away, but the eschar should not be forcibly removed prematurely. If it is forcibly torn away, bleeding will result because of loss of the underlying thin epithelium, with the attendant risk of scarring. As the eschar separates, the exposed epithelium is treated with steroid cream. For this purpose, I prefer 0.01% fluocinolone acetonide (Synalar) cream. This rapidly reduces the erythema initially seen and, I believe, minimizes the possibility of hypertrophic scarring. Steroid cream is used four times a day. By the ninth day, all eschar is gone, and the steroid cream is used for 5 to 7 additional days. Application of the steroid is interspersed with moisturizer application. Thereupon, at the end of this period of time, makeup is permitted. A nonallergic type of foundation is advocated, and for this purpose, I favor Clinique. Moisturizers are encouraged morning and evening, permanently. Sunscreen filters beneath the makeup are a sensible precaution.

Some patients have persistent periods of burning, itching, or tightness. They should protect their skin against excessive drying by heat or wind

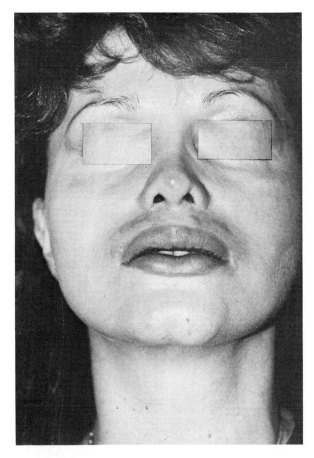

Fig. 35-15. Hypertrophic scarring secondary to peel. This is not amenable to excision, and best treatment is conservative—by pressure or intracicatricial steroid injection.

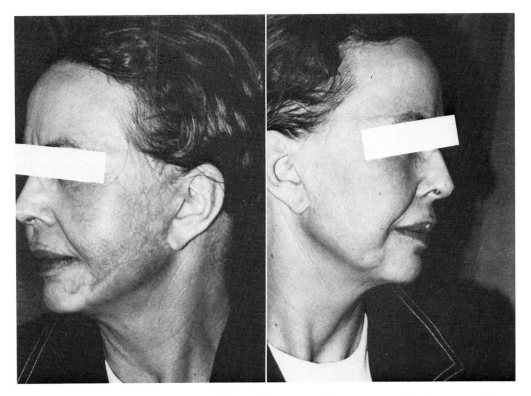

Fig. 35-16. Scars secondary to peel by totally untrained lay operator. Best treatment is by serial excisions.

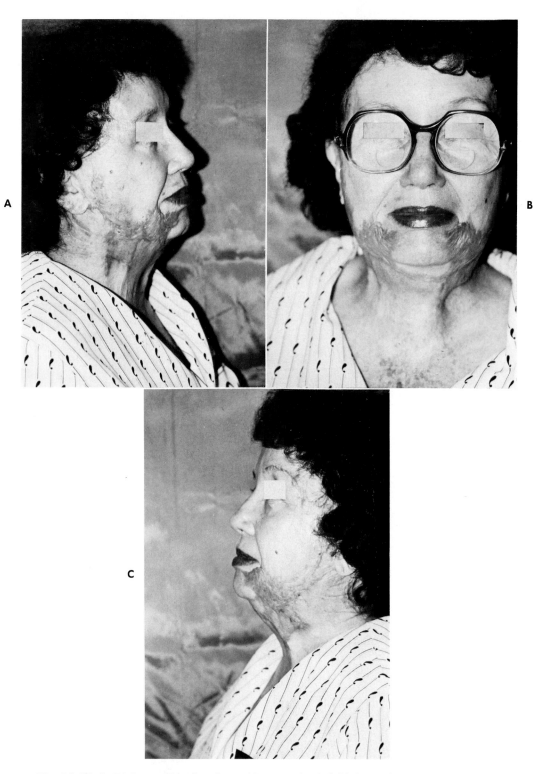

Fig. 35-17. A, Right profile of patient with extensive keloidal scarring and contractures secondary to peel by itinerant practitioner, whereabouts unknown. **B,** Frontal view, same. **C,** Left profile, same.

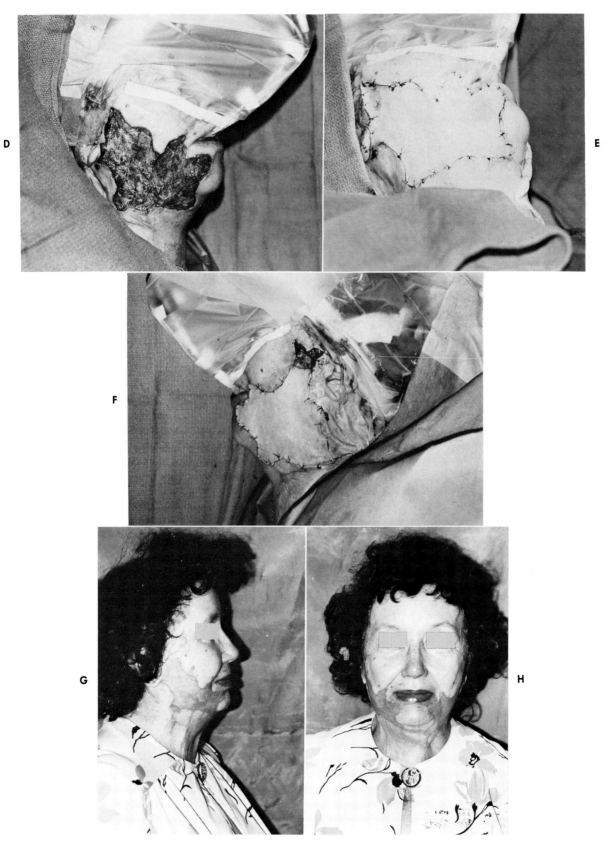

Fig. 13-17, cont'd. D, Excision and release of right face and neck showing resultant defect. **E,** Thick split-skin graft was applied from abdomen 48 hours following excision with complete hemostasis. **F,** Excision and revision of left face and neck showing resultant defect. **G,** Right profile, 100% graft take **H,** Frontal view, same.

Continued.

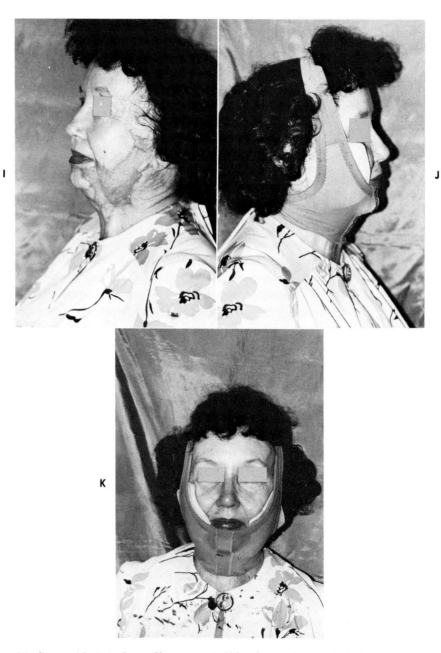

Fig. 35-17, cont'd. I, Left profile, same. **J,** Side view. Jobst mask is in place with underlying foam rubber used initially to soften and flatten scar and later to keep graft smooth. **K,** Frontal view, same.

and be educated in the increased use of moisturizers. These symptoms usually cease within several months. All patients I have seen who complain of these symptoms for longer periods of time are usually schizophrenic in nature.

Finally, patients should be discouraged from using oily makeup in the early postoperative period, or excessive milia will result.

TREATMENT OF COMPLICATIONS

If discrete hypertrophic or keloidal scarring occurs, treatment is best delayed until the tissues have fully recovered from the trauma and the insult of the burn has resolved, which takes 6 to 12 months. During this time conservative measures, including the application of topical steroid creams, intracicatrical steroid injections, and localized mild constant pressure may save the day. Pressure can be applied with elastic devices (e.g., elastic ribbon, tape, or Jobst masks) (Figs. 35-15 and 35-17, *J, K*). If scarring is extensive, serial excisions may be required (Fig. 35-16).

If the scarring is too extensive for the above, and functionally debilitating contractures have occurred, only excision and release of contractures followed by thick split-skin grafting, large rotation flaps, or free flaps will unfortunately serve, depending on the extent of the problem (Fig. 35-17).

CONCLUSION

In conclusion, the chemical peel is a modality that is unsurpassed for the improvement of fine lines and wrinkles of the complexion. It is emotionally demanding on the patient and challenging to the surgeon. Active, scrupulous wound care is essential to minimize serious complications.

REFERENCES

1. Baker, T.J., Gordon, H.L., and Seckinger, D.L.: A second look at chemical face peeling, Plast. Reconstr. Surg. **37**:487, 1966.
2. Litton, C.: Chemical face lifting, Plast. Reconstr. Surg. **29**:371, 1962.
3. Seropian, D.: Personal communication, October 1982.
4. Spira, M., et al.: Complications of chemical face peeling, Plast. Reconstr. Surg. **54**:397, 1974.
5. Truppman, E.S., and Ellenby, J.D.: Major electrocardiographic changes during chemical face peeling, Plast. Reconstr. Surg. **63**:44, 1979.

Chapter 36

Complications of dermabrasion

Norman E. Hugo

Although the incidence of complications following dermabrasion is not high, every effort should be made to minimize them. The complications can be divided into immediate and delayed.

IMMEDIATE COMPLICATIONS

Immediate complications include pain, infection, and milia. Pain occurs in about 2% of patients following dermabrasion. The dermabraded area in these patients does not appear to be significantly different from others that are painless, yet these patients complain bitterly of severe, burning pain. Often they have a neurotic personality and drink alcohol excessively. The complaints usually persist until the scab has fallen off. There is no universally effective remedy, although cold packs, diazepam, and petrolatum ointment have been effective in helping these patients through the 10 or so days that they are under duress.

Infection is fortunately quite rare and is usually from *Staphylococcus aureus*. It should be treated with topical antibiotics such as bacitracin and kept under close watch to ensure that it does not become a deep infection with destruction of regenerating epithelium and resulting deep scars. A patient suspected of having an infection should have an immediate culture and sensitivity done so that effective antibiotics can be instituted. Tepid saline soaks to accelerate removal of the eschar may be helpful.

Milia are more of a nuisance than a complication. They arise when the pilosebaceous glands are occluded by regenerating epithelium. Nicking these with a no. 11 scalpel blade* is effective treatment. Occasionally remnants of buried epithelium will give rise to inclusion cysts, which are treated in similar fashion.

DELAYED COMPLICATIONS

The delayed, or chronic, complications include persistent erythema, hypopigmentation, and hyperpigmentation.

Erythema may persist for as long as a year and may be confused with hyperpigmentation. The persistent hypervascularity may be covered easily with cosmetics and should not interfere with routine activities. It may be differentiated by gently pressing on the area and noting the decrease in color. It subsides spontaneously.

Hypopigmentation is an expression of dermabrasion deep into the dermis and the subsequent absence of the basal layer's pigment. It is uncommon and usually less severe than the depigmentation seen after a chemical peel.

Hyperpigmentation is most often the result of oral contraceptives or too-early exposure to sunlight after dermabrasion. A patient should have stopped taking birth control pills for several months before dermabrasion is attempted. Obviously, this is not a consideration in the older age group. Postponement of sun exposure for a year is usually sufficient and can be accomplished by sun-blocking agents and minimal exposure during recovery. If hyperpigmentation does occur, it may be treated by applying hydroquinone (4%) to the area.

---

*EDITOR'S NOTE: Or a hypodermic needle. (B.L.K.)

Chapter 37

Combined chemical face peel and dermabrasion

Charles E. Horton,
Albert F. Fleury, Jr.

The use of the chemical face peel procedure for treatment of fine wrinkling of facial skin associated with aging has become more frequent since its reintroduction in the medical literature in the 1960s by Brown, Kaplan, and Brown[11]; Ayers[1,2]; Baker[4]; Litton[19]; and others. Gilles and Millard[15] reported occasionally using carbolic acid in the management of fine wrinkling of the face. Even at present, lay operators still perform chemical "facial rejuvenation" in their parlors—sometimes with disastrous results. Phenol has been the agent most commonly used. Numerous authors have reported on the techniques and complications of phenol skin tightening, extolling its safety and efficacy, but also warning of potential complications.[5-7,9,20] As a result, chemical face peeling has now become an acceptable treatment modality for the plastic surgeon treating the aging face.

Kromyer in 1905 was the first to introduce the principle of surgical planing of the skin.[12] The technique of abrasive treatment of facial scarring was reintroduced to the plastic surgery literature by Iverson[17,18] in 1947. Mechanical dermabraders were soon developed. Since that time, dermabrasion has been advocated for the treatment of traumatic facial tattoos, as well as scarring secondary to acne and trauma, and in the elimination of fine facial wrinkling associated with aging.[16-18,21]

Dupont et al.[14] in 1972 and Stagnone[23] in 1977 first described the combined use of a chemical peel and dermabrasion on the same area at the same time for acne scars. The combined use of a chemical face peel and simultaneous mechanical dermabrasion for the treatment of fine facial wrinkling has been used by us since 1973 in over 200 cases.

PHYSIOLOGICAL AND HISTOLOGICAL EFFECTS OF PHENOL

When phenol is applied to the skin, it exerts a local effect and a systemic effect.[12] Following the initial application to skin, phenol is rapidly absorbed into the bloodstream. Once absorbed, it is detoxified by either (1) oxidation to hydroquinone and pyrocatechin, or (2) renal excretion unchanged or conjugated with glycuronic acid. The toxic effect of absorbed phenol is manifested primarily in the kidney, liver, medullary centers of the brain, and myocardium. Toxic levels can result in vasomotor collapse, convulsions, and respiratory failure. Phenol appears to have a direct toxic effect on the myocardium and blood vessels. Truppman and Ellenby[24] noted cardiac arrhythmias in 10 of 43 patients undergoing chemical face peels. They reported premature ventricular contractions, bigeminy, paroxysmal atrial tachycardia, and ventricular tachycardia. Arrhythmias were found to be more prevalent in patients who had more than 50% of the face treated in less than 30 minutes. A toxic level for phenol has not been established. Blood levels as high as 23 mg/dl have been recorded in a man surviving oral phenol injection. Using a total of 3 ml of phenol, Litton[19] recorded a maximum concentration of 0.63 mg/dl 1 hour following a full face peel. Ayers[1] reported transient albuminuria and granular casts in the urine without permanent renal damage following topical application of phenol.

The application of phenol to intact skin causes destruction and "regeneration" in two anatomical areas. There is destruction in both the epidermis and the papillary dermis followed by "regeneration" or healing to some degree of each of these elements.

When phenol is applied, the skin turns white within seconds. Histologically, there is initially keratocoagulation and epidermolysis, and cellular destruction extends into the upper papillary dermis. The destroyed keratin and epidermis combine with a proteinaceous exudate to form a crust. Epidermal regeneration by epidermal cells lining pilosebaceous glands, sweat glands, and hair follicles begins as early as the second day and is usually complete by the seventh day. Several changes are noted in the regenerated epidermis. There is cellular crowding and high cellularity of the basal layer with marked diminution of the number of melanin granules.[2,4,13,19] The sequence of epidermal regeneration is the same as is seen in the healing of a split-thickness skin graft donor site or partial-thickness burn.[13]

Ayers[1] and others have demonstrated that the depth of phenol destruction is 0.3 to 0.4 mm and have suggested that the effect of destruction is confined to the papillary dermis. The reticular dermis is probably not affected. Forty-eight hours after the application of phenol, Litton[19] noted coalescence of collagenous fibers of the stratum papillare associated with a marked hyperemia and inflammatory response. New blood vessels were noted. At 3 weeks fibroblasts and new collagen appear. The increase in vascularity persists. By 3 months the collagen is mature but has a more rigid, tight horizontal appearance than untreated collagen. Several authors believe that there is a persistant increase in vascularity. Some investigators have felt that new collagen formation may be accompanied by the appearance of regenerated elastin or elastin-like fibers. However this is an inconsistent finding and may be secondary to the stain used.[8,10] Most authors agree that the youthful appearance of the skin following a chemical peel is due to the nature of the new collagen in the papillary dermis and the increase in vascularity.

Healing following dermabrasion has been extensively studied by Ayers, Wilson, and Huekart.[3] They have noted no significant difference in the healing of the dermabrasion wound and the peel wound. Others believe that the changes in the papillary dermis are not as pronounced in dermabrasion.[16,25]

INDICATIONS

A chemical peel is indicated for the treatment of fine wrinkling of the skin that is not corrected by surgical face-lift procedures. This is most commonly seen in the perioral area but can occur in all areas of the face.

The role of a peel for prophylaxis against keratosis and skin cancer is not well established. Peel removal of keratotic skin with dermabrasion and/or a peel has been a beneficial treatment in our hands and will decrease the number of abnormal skin eruptions for 2 to 5 years. New growths appear in the treated areas, but the number and severity of the lesions seems diminished.

Peeling is not as effective for treating the pitted scars of acne, which apparently respond more favorably to dermabrasion. It does not help deep wrinkling or drooping of the skin, which responds more favorably to the surgical face-lift procedure. The lower cervical areas tend to respond poorly to peeling because of skin pigment changes. Peeling is ineffective in the treatment of port wine stains and nevi, which lie deeper in the dermis.

Dark-skinned individuals are poor candidates for the peel procedure because of permanent depigmentation. Fair-skinned people are good candidates because the pigmentation changes are not as pronounced.

Revision of uneven scars is generally managed better by dermabrasion.

TECHNIQUE FOR THE STANDARD PEEL

The chemical face peel may be performed alone or in conjunction with surgical rhytidectomy. If done with the surgical face-lift, the peel must be confined to areas that are not undermined, to avoid embarrassment of the vascular supply to the flaps.

Although various strengths of phenol have been used, we prefer the formula described by Baker[4]:

3 ml USP phenol
3 ml tap water
8 drops liquified soap
3 drops croton oil

Soap acts to decrease the surface tension and makes application more even. Croton oil is advocated as a nonspecific skin irritant.

The solution must be mixed fresh each time. The skin is washed with surgical soap and scrubbed with diethyl ether, which removes the surface oily residue. Ordinary cotton-tipped applicators are used to apply the solution to the face.

No anesthesia is required because of the local anesthetic properties of phenol. If the entire face is to be peeled, the procedure is usually started on the forehead. Immediately on contact with the solution, the patient experiences a burning sensation, which rapidly subsides. The skin turns frosty white and then takes on a red hue. Waterproof adhesive tape is meticulously applied to all treated areas. The mask remains for 48 hours and is then carefully removed. Removal of the tape is usually quite painful.* Following exposure of the skin, the surface becomes moist and edematous. No attempt is made to cleanse the proteinaceous debris. The entire area is covered with thymol iodide powder, which forms a thick crust. After removal of the tape and the formation of the crust, the patient applies Neosporin ointment to the entire crust. On the seventh to eighth day the crust separates, leaving regenerated epidermis behind. Initially the skin is erythematous and smooth. After this reaction resolves, makeup can be worn, usually within 3 weeks following the procedure.

The skin is dry after crust separation and requires oil. Itching may be severe. Lanolin products are needed to moisten the skin for several weeks following the peel. For the first 1 to 2

---

*EDITOR'S NOTE: And requires heavy sedation. (B.L.K.)

weeks, Crisco seems to sooth the skin better than oily creams. Patients are advised to avoid exposure to the sun for 3 months.

TECHNIQUE FOR DERMABRASION

Following local infiltration or general anesthesia, the area to be treated is mechanically abraded with one of the commercial mechanical demabraders or by hand brushing. The epidermis and upper layer of the papillary dermis are removed. There may be rather profuse bleeding, but this is easily controlled with epinephrine soaks. The area that has been treated is left open to form a crust of proteinaceous exudate. Neosporin ointment is applied to the crust, which spontaneously separates in 5 to 7 days, leaving regenerated epidermis behind. The skin should be cared for in the same fashion as following a chemical peel.

TECHNIQUE FOR COMBINED PROCEDURE

In the combined chemical peel and dermabrasion (peel-abrasion) procedure, Baker's formula is applied in the routine fashion. The face is peeled in anatomical units: the forehead and upper lids, the cheeks and lower lids, and the perioral area. When the lower face is being peeled, the solution

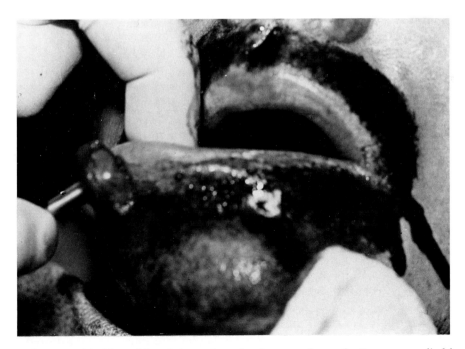

Fig. 37-1. Hand-held steel brush is used to abrade around mouth. Pressure applied by placing finger inside lips is helpful.

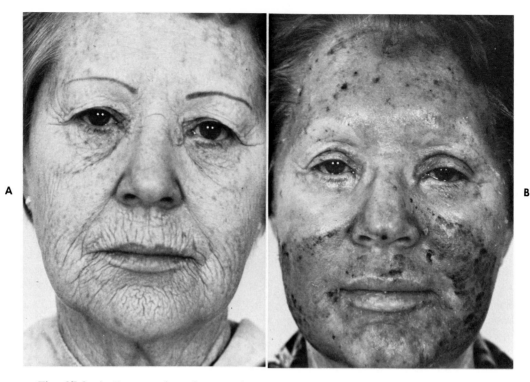

Fig. 37-2. A, Preoperative photograph. **B,** Appearance 10 days following peel-abrasion.

should be applied to just below the mandible to avoid a visible line of sharp demarcation. For the same reason, the peel should be carried onto the lip vermilion. One to two minutes after application of the peel solution, the treated area is briskly abraded either mechanically or by hand. Placing a finger in the mouth and tensing the lip or cheek allows more precise depth control (Fig. 37-1). This removes all necrotic debris. No anesthesia other than the phenol is used. Bleeding is controlled with epinephrine soaks. The area is left open so that within 2 hours the proteinaceous exudate forms a crust similar to that of a routine dermabrasion procedure. One to two days later, applications of Neosporin ointment to the crust are begun. After 7 to 9 days the crust separates, leaving the newly regenerated epidermis behind (Fig. 37-2). As with a peel or dermabrasion alone, in the first 2 weeks after separation of the crust, pruritis is a particular problem, for which the application of Crisco has been found to be helpful. Later a regular moisturizing cream is used. The smooth skin that results often creates difficulty in applying makeup; however Este Lauder and Clinique brands appear to be satisfactory to most patients.

DISCUSSION

Although both dermabrasion and peeling are effective in removing fine wrinkling, it is generally agreed that the chemical face peel gives a longer-lasting result. Reasons for this are unclear. Some believe that the changes in the papillary dermis are different after a chemical face peel.[3,16] However, Ayers has not found this to be true. Other advantages of a peel over dermabrasion are that it may be done without the use of an anesthetic, which dermabrasion requires. It seems to be accepted better by patients than surgical planing.

Disadvantages of the chemical peel are that it results in a permanent depigmentation of the skin, whereas dermabrasion does not seem to do so.[16] The removal of the adhesive tape after a peel is exceedingly painful for the patient. Accurate depth control is difficult with a chemical peel. With dermabrasion the operator has more precise control. Infection may occur under the tape. At times linear scars result from uneven tape application. Occasionally a peel has been noted to be uneven. Some think that this may be secondary to pooling of phenol-concentrated exudate underneath the tape.

With standard dermabrasion removal of tape

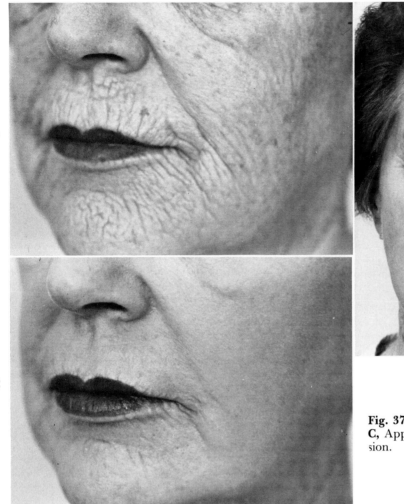

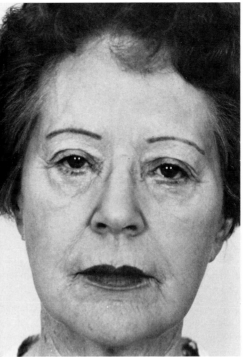

Fig. 37-3. A, Preoperative photograph. **B** and **C,** Appearance 3 months following peel-abrasion.

Table 37-1. Advantages and disadvantages of the chemical peel, dermabrasion, and peel-abrasion

	Chemical peel	*Dermabrasion*	*Peel-abrasion*
Advantages	Lasts 5 to 7 years No anesthesia is required Well tolerated by patients	Depth control is precise No tape is necessary Permanent depigmentation is not as significant	Lasts 5 to 7 years No tape is necessary No additional anesthesia is needed Phenol facilitates dermabrasion Depth control is more precise Debridement of necrotic tissue Less pain Less swelling
Disadvantages	Permanent depigmentation of skin Removal of tape is painful May be infection under tape May be scars produced by tape Depth control is not precise	Lasts 2 to 3 years Requires additional anesthesia	May be permanent depigmentation of skin

and problems associated with tape are obviated because no tape is used. Depigmentation, as noted with peeling, is minimized. Depth control is more precise. However, it does require local or general anesthesia.

Combining dermabrasion and peeling retains the advantages of the peel but eliminates many of the disadvantages (Table 37-1). The phenol provides its own anesthesia. In addition, the phenol makes the skin somewhat firm and leathery, which facilitates dermabrasion by decreasing the tendency of the skin to catch and roll on the dermabrader. Depth control of the peel is more precise. The problems associated with tape removal are not encountered, because tape is not used. Infection has never occurred. Streaking of the treated area is not a problem, because all of the peeled area is abraded equally. Dermabrasion of necrotic tissue is similar to early tangential excision of a partial-thickness burn. Clinically, there appears to be much less edema and much less pain. The results appear to be as long lasting as those obtained with chemical face peeling alone, although not more so. The depigmentation seen following peel-abrasion is the same as that with the peel alone.

Histologically, we see the same changes following the combined procedure as those described with the other individual procedures.

As with the peel, the combined procedure can be performed on the entire face or on selected anatomical segments. The full face is not peeled and dermabraded at the same time that a surgical face-lift is being done, to avoid damage to the skin flaps. However, a circumoral skin peel–dermabrasion is frequently combined with a surgical face-lift.

If the eyelids are peeled, no accompanying dermabrasion is done. They are not taped but are left open for healing. If the lower lids are peeled, little or no skin excision is done to avoid ectropion.

We have found that the combined peel-abrasion procedure corrects fine facial wrinkling in most patients (Fig. 37-3). It can be repeated. More precise control of depth, less potential for infection beneath tape, less tape streaking, and a marked decrease in postoperative pain and edema following the combined procedure make it the operation of choice in most patients considering a peel or dermabrasion for cosmetic correction of fine facial wrinkling.

REFERENCES

1. Ayers, S. III: Dermal changes following application of chemical cauterants to the skin, Arch. Dermatol. **82:** 578, 1960.
2. Ayers, S. III: Superficial chemosurgery in treating aging skin, Arch. Dermatol. **85:**125, 1962.
3. Ayers, S., Wilson, W., and Huekart, R.: Dermal changes following abrasion, Arch Dermatol. **79:**553, 1959.
4. Baker, T.J.: Chemical face peeling and rhytidectomy, Plast. Reconstr. Surg. **29:**199, 1962.
5. Baker, T.J., and Gordon, H.L.: Chemical face peeling and dermabrasion, Surg. Clin. North Am. **51:**387, 1971.
6. Baker, T.J., and Gordon, H.L.: Chemical peeling as a practical method for removing rhytides of the upper lip, Ann. Plast. Surg. **2:**209, 1979.
7. Baker, T.J., Gordon, H.L., and Seckinger, D.L.: A second look at chemical face peeling, Plast. Reconstr. Surg. **37:**487, 1966.
8. Baker, T.J., et al.: Long term histologic study of skin after chemical face peeling, Plast. Reconstr. Surg. **53:**522, 1974.
9. Batstone, J.H.F., and Millard, D.R.: An endorsement of facial chemo-surgery, Br. J. Plast. Surg. **21:**193, 1968.
10. Bhangoo, K.S.: Histologic changes following chemical face peeling, Plast. Reconstr. Surg. **54:**599, 1974.
11. Brown, A.M., Kaplan, L.M., and Brown, M.E.: Phenol induced histologic skin changes: hazards, techniques and uses, Br. J. Plast. Surg. **8:**158, 1960.
12. Campbell, R.M. Surgical and chemical planing of the skin. In Converse, J.M., editor: Reconstructive plastic surgery, ed. 2, Philadelphia, 1977, W.B. Saunders Co., p. 442.
13. Converse, J.M., and Robb-Smith, A.H.T.: The healing of surface cutaneous wounds: Its analogy with the healing of superficial burns, Ann. Surg. **53:**522, 1974.
14. Dupont, C., et al.: Phenol skin tightening for better dermabrasion, Plast. Reconstr. Surg. **50:**588, 1972.
15. Gilles, H.D., and Millard, D.R.: The principles and art of plastic surgery, Boston, 1957, Little, Brown & Co., p. 403.
16. Hugo, N.E.: Videotape discussion on dermabrasion procedures. In Goulian, D., and Courtiss, E.H., editors: Symposium on surgery of the aging face, St. Louis, 1978, The C.V. Mosby Co.
17. Iverson, P.C.: Surgical removal of traumatic tattoos, Plast. Reconstr. Surg. **2:**427, 1947.
18. Iverson, P.C.: Further development in the treatment of skin lesions by abrasion, Plast. Reconstr. Surg. **12:**27, 1953.
19. Litton, C.: Chemical face lifting, Plast. Reconstr. Surg. **29:**371, 1962.
20. Litton, C., Fournier, P., and Copinpin, A.: A survey of chemical peeling of the face, Plast. Reconstr. Surg. **51:**645, 1973.
21. Smith, F.: Mechanical abrasion to remove pits, foreign bodies, scars, etc., Plast. Reconstr. Surg. **14:**236, 1954.
22. Spira, M., et al.: Chemosurgery—a histologic study, Plast. Reconstr. Surg. **45:**247, 1970.
23. Stagnone, J.J.: Dermabrasion, a combined technique of chemical peeling and dermabrasion, J. Dermatol. Surg. Oncol. **3:**217, 1977.
24. Truppman, E.S., and Ellenby, J.D.: Major electrocardiographic changes during chemical face peeling, Plast. Reconstr. Surg. **63:**44, 1979.
25. Wood-Smith, D., and Rees, T.D.: In Rees, T.D., and Wood Smith, D., editors: Cosmetic facial surgery Philadelphia, 1973, W.B. Saunders Co.

Editorial comments
Part VI

Surgery of the surface is as important to over-all facial rejuvenation as is the finish to a fine piece of furniture. One of the problems in aesthetic plastic surgery of the face is the fine wrinkling that occurs with time, heredity, gender (the fine wrinkles that can occur in the female upper lip, even in younger women), mode of living (chronic sun and wind exposure), and habits (smoking?). Obviously, the surgical face-lift is not sufficient to correct these surface problems. The plastic surgeon has the three modalities discussed in this part available for treatment of this problem, namely chemical peel, dermabrasion, and combined peel and dermabrasion.

The chemical peel, as we know it, is a modality that goes back well over half a century. Dr. H. Otto Bames of Los Angeles discussed the phenol peel with taping (as well as the resorcinol peel) in 1927,* and he indicated that the method had been in use prior to the time of his writing. He also mentioned some of the results and complications of face peeling, including "a clear, almost parchment-like complexion," phenol poisoning, chronic nephritis, scarring (especially in the neck), and scar contracture. It appears that Cora Galanti, one of the early lay peelers in California, was not the first to invent the phenol formula, as we had been led to believe by her son and others closely associated with her.†

I agree with Dr. Fredricks that the chemical peel is unsurpassed as an effective, long-term treatment for facial wrinkling, because it not only treats the surface, but effects long-term changes in the underlying framework of the skin. On the other hand, as every plastic surgeon knows, it is not a substitute for a face-lift operation, just as collagen injections cannot take the place of a surgical face-lift. The trade-off of a chemical peel is a permanent color change, a lightening of the treated skin, which obligates the patient to wear makeup to compensate for it. Patients who are accustomed to wearing makeup are happy to accept this trade-off. The color change may be more of a burden to the patient who likes to wear little or no makeup and who may be an outdoors, sports-oriented person. Also, there is aways the demarcation line where treatment was stopped, which precludes a face peel for most dark-complexioned individuals.

Dermabrasion will also treat fine wrinkles, but its effects are not as long lasting, since it does not produce the deeper skin changes that the chemical peel accomplishes. On the other hand, it does not usually produce permanent lightening of the skin. For women who will not accept the permanent color change that accompanies face peeling, dermabrasion may be the treatment of choice, particularly in limited areas such as the lips and perioral region. Patients who want to maintain their smoother skin appearance must be made to understand that they will require repeated dermabrasions every few years. This does not seem too much to ask of patients who shun permanent color change, particularly in view of the fact that the effects of surgical face-lifting are not permanent (the operation must be repeated for those patients who want to maintain their facial rejuvenation).

Dr. Fredricks has wisely pointed out that skin will not tolerate simultaneous surgical lifting and peeling and will usually respond to such combined insults with necrosis, slough, and scarring. On the other hand, I will not hestitate to do light, localized dermabrasion over areas that have been

---

*Bames, H.O.: Truth and fallacies of face peeling and face lifting. In Stignell, G., editor: Medical journal and record: a national review of medicine and surgery, vol. 126, New York, July-December 1927, A.R. Elliott Publishing Co.
†Litton, C.: Personal communication, 1976.

elevated as flaps, such as abrading forehead frown lines after a forehead lift. Dermabrasion is only a momentary trauma, without the prolonged thermal insult of chemical peeling, and I have seen no adverse results from such limited, momentary combined treatments.

When discussing chemical face peeling, we owe special acknowledgment to Drs. Thomas Baker and Howard Gordon, who for many years have introduced thousands of plastic surgeons to the procedure through their annual Cedars of Lebanon Hospital symposiums. I wish I had had the benefit of such demonstrations when I first started doing the procedure many years ago, before these symposiums began. The memory of my first shocked look at the gray, exudating skin as I removed the tapes is still very strong, as was my gratitude for my youthful, resilient coronary arteries.

As Dr. Fredricks points out, a chemical peel should be done no less than 6 to 8 weeks (some say at least 3 months) after a surgical face-lift. It may also be done prior to the face-lift, as Dr. Diran Seropian has done for many years.* He believes that the reduction of the elastic stretch of the skin after a chemical peel makes the subsequent surgical face-lift last longer. He also believes that the slight residual edema of the peel makes the surgical face-lift dissection a little easier. (He will do a face-lift about 3 months after a peel.) Dr. Seropian also points out that occasionally patients have been so satisfied with the results of the face peel alone that they have not gone on to have their surgical face-lifts until many months later.

Certain precautions discussed by Dr. Fredricks deserve emphasis. It is prudent to keep the container for the peel solution below the level of the patient's head, so that if it spilled, no harm will result. It is also wise to have sterile saline solution immediately available in case it is needed to irrigate the eyes.

Cardiac arrhythmias are known to occur with the application of phenol solutions to the skin. Therefore, for anything more than application over a small area (such as the eyelids or lips), one should have a cardiac monitor, a good intravenous infusion, and appropriate medications available to treat possible arrhythmias. Also, application of the solution should be spread out over a period of time to avoid excessively rapid absorption of phenol. It is wise to paint a given area and tape it before going to the next area, rather than applying the phenol to the entire face in one step.

In my own practice, I do my full face peels with the patients under light general anesthesia, which provides at least two advantages. It eliminates the initial pain of application of solution and taping for the patient. It also provides me with the presence of an anesthesiologist, who can concentrate on monitoring the patient and can administer appropriate therapy should any arrhythmias occur. I also like to anesthetize the face with *blocks* of long-acting local anesthetics such as bupivacaine (Marcaine) or etidocaine (Duranest). (CAUTION: Do not inject epinephrine-containing solutions into areas that will have phenol applied to them; the vasoconstriction combined with the chemical peel may be more than the skin can bear and still survive.)

Dermabrasion itself is not free of complications, but, as shown by Dr. Hugo, most can be avoided, or if necessary, treated. Although it does not have the long-term result that the chemical peel provides for facial wrinkles, I believe it is the treatment of choice for most scars resulting from acne.

Although I was educated to believe that dermabrasion had to be done at high speed, I now find that this is not so. I can obtain as good results from low-speed rotary instruments, such as the battery-powered Mini-brader* with a wire brush. This provides the advantage of maneuverability, low cost, relatively quiet operation, and decreased risk of gauging or burning the skin if applied too long or with too much pressure.

I was also educated in the tradition of having a crust form over the dermabraded area and allowing it to remain in place until it fell off or was softened by ointment application starting several days later. At the Educational Foundation Symposium at Lake Tahoe in 1979, I learned from one of the other faculty members, Dr. Norman Orentreich of New York, that one could obtain just as good results by commencing ointment application immediately and continuing it until full healing occurred, without ever having a crust form. Patients seem more comfortable with this type of treatment than when their faces are immobilized under a stiff crust. Also, by using Poly-

---

*Seropian, D.: Personal Communication, 1983.

*Concept, Inc., Clearwater, Fla.

sporin ointment instead of Neosporin ointment, I find that there are fewer allergic reactions to the ointment.

I have adopted the combined face peel and dermabrasion (or peel-abrasion) technique described by Drs. Horton and Fleury as my procedure of choice for facial wrinkles. I have used it ever since Dr. Horton introduced it to me at the Educational Foundation Symposium on Surgery of the Aging Face in Denver in 1976.

Although Dr. Fredricks disagrees, I believe that I can obtain the same clinical results with peel-abrasion that I used to get from the traditional peel with application of tape. I must confess that I never liked the taping part of the treatment, perhaps because as a surgeon I had no control over what was going on under the tapes, whereas I can control what I do with the dermabrasion brush. I have abandoned the use of taping and now use the peel-abrasion technique exclusively, where I formerly would have applied tape. My postoperative care is identical to that of straight dermabrasion, namely, application of Polysporin ointment several times a day until complete healing takes place.

B.L.K.

INDEX